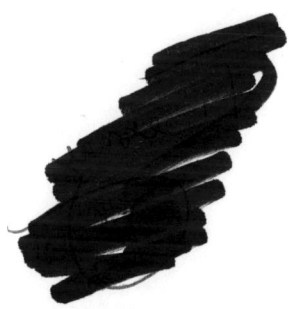

MEDICAL TERMINOLOGIES
Classical Origins

OKLAHOMA SERIES IN CLASSICAL CULTURE

Oklahoma Series in Classical Culture

Series Editor

A. J. Heisserer, *University of Oklahoma*

Advisory Board

David F. Bright, *Iowa State University*
Nancy Demand, *Indiana University*
Elaine Fantham, *Princeton University*
R. M. Frazer, *Tulane University*
Ronald J. Leprohon, *University of Toronto*
Robert A. Moysey, *University of Mississippi*
Helen F. North, *Swarthmore College*
Robert J. Smutny, *University of the Pacific*
Eva Stehle, *University of Maryland at College Park*
A. Geoffrey Woodhead, *Corpus Christi College, Cambridge/ Ohio State University*
John Wright, *Northwestern University*

MEDICAL TERMINOLOGIES

Classical Origins

By
John Scarborough

University of Oklahoma Press : Norman and London

For Yasemin

By John Scarborough
Roman Medicine (London, 1969; Ithaca, 1976)
Facets of Hellenic Life (Boston, 1976)
Symposium on Byzantine Medicine (ed.) (Washington, D.C., 1985)
Pharmacy's Ancient Heritage: Theophrastus, Nicander, and Dioscorides (Lexington, 1985)
Folklore and Folk Medicines (ed.) (Madison, 1987)
Medical Terminologies: Classical Origins (Norman, 1992)

Scarborough, John.
   Medical terminologies : classical origins / by John Scarborough.
     p. cm.—(Oklahoma series in classical culture ; vol. 13)
   Includes bibliographical references and index.
   ISBN 0-8061-2443-1
   1. Medicine—Terminology. 2. English language—Medical English—Etymology. I. Title.
   [DNLM: 1. Nomenclature. W 15 S285m]
   R123.S312 1992
   610′.14—dc20
   DNLM/DLC
   for Library of Congress   92-54139
                                                                                                CIP

Medical Terminologies: Classical Origins is Volume 13 of the Oklahoma Series in Classical Culture.

The paper in this book meets the guidelines for permanence and durability of the Committee on Production Guidelines for Book Longevity of the Council on Library Resources, Inc. ∞

Copyright © 1992 by the University of Oklahoma Press, Norman, Publishing Division of the University. All rights reserved. Manufactured in the U.S.A. First edition.

CONTENTS

Preface	ix
Abbreviations	2
1. Special Vocabularies in Medical and Other English: Why There Are Jargons	3
2. Botany	14
3. Invertebrates: Protozoa to Molluscs	30
Some Numbers for Perspective	34
The Animal Kingdom and the Invertebrates	35
4. Arthropods	70
The Myriapods	82
The Insects	85
Greek and Latin for Insect Names	90
Spiders and their Cousins	119
5. Bones	124
Some Bones of the Skull	126
Some Vertebrae	127
Bones of the Pelvis	129
Some Other Bones	131
Bones of the Leg and Foot	134
6. Nerves	141
The Brain and Its Parts	145
The Cranial Nerves	149
Nerves of the Body	153
7. Muscles	158
Muscles and Anatomy	160
Three Muscles and Their Names: Gastrocnemius, Sartorius, Stapedius	165
A Sampling of Muscles: Names and What They Say	168
8. Breathing and How It Works	173
9. Eating, Digestion, Elimination	183
To Eat, To Digest, To Eliminate: The Parts	188
10. Sex	196
Sexual Anatomy: The Parts (Female)	210
Sexual Anatomy: The Parts (Male)	211

11. Vascular Matters: Heart and Blood, "The Liquids of Life"	213
The Four Elements	224
The Four Qualities	225
The Heart as Muscular Pump	228
Heart and Vascular Anatomy	232
12. Some More Fluids: The Endocrine Glands, Hormones, and Lymph	236
The Endocrine Glands	241
The Lymphatic System	247
13. The Human Context: Sight, Sound, Voice, and Touch	249
The Eye and Its Parts	251
The Ear and Its Parts	253
Speaking	254
Touching	260
Appendices	
1. Greek and Roman Numbers	263
2. The Greek Alphabet and the Transliteration of Greek into Roman Letters	268
3. Pronunciation of Greco-Latin Terms	268
4. Some Abbreviated Paradigms	269
Bibliography	
On Gaining More Information	274
Texts and Sources	277
Secondary Works	281
Index	288

PREFACE

WHEN students begin their long intellectual treks toward one of the medical professions, an initial barrier they encounter is the often opaque and specialized vocabulary that is the "language" of the medical and biological sciences. Too frequently, freshmen and sophomores indulge in frantic memorization-binges, perhaps never to understand or comprehend what these generally multisyllabic terms might mean in their own right. On reaching medical school or another of our professional institutions that train physicians, pharmacists, nurses, or any of the other medical occupations, students encounter those same terms again, this time learning what the terms mean through repeated use and through the essentials of clinical and laboratory contexts. Yet too few of our justly esteemed medical specialists know why they speak the "lingo" they do, which sometimes leads to confusion and imprecision in writing and in the necessary communication with patients. Moreover, the language of the medical sciences is now changing (even while retaining many derivations from Greek and Latin) very rapidly, so that precision becomes even more of a necessity in speaking and writing.

In teaching the large "med terms" course here at the University of Wisconsin, I quickly discovered that several approaches helped my students understand not only the terms but also why learning them precisely was so necessary. Repetition in varying contexts (history, philology, "straight" medicine, entomology, botany, etc.) apparently allows the intellect to associate a single concept within several different topics, and the multiple associations reinforce concise recollection. And—as a number of students have said to me—the use of "real" sentences and "real" science and history gives them an assurance that what they are learning fits a "real" subject, as contrasted with the vacuous and artificial "memorize-these-words-for-the-next-exam" instructions all too common in beginning courses of comparative anatomy, or biochemistry, or the dozens of other "weeder" courses taken by premedical students in American universities and colleges. As one of my wittier students put it so well: "We've been taught to regurgitate it all back. That's one of your Greek-type words for 'vomiting it up,' isn't it?" That student guessed the wrong language but had exactly the right idea (*regurgitare* is medieval Latin ["to give back something not fully assimilated"]). Once "regurgitated" for an exam, the information was lost.

Medicine's future will certainly involve greater interdisciplinary efforts among specialists in the hundreds of particular subjects now classed as separate in research, and my students appreciated the introductions to the kindred vocabularies of protozoology, medical entomology, and some aspects of botany and pharmacy, as well as the pleasant quandaries of terms in biochemistry and endocrinology. In each of these topics, along with the traditional "systems of the body" chapters that follow, I continually reminded my students that these subtopics were selected examples of how the vocabularies "worked" and that I expected them to seek precision of meanings in their chosen fields long after they left the University of Wisconsin. Investing in a good, unabridged dictionary remains one of the best expenditures any medical professional can ever make, and I warned that the words I chose to use were my personal choices from thousands of such terms in each of the medical or biological specialties.

Translations from Greek to Latin, as found in the text, are my own unless otherwise specified. Greek and Latin texts are cited in the traditional manner (that is, not by volume and page as would be usual for modern works but by "book" [the Roman numeral] and subsections; good translations, which one will find in the Loeb Classical Library or other series of English translations of Greek and Latin writings, will always have these book and subsection numbers, along with page numbers for the volume itself). The major exception I make is with the works of Galen; I cite the volume and page from the twenty-volume edition of the Greek texts edited by C. G. Kühn (unless there are better editions of particular tracts).

A final caveat: medical students often assume that if they learn what the Greek or Latin names mean, they will automatically know what the terms mean in modern medical English. Sometimes, this is quite right, but very frequently indeed, the modern Greco-Latinate term is an adaptation of the ancient meaning or merely an obscure nuance rarely (if ever) used in classical antiquity. So a medical scientist should not presume, for example, that a *tibia* always meant what it designates today. In their own way, Greek and Latin as living languages were as supple and multi-layered as is English, and in spite of what one gains from abridged Latin-English dictionaries, there are occasionally several major meanings encompassed by a single word. At the same time, I would urge readers to do what my students enjoy doing when they first meet previously unknown Greco-Latinate words or phrases: make reasonable guesses from what is already in a working vocabulary—sometimes the results are surprisingly accurate. I suggest some of the process of how Latin-like words become technical terms in English (and thus recognized for what they are) in chapter 11, "Vascular Matters." Students are always pleasantly surprised at how they can "read" or at least gain the gist of the Latin of William Harvey from the early seventeenth century.

JOHN SCARBOROUGH

Madison, Wisconsin

MEDICAL TERMINOLOGIES
Classical Origins

Abbreviations

Aristotle, *GA, HA,* and *PA*: Aristotle, *Generation of Animals, Enquiry into Animals* (traditionally cited by its Latin title, *Historia animalium,* thus *HA*), and *Parts of Animals.* A number of edited texts and translations by various scholars are available, including those in the Loeb Classical Library, published by Harvard University Press.

CMG: Corpus Medicorum Graecorum. A series of edited Greek texts of Greek and Roman medical works, published in Leipzig (B. G. Teubner) before 1940 and in Berlin (Akademie-Verlag) since 1950.

Dioscorides, *Materia Medica* or *MM*: Max Wellmann, ed. (Greek text only), *Pedanii Dioscuridis Anazarbei De materia medica,* 3 vols. (Berlin: Weidmann, 1906–14; reprint, 1958). There is no reliable English translation.

Galen, ed. Kühn or simply K.: C. G. Kühn, ed. (Greek texts with Latin renderings), *Claudii Galeni Opera omnia,* 20 vols. in 22 parts (Leipzig: Cnoblichius, 1821–33; reprint, Hildesheim: Georg Olms, 1964–65). The Latin translations footing the Greek texts are often quite untrustworthy.

LSJ: Henry George Liddell, Robert Scott, and Henry Stuart Jones, with assistance of Roderick McKenzie, *A Greek-English Lexicon,* 9th ed with supplement (Oxford: Clarendon Press, 1968).

OED: The Compact Edition of the Oxford English Dictionary, 2 vols., complete text reproduced micrographically (Oxford: Clarendon Press, 1971).

OLD: P.G.W. Glare, ed., *Oxford Latin Dictionary* (Oxford: Clarendon Press, 1968–82 as issued in eight fascicles; full edition, 1983).

Pliny, *NH*: Pliny the Elder, *Natural History.* Latin text edited with English translation by H. Rackham, W.H.S. Jones, and D. E. Eichholz, in the Loeb Classical Library, 10 vols. (Cambridge, Mass.: Harvard University Press, 1942–63).

Theophrastus, *HP*: Theophrastus, *Enquiry into Plants* (traditionally cited by its Latin title, *Historia plantarum,* thus *HP*). Greek text edited with English translation by A. F. Hort in the Loeb Classical Library (London: William Heinemann, 1916), reprinted several times by Harvard University Press. Theophrastus, *On Odors,* is also in this edition (with translation by Hort).

CHAPTER 1

SPECIAL VOCABULARIES IN MEDICAL AND OTHER ENGLISH: WHY THERE ARE JARGONS

EVERY speaker and reader of English comes to the medical and biological sciences equipped with a vocabulary of words, phrases, and clichés very well suited for ordinary conversation or for reading newspapers, magazines, and most works of fiction. Yet even in their most elementary forms, the sciences present a specialized vocabulary, words and terms that must be mastered before one can proceed beyond what might be called merely "descriptive." Middle-school children in America receive bits and pieces of this specialized jargon as they learn the names of the elements from the periodic table or when they learn fundamental basics of such subjects as astronomy, botany, or entomology. They soon learn that the word *bug* is replaced by *fly, beetle, locust,* and hundreds more of the nonscientific "common names" suggesting particulars of the insect world. They also soon comprehend that among the "trees" there are oaks, maples, beeches, walnuts, and so on, each distinguished by leaf shapes, bark textures, fruits, and growth patterns.

Students may learn that study according to differences in shapes of leaves is called morphology. Visually such terms are labels, easily pictured through repetition in the mind's eye, a greatly dissimilar intellectual process from that required when children begin to memorize the abstractions that are the names for chemical elements. Can one visualize oxygen? Helium? Xenon? Molybdenum? Some, like iron, sodium, aluminum, gold, zinc, and lead, may seem familiar enough, but a perceptive child will always ask why water and wood are not elements. Thus even at this elementary level, children introduced to the vocabulary of science must deal with abstractions, and each term's "history" (that is, its etymology) forms an essential basis to answer that child's "why." Or put another way, when children are taught some of the essentials of why such names are given to the basic blocks of the natural universe, they recognize early that rote memorization is *not* science at all but that names and terms always signify something else, something more: a connection with another time, a choice made by someone in the past to specify particulars about this special substance.

Scientific terms often reflect an effort to ensure an exact meaning, so that this word will mean one thing and only one thing. If one writes *beetle,* this can mean in ordinary English several hundred thousand particular beetles, whereas if one writes *lucanid beetle,* one has narrowed the beetles down to the few hundred beetles that display "stag-like horns." All of the sciences mirror this constant attempt at precision, and English has a common stock of foreign terms adapted into the spoken and written languages, a common stock that includes deeply rooted stores of classical Greek and Latin. Both "common" English and scientific English borrow heavily from these so-called dead languages; sometimes these loan-words are so ordinary that their classical roots are unnoticed, while other words spring out as obvious adaptations or borrowings from Latin or Greek. To be sure, English continuously mooches terms from living languages, but classical Latin and Greek have given our tongue subtle variations and shadings of meaning since the Middle Ages, and English enjoys a supple structure well suited for science as well as colorful speech. This pliable vocabulary, composited from varied historical roots, can be illustrated by two kinds of writing in English, set in tandem: the first is from science fiction, a very popular genre among all ages and educational levels throughout the world; the second example comes from a modern textbook of human anatomy. In each instance, Latin and Greek terms (or those derived from Latin or Greek) may surprise initially by their frequency.

> Then she was in my arms and it seemed strange that she should be there: this woman who had stepped out of a long, black car in this Wisconsin evening across two decades of time. How hard it was to equate her with the gaily laughing girl of that Mideastern dig, where we had slaved together to uncover the secrets of an ancient tumulus that, finally, turned out to be of slight importance—I digging and sifting and uncovering, while she labeled and tried somehow to identify the shards and other prehistoric junk laid out on long tables. That hot and dusty season had been far too short. (Simak, *Mastodonia,* 5.)

The heart first appears in the embryo as a longitudinal tube with branching ends. The branches at the head end are the aortic arches; those at the tail end are the great veins. As development proceeds, the venous connections of the heart stay put in the celom wall, but the aortic arches grow and elongate. The cranial end of the heart tube therefore moves down into the thorax, where the hypaxial body wall closes over it. The heart thus becomes increasingly S-shaped and winds up as a twisted bag hanging from a crown of vessels near its cranial end. (Cartmill, Hylander, and Shafland, *Human Structure*, 101.)

Each author (or team of authors) has chosen words and phrases with explicit purposes and careful intentions. Simak, as a writer of widely popular science fiction, desires to impart moods and seeks to express contexts sparingly yet clearly. He also hopes to convey impressions of motion, across both space and time, one of the more difficult tasks faced by all writers of fiction. By contrast, the authors of *Human Structure* wish to describe objects as clearly as possible, and simultaneously to provide a description of embryonic changes as exactly as credible, so that students of anatomy will comprehend growth and change in the early heart. Both kinds of writing attempt that description of motion or change as clearly as possible, but Simak's fiction aims for a loosely woven context of time (a mood), whereas Cartmill and his colleagues must employ words that are much meatier and exact. The contrast between fiction and good anatomy is signaled by the Greco-Latinate terms found in Simak's paragraph, as distinguished from the greater number of such words contained in the paragraph from *Human Structure*.

Simak's paragraph has 108 words. Prominently important are those expressions derived from Greek or Latin, in particular:

arms: from Middle English, derived from Latin *armus* ("shoulder"), in turn related to the Greek *harmos* ("joint").

strange: from Middle English, derived from Old French *estrange,* in turn from Latin *extraneus;* original meaning was "superfluous" or "extraneous."

long: from Middle English and Old English, probably derived in common from the Icelandic *langr* and Latin *longus.*

car: from Late Latin *carrum* ("wheeled vehicle").

decades: from Late Latin *decas* ("collection of ten"), derived from Greek.

equate: from Middle English, derived from Latin *aequatus* = *aequus*.

slaved: from Middle English, derived from Medieval Latin *Sclavus* ("Slav").

secrets: from Middle English, derived from Old French *secret*, in turn from Latin *secretus* (*se* + *cernere* [*cernere* "to sift"]).

ancient: from Old French *ancien*, derived from Vulgar Latin *antianus* = *ante* + *anus* ("before the [or a] year").

tumulus: Latin "mound" or "swelling"; = *tumere* ("to swell") + *-ulus* (a suffix of place).

finally: adverb from adjective [final; from Middle English, derived from Latin *finalis* = *finis* ("end") + *-alis* (a suffix for "pertaining to").

importance: from Medieval Latin *importantia* (*importans*, "weighing"), from classical Latin *importare* ("to bring in," or "to cause," or "to bring an action [in court]") = *im-* (variant of *in-* occurring before *b*, *m*, and *p*; prefix denoting motion "in" or "into") + *port-* (basic Latin root from *portare* ["to carry"]) + *-ance* (suffix used to form nouns from adjectives in *-ant*, or from verbs [for example, "appear" and "appearance"]). Often the Latin *-antia* becomes Englished as *-ancy*.

identify: from Late Latin *identificare*, coined from Latin *identidem* ("repeatedly," that is *idem* + *-ti-*); the Late Latin noun became *identitas*. In most references, "Late Latin" frequently means "Renaissance Latin."

Prehistoric: from Latin *prae-* + *historicus* (derived from Greek *historikos* ["inquired" or "searched out"]). The root is *historia* (Greek), so that the original meaning (in Latin) was "before inquiry."

tables: from Old English as a variant derived from the Latin *tabula* ("plank" or "tablet").

season: from Middle English, derived from Latin *satio* ("a sowing"); in Vulgar Latin, *satio* came to mean "sowing time."

Of 108 words used by Simak, an important 16 (*long* occurs twice) have Greek or Latin roots or derivations (just under 15 percent of the total). The remainder are generally Anglo-Saxon, or

SPECIAL VOCABULARIES 7

German, or various Scandinavian etymologies, with the obvious exception *Wisconsin,* descended from a French corruption of an Indian name (the exact origin or tribe is disputed among specialists). Ordinary English, however, gains a rich panoply of nouns, verbs, pronouns, adjectives, and adverbs from Anglo-Saxon, Old and Middle English, German, and Scandinavian words, and for normal conversation or for general fiction, *woman, dig, slight, shards, junk, hot, dusty,* and *short* are quite sufficient. Suppose, on the other hand, that one wants to know which arm (or which part of an arm), what kind of automobile, or what particular type of heat, dust, evenings, mounds, or junk: one could write "colored shards" (*color* is straight Latin), or red or yellow shards; one could also say "Ford" or "Buick" or "Studebaker" (with a specific year, as in "a '52 Ford"), exact names bringing to mind innumerable details of style, grills, tail-lenses, curvatures of windshields, and the like. Perhaps a reader might be curious where the "Mideastern dig" took place, so that an author might supply "Upper Egypt," "the Jordanian banks of the Dead Sea," "in the semiwilderness of Cilicia Tracheia," or "in the shadows of Roman Palmyra." Yet Simak chooses not to overload his paragraph with too many particulars, and the reader moves swiftly with the author into a carefully crafted mood as contrasted with detailed descriptions of setting, place, or even special aspects of the car, the woman, or her past experience as an archaeologist somewhere in the Middle East. Simak's spare use of specific descriptives is perfectly appropriate for his purposes, and there is appreciation for the lack of needless details to clutter the progress of his narrative. This is good, straightforward English, and Simak intentionally limits his employment of Greco-Latinate terms. English words derived from Greek or Latin tend to be those of several syllables, whereas "Anglo-Saxon" is generally clipped, short, and pithy.

Yet even as Simak prunes his vocabulary, there are odd flashes of curiosity about exact items that might aid the reader to become more infused with the mood Simak wishes to impart. Perhaps the car ought to carry a name and year. Maybe those shards require some detail of color, texture, and possibly taste (occasionally, experienced archaeologists taste potsherds to ensure accurate matches of scattered fragments of pottery). Simak chooses not to provide these bits of information, and his prose is smooth and seamless, quite in keeping with the skills displayed by practiced writers of fiction in modern English. This technique, however, would not work if Simak were composing a story depending on the details of a game of chess, in which technical terminologies are essential. Likewise, a story that took as its focus or setting a game of baseball would demand technical expertise by the author, since *home runs, outs, double plays, stalls, mound,* and so on have specific meanings in baseball—and only baseball. This is a jargon of technical vocabulary, much like the jargons of tennis, football (American), stamp collecting, automobile mechanics, breeding racehorses or dairy cows, collecting Golden Age comic books—in fact *all* specialized activities have their technical terms. In medical diagnostics, to say that an illness is "short" is to say that it is not long, so that medical terminologies by definition demand precision, founded in part on the context of connected description and in part on word choices that mean one thing and only one thing. The paragraph from *Human Structure* (which has 99 words) illustrates how Greco-Latinate terminologies beautifully serve this essential requirement of exact meaning:

appears: from Middle English, derived from Latin *apparere* ("to attend in public") = *ap-* + *parere* (*ap-* is a variant prefix of *ad-*, used before *p* ["toward"] + *parare* ["to be visible"]).

embryo: Greek *embryon;* the root is *-bryein* ("to swell").

longitudinal: Latin *longitudo* ("length") + *-alis* (Englished as *-al;* suffix for "pertaining to").

tube: Latin *tubus* ("pipe").

branches: from Middle English, derived from Latin *branca* ("paw").

aortic: adjective of *aorta;* Greek *aortē* ("an artery springing from the heart"), but ordinarily in ancient Greek, "a strap to hang anything to," for example a belt for a sword as in Homer, *Odyssey,* XI, 609.

arches: Latin *arcus* ("arc").

vein: Latin *vena,* through Middle English and Old French.

connections: Latin *con[n]exus* ("combination") = *con-* (a variant of *com-* before a consonant [except *b, h, l, p, r,* and *w*], in turn a variant of Latin *cum* ["with" or "together"]) + *nexus* ("grip" or "entwining," or "obligation" [in Roman law]). The suffix *-ion* denotes action or condition in words of Latin derivation in English.

SPECIAL VOCABULARIES 9

celom [usually *coelum*; pronounced "seelum"]; from the Greek *koilōma* ("cavity").

elongate: the root is *longus* (Latin) + the prefix *e-* (or *ex-* ["from" or "out of"]) + the suffix *-atus* (Englished as *-ate*), which suggests an action "in progress" or "in process." In chemistry, however, *-ate* names a salt of an acid, whose name ends in *-ic*, for example "sulfuric" and "sulfate."

cranial: Medieval Latin *cranium*, derived from the Greek *kranion* ("skull").

thorax: Greek *thōrax* ("that part of the body covered by a breastplate or scale armor"), which is the chest or the trunk. Englished adjectives appear as "thoracic" or "thoracico-" or "thoraco-." In entomology, however, the "thorax" designates that part of the insect body between the head and the abdomen.

hypaxial: Greek *hypo-* ("below" or "beneath") + Latin *axis* ("axle"). Here *hypaxial* would mean "below the central line of the body or any of its parts."

increasingly: Middle English derived from Latin *increscere* ("to grow into" or "to increase").

crown: from Middle English, derived from Latin *corona* ("wreath" or "crown").

vessels: from Middle English through Old French, derived from the latin *vascellum* ("small urn" or "small dish").

Of the 99 words in the paragraph from *Human Structure,* an important 17 are Latinate or direct borrowings from the Greek. Of these 17 words of Latin or Greek derivation, 6 are repeated at least once, with *cranial* used three times, so that 35 of the 99 words (or slightly over 35 percent) are either Latin or Greek. Cartmill, Hylander, and Shafland intend an "updated" anatomy text, using as many "English" terms as possible, yet over one-third remain those of a traditional and classical derivation. Comparison with the more standard account of early embryonic development of the heart in Gray, *Anatomy of the Human Body,* 568–76, shows how Cartmill and his colleagues have Englished a Latin-infused text, with a decrease in Latin and Greek words by about 40 percent. The authors of *Human Structure,* however, remain securely dependent on the Greco-Latinate vocabulary for precise description, even after ruthless pruning and tasteful substitution of multisyllabic terms with the more forceful and vivid words of a common English.

In spite of the frequent comments by literary critics, words derived from Greek and Latin origins are often as sharp and vivid as those specifically designated as Anglo-Saxon or Middle English. This is especially true when there is a requirement for a particular term in order to distinguish something from all other things of similar structure or function. If an author writes "a dusty road," this could be any dusty road anywhere in the world, and the only distinguishing feature of this universal road is its hazy, puffy, dry, and powdery feel or look. *Dusty* does incorporate all these specifics, but only in a vague manner. Suppose one wrote "a road mired in the dusty powder of the summer's drought." By adding *mire* in this context, one now has the sense of something deep or even mossy, since the word usually occurs in connection with mud or slime, but such is the flexibility of English that one can become mired in dust as easily as muck. Including *powder* adds an important aspect of vivid description because of the force of the Latinate term (*powder* comes into English from Middle English through Old French's *poudre,* in turn from Latin's *pulvis*), which is why detective fiction overuses the word *pulverize*. And *summer* tells instantly an all-important "when" for the phrase ("summer" and its German cognate *Sommer* ultimately are linked to the ancient Sanskrit *samā* ["half-year"], indicating why terms for seasons are so evocative). To be sure, an editor might sniff "too many words" when reading "a road mired in the dusty powder of the summer's drought," but that editor would also recognize how the writer had attempted to amplify "a dusty road" into something more vivid. *Powder* and *summer,* with their deep etymologies, certainly provide forcefully vivid contexts, and perhaps a reader might now ask, "Where?" Kansas or maybe Zimbabwe would do, depending on what the author was trying to develop as a story.

When scientists coin new words, they indulge in a similarly intellectual exercise as they attempt to refine particulars. Frequently, they draw terms or fragments of words from the large stock of ancient Greek or Latin nouns and adjectives. Why Latin and Greek? There are a number of salient reasons, but most important is a combination of Latin's widespread underpinnings of several modern European languages (the Romance tongues, especially French, Italian, Spanish, Portuguese, and Rumanian) and Latin's once universal function as the language of learning, coupled with the basic fact that classical Latin and Greek are "dead languages" (that is, they are no longer spoken). Greek and Latin words become for the sciences the ordinary quarry for coinages as researchers try to name what they have discovered, and to ensure that the name applied is understood by everyone in the subspecialty. The following is reflective of this continuous process:

In 1964, Vladimir Prelog and his research personnel at the Eidgenössische Technische Hochschule in Zürich called [some] red-brown metabolites . . . "siderochromes." In Greek, *sideros* is the word for "iron" and *chroma* means "color." At the University of California at Berkeley in 1973, John Neilands suggested that "siderochromes" should not be confined to hydroaxamate structures but ought to embrace other iron compounds with similar biological functions. During the same year, Charles Lankford of the University of Texas felt that a class name based on color isn't such a red-hot idea; what if someone discovered a colorless example? He prefers "siderophore"; *phorein* is from a Greek verb meaning "to carry." A 1984 review about siderophores told us this onomastic difference was ironed out. (Nickon and Silversmith, *Organic Chemistry,* 145–46.)

Aside from Nickon and Silversmith's fondness for puns (their very family names are almost unintentional puns in their own right), note that Prelog (who won the Nobel Prize in chemistry in 1975) and his Swiss colleagues coined their new term from a combination of two Greek words; note too that the Berkeley chemist proposed that the new term ought to incorporate a broader class of substances than first suggested; and finally, notice how a Texas scientist pointed out why the Prelog term might not be useful if future substances chanced to be without color. A new coinage (again using a Greek word) entered the literature, but both the Prelog proposal and the nomenclature suggested by Lankford were understood because of their common roots in Greek. If, by contrast, Prelog had proposed a German term, or Neilands and Lankford had suggested English, the international community of organic chemists might not have comprehended Prelog's original discovery, and that same community of scientists certainly would not have been able to understand why Lankford's alternative term would better account for future discoveries. Classical Greek provided the base, even in the most modern of laboratory descriptives, and Prelog's stature as an international figure in organic chemistry reinforced this common custom of coinages from Greco-Latinate roots. Even the account by Nickon and Silversmith acknowledges the ordinary employment in the sciences of Greco-Latinate terminologies: *hydroaxamate* and *onomastic* are key words, derived from roots in Greek. *Hydro-* emerges from the Greek *hydōr* ("water") and is here joined with an *amine* form (ultimately derived from the Greek *ammoniakos* ["of Ammon"]), and *onomastic* is the Englished form of the Greek *onomastikos,* the adjective of *onoma* ("name"). Nickon and Silversmith use these terms without comment.

"ROOTS," PREFIXES, AND SUFFIXES

Simak's *Mastodonia,* the selection from *Human Structure* by Cartmill and colleagues, and the paragraph from Nickon and Silversmith's *Organic Chemistry* all illustrate the use and meanings of various Latinate or Greek-derived terms. Such words often are combinations of a fundamental "root" augmented by either a prefix or a suffix, or both. Some of the brief etymologies given for particular words indicate how each part of the "new" term adds a piece to the exact meaning of the word as it might be used in modern, technical English. Some medical and scientific terms combine more than one root into a single word, for example *neuropathology,* with three roots (one can, of course, argue that *neuro-* is the prefix and that *-logy* is the suffix, but for purposes of illustration, each part of this term will be counted as a root):

> *neuro-:* from the Greek *neuron* ("thong" or "tendon"), and in Hellenistic and Roman medical Greek, a "cord which transmits an impulse."
>
> *-patho-:* from the Greek *pathos* ("that which happens" and, in a bad sense, "misfortune"); in ancient Greek, *pathos* often means "passion" or "emotion" (and thus a "disturbance of the soul"), so that later Greek uses *pathos* to mean "suffering" and by implication—depending on context—"disease."
>
> *-logy:* from Greek *logos* ("reason," "word," "speech," "reckoning," "subject matter," and several other related meanings); in later

Greek, *logos* often came to mean something akin to "reasoning about a subject," thus leading to the common coinage seen here, "the study of, or knowledge of, a subject."

Thereby, *neuropathology* is the "study of" or "knowledge about diseases of the nervous system," a translation easily gained from comprehension of the three Greek roots in the word.

CHAPTER 2

BOTANY

> 'Tis but thy name that is my enemy;
> Thou art thyself though, not a Montague
> What's Montague? it is nor hand, nor foot,
> Nor arm, nor face, nor any other part
> Belonging to a man. O, be some other name!
> What's in a name! that which we call a rose
> By any other name would smell as sweet
> —WILLIAM SHAKESPEARE, *Romeo and Juliet*

ONE of the greatest revolutions in the history of humankind was the change from hunting and gathering to the domestication of certain animals and plants, ensuring food supplies generally not subject to the vagaries of herd migrations and to the limited quantities of seeds and fruits collected in the wild. From the beginnings, each culture and tribe had its names for important plants and animals, and if the Neanderthals who lived at Shanidar in Iraq in about 30,000 B.C. understood the healing properties of specific herbs, they certainly gave the plants particular names, perhaps suggestive of shape, color, or use as drugs. Yet a variation in plant names from culture to culture caused confusion from earliest times, and we still remain uncertain about specifics of botanical lore among the civilizations of ancient Mesopotamia, although scholars of the cuneiform scripts have made learned guesses about which herbs, roots, seeds, and plants were prominent along the Tigris and Euphrates some five thousand years ago. Such guesses are based on cognates in Arabic, Coptic, Aramaic, Syriac, and similar languages that resemble extinct earlier tongues, written in the cuneiform scripts.

A modern example of this curious confusion of botanical names as they cross even the thinnest of cultural lines is what Americans call "wheat" and the English call "corn." In any text from Britain on ancient history, there are frequent mentions of the "corn trade" in the Roman Empire, a literal impossibility to an American reader, since "corn" was discovered in the New World by Spanish explorers after 1492—and then taken back to Europe, where it became an important food crop. It turns out that British English's *corn* is American English's *wheat* and that British English's *maize* is American English's *corn*. The common terms in both Englishes generate confusion, but if one digs out the scientific names of wheat (*Triticum* spp.) and corn (*Zea mays* L.), there is instant clarity, thanks to the modern binomial system of botanical nomenclature used internationally. One quickly sees that *Zea mays* L. is called "Indian corn," "maize," or (rarely) "corn" in England and that *Triticum* spp. (the English "corn") include wheats, emmers, and spelts of about twenty species (spp.) grown throughout the world as a major cereal crop.

In choosing *Triticum* as the standard name for the genus of wheats in the grass family (*Gramineae* [from the Latin *gramen*, gen. *graminis*, "grass"]), agricultural botanists went back to the word among the Romans for durum wheat, a hard and semi-translucent emmer and the favored species in Italy for making macaroni and spaghetti (the hulled wheat makes flours known as semolina and farina). *Triticum* occurs quite early in Latin literature, with instances of *triticum* as durum wheat appearing in the works of Ennius (239–169 B.C.) and Plautus (fl. 200 B.C.); *triticum* also meant the "threshed grain of wheat" and "wheat" (as a commodity) in Plautus's day, and by the time Cato the Elder (234–149 B.C.) put down his *De agri cultura* in about 160 B.C., the word was the ordinary one for "wheat." Today's botanical nomenclature for durum wheat is *Triticum durum* Desf., indicating how plants gain their scientific names in a manner much like the coinages in the other sciences: the neo-Latin means "hard wheat" (which is what it is, in comparison with other species of *Triticum*, for example *Triticum aestivum* L., our "common wheat" with its high gluten content), and the nonitalicized "Desf." trailing the Latin coinage is the abbreviation of the name of the person whose nomenclature for the plant is the one generally accepted internationally among botanists, in this case R. L. Desfontaines (1750–1833), a famous French botanical scientist. Yet, as any professional botanist will grumpily warn amateur gardeners, quite often there are fierce debates among botanists over just this question of which Latinate name *will* be accepted, and the nomenclature for "common wheat" is a case in point. That nonitalicized capital "L." after *Triticum aestivum* stands for Carl Linnaeus (1707–78), whose brilliantly conceived *Species plantarum* (1st ed., 1753) is the fountainhead of modern binomial nomenclatures for plants and whose *Systema naturae* (10th ed., 1758) is the beginning of zoological nomenclatures in modern biology. But should one look up the Latin names for "common wheat," one will find *Triticum vulgare* Vill. and *Triticum sativum* Lam., among several; one will also find notes on how the name *Triticum aestivum* has been emended in nineteenth- and twentieth-century botanical debates, so that there *is* general agreement that the genus shall be known as *Triticum,* but the species name will depend on which authority the botanist has chosen to follow, as listings are given. Employing *Triticum vulgare* Vill. indicates a botanist prefers the Latin meaning literally "common wheat" according to the name given by D. Villars (1745–1814), but if the name is given as *Triticum sativum* Lam., then the meaning is "cultivated wheat" on the authority of the famous eighteenth-century French botanist and zoologist Jean-Baptiste de Lamarck (1744–1829). *Triticum aestivum* translates as "summer wheat," which is not much more satisfying than other names, but in honor of Linnaeus's work, botanists frequently choose this binomial in preference to any of the more modern suggestions in botanical Latin

By contrast, American English's "corn" and British English's "maize" or "Indian corn" always carry the label *Zea mays* L. Only a single species is involved, and Linnaeus's name has satisfied everyone since it appeared in the *Species plantarum* of 1753 (pp. 971–72). Linnaeus's Latin summarizes why the name has endured; as he writes, *Frumentum indicum Mavs dictum* and *Habitat in America:* the Indians call it "Mays," and it is native to the New World. But why *Zea*? The Latin for "wheat" had already been used by Linnaeus (pp. 85–87, under which he has seven species [the first listed is *Triticum aestivum*]), but some earlier botanists had pulled over the Greek *zeia* (Latinized as *zea*) as an alternative name for certain varieties of wheat, so that this Greco-Latinate term was now free for use elsewhere in Linnaeus's binomial system of naming plants. In Greek, *zeia* usually meant "one-seeded wheat" (beginning with Homer [c. 800 B.C.) in the *Odyssey,* IV, 41), which Linnaeus had firmly named *Triticum monococcum,* the Latin for "one-seeded wheat" (*Triticum monococcum* L.—the Linnaean name has survived intact—is the common einkorn of Italy, Germany, and Switzerland). So a "new wheat" (which Indian "Mays" was not) could bear the Greek *zea,* to distinguish it from the seven species of *Tritica*. And if one notices that Indian name, "Mays," one then understands why the English call Indian corn "maize," a word stemming ultimately from Hispaniolan Taino and which came into Spanish as *maiz* and thence into mid-sixteenth-century English as *maize*. "Corn" on both sides of the Atlantic is *Zea mays* L., even though the only accurate part of the Latinate binomial is "mays," which is more-or-less what it was called by native Americans in the West Indies before the arrival of the Spanish.

If *wheat* and *corn* are imprecise as they occur in the common speech of Britain and the United States, this illustrates why common names for plants might engender confusion and why Linnaeus's concept of a binomial nomenclature has become so essential in the biological sciences since the eighteenth century. As in the case of the name for corn (American), many Latinate names for plants do not reflect exactly what they are, but inaccuracies are more than compensated by the manner in which the international scientific community can use these names to mean one plant and only one plant. *Dandelion* in American English immediately brings to mind a full image of a low-growing lawn flower with a bright yellow top, which produces fluffy seeds loved by children as they blow them into the summer breezes to watch them float gently away. This lovely image may warm childhood memory, but does it provide an exact name? In the United States, many larger, flowering bushes are termed *rhododendrons*, but are they all the same species as the state flower of West Virginia? One knows exactly what a *tomato* is—or does one? And just what is a *jack pine*? An *oak*? Are all *tulips* alike? And *maples*? *Elms*? And how does one describe the useful, lawn-growing *plantain* or the widely dispersed *Jimsonweed*? If Shakespeare's question implied in "What's a name!" is extended to a logical end, we find that there are some names suggestive of some qualities of a flower or plant (Shakespeare chooses the rose, wisely observing that only a rose would ever smell like a rose) but that common names for plants and flowers are generally context-bound, culturally limited labels that do not transfer or translate well across linguistic or cultural boundaries. Scientific nomenclatures, using coined Greek or Latin terms, seek to obviate confusion, illustrated by the dandelion, the rhododendron, and the Jimsonweed.

Our *dandelion* is an anglicized form of the medieval French *dent de lion* ("tooth of a lion"), which is the French form of the medieval Latin *dens leonis* (meaning also "tooth of a lion"). When Linnaeus provided his nomenclature for this very common plant, frequently employed in herbal preparations, he chose to preserve the older descriptive of "lion-tooth" (which applied supposedly to the shape of the leaves) and wrote *Leontodon taraxacum* as the binomial (*Species plantarum,* 798). *Leon-* is the "lion," but *-odon* is Greek, not Latin, for "tooth" (*odous* is the nominative singular form, *odontos* the genitive singular), so that Linnaeus has again used a combined Greco-Latinate coinage to express what an earlier purely Latin name had said. The *taraxacum* is a Latinized coinage from a Persian word meaning "bitter herb," and thereby Linnaeus has acknowledged the dandelion's widespread use in eighteenth-century herbal pharmacology by adapting a term from a Near Eastern language into a Latinized form. Later botanists, however, believed that Linnaeus's name did not quite describe the dandelion, and if one looks up the usual nomenclature in a modern guide to flowers, one will normally find *Taraxacum officinale* Weber (sometimes followed by *Leontodon taraxacum* L.). "Weber" stands for G. H. Weber (1752–1828), who suggested this new name, which seemed to say more about the dandelion than merely the "lion-toothed bitter herb" in Linnaeus's coinage; Weber's nomenclature means "the bitter herb of the druggists' shops" of the day, indicating how common were dandelion concoctions in European drugs of the early nineteenth century. The *officinale* says that this is *the* bitter herb, which is dandelion, sold in the drug shops, and the adjectival *-ale* agrees in gender (neuter) with the Latinized Persian word ending in *-um* (if Linnaeus had chosen a masculine *Taraxacus* or feminine *Taraxaca,* the adjectival would appear as *officinalis*). Classical Latin's *officina* normally meant "workshop," that is, where something is made or manufactured, so that the *officinale* of the modern binomal nomenclature for "dandelion" also tells something of its preparation in the druggists' establishments of eighteenth- and nineteenth-century Europe and thus is known as an "officinal" medicine. This meant simply that apothecaries stocked the substance as a matter of course, and the most widely used of such drugs often became part of the listings in the pharmacopoeias of the nineteenth century. No longer a recommended drug in American pharmacy, the dandelion still enjoys a respected reputation in folk medicine as a diuretic and mild laxative and as a coffee substitute (the roots). Although somewhat dated in the meaning of its name, *Taraxacum officinale* Weber is thereby known internationally as one plant and only one plant in the family of plants called Compositae (from the Latin *compositus* ["compound"] but in modern botanical Latin meaning "with flowers in a head"), often called the "Daisy family."

A second example of how botanical nomenclatures, coined from Greek and Latin (or Latinized words from other languages), reduce confusion in modern botany is the name for "rhododendron": *Rhododendron maximum* L. The common name in this instance mirrors part of the scientific name, but both have origins in the Greek *rhodon* ("rose," a flower characteristic of the island of Rhodes) and the Greek *dendron* ("tree"); the common name means "rose-tree," and the botanical Latin is "largest rose-tree." *Rhododendron maximum* L. is the "great laurel" or "rose bay" or simply "great rhododendron" of temperate North America, and anyone who knows the hills of West Virginia or Kentucky will recall these flowering shrublike trees in summer settings of mountain creeks and waters trickling down ledges of sandstone coupled with odors of wet humus. Even if one noted that the "great laurel" has leaves throughout the winter and that these leaves are leathery and occasionally downy on the undersides, there would remain some uncertainty, since there are almost six hundred species of "rhododendrons" throughout the world (although only two in North America have evergreen-like leaves). Moreover, others with memories of similar "laurels" and "azaleas" in the southern states would picture different plants altogether, since most "azaleas" have leaves like the "rhododendrons," but "azaleas" lose their leaves in the winter. Even flower descriptions are unhelpful, because the genus *Rhododendron* (which includes the azaleas) generally has large and showy flowers, with five-lobed and funnel-shaped corollas, and are usually radially symmetrical. As exact-sounding as is the description, it can apply to many species with genus *Rhododendron*. Again, once a special and necessarily unique botanical binomial name is attached to the "great laurel" (or whatever common name would be used, depending on regional preferences), there is no doubt regarding *Rhododendron maximum* L. The binomial may not "describe" the plant too well, but the nomenclature ensures exact identification.

Rhododendrons and azaleas are among the nearly six hundred species in the family Ericaceae (a botanical Latin coinage from classical Latin's *erica* ["heath" or "broom"] adapted from the Greek *ereikē*).

The infamous "Jimsonweed" is a third illustration of why Latinized binomials provide exact identities for plants while the common names frequently perpetuate confusion. A popular musical-cowboy lyric of the late 1940s ran "I'm back in the saddle again / Out where a friend is a friend / Where the lonesome cattle feed on the lowly Jimson weed," as if anyone who tuned in to the Gene Autry radio hour in those days knew exactly what a "Jimsonweed" was. If range cattle did consume this plant, they might have perished, or as a standard handbook on noxious plants puts it, "Losses have been reported in the world literature in all classes of livestock, including ostriches" (Kingsbury, *Poisonous Plants*, 281). Depending on where one is in the United States or Mexico, or South America, or Eurasia ("Jimsonweed" is cosmopolitan), it is called "devil's apple," "thorn apple," "Jimsonweed," "stinkweed," "datura," "stramonium," and "angels' trumpets" among a number of common names. The ordinary American name for this beautiful flowering annual, "Jimsonweed," has its own curious history. "Jimson" is a contracted form of "Jamestown," the famous first permanent English settlement in Virginia (1607), but "Jamestown weed" did not attain notoriety until the last phases of Bacon's Rebellion (1673–76). King Charles had sent one thousand soldiers to aid Governor William Berkeley in putting down the revolt, but some of the European fighting men became ill from eating "the JamesTown weed (which resembles the Thorny Apple of Peru, and I take it to be the plant so call'd)," as is related in the contemporary account by Robert Beverly in *History and Present State of Virginia*. Nat Bacon had died earlier from dysentery, and the soldiers recovered from their mistaken use of what looked like an edible potherb. Since 1676, this "thorn apple" (another quite common name for the plant) has carried "Jimsonweed" as its label, from Beverly's recounting of symptoms of ingestion at Jamestown, which states that "the Effect . . . was a very pleasant Comedy," clearly delirium.

Linnaeus's nomenclature for the Jimsonweed was *Datura stramonium*, and he assumed that the plant was native to the New World even while he added *nunc vulgaris per Europam* ("now common throughout Europe": *Species plantarum*, 179), a problem still argued by botanists and pharmacologists (the origin of *Datura stramonium* L. remains disputed). Linnaeus's Latinate coinage is a fascinating blend of Latin, Hindi, and probably French: *Datura* is borrowed directly from the Hindi *dhatura* (ultimately derived from the Sanskrit *dhattūra*), meaning "thorn apple," and Hindi's *dhat* was the poison prepared from the plant (folklore recorded how a thief who might use such a preparation in his trade [the victim would be drugged with this substance] was termed a *dhatūrea*); *stramonium* is a Latinized form of the French *stramoine* or perhaps the Italian *stramonio*, which had come into seventeenth-century technical English as *stramonium*, meaning in all three languages "thorn apple" (in French also "stinkweed"), and the Linnaean gist in the adaptation is "spiky-fruited," quite appropriate for the matured seedpods that succeed the beautiful trumpet flowers in the growing cycle of the Jimsonweed. Popular names of this very common, widely known, and generally recognized "weed" merely confuse exact identity, and when Linnaeus chose the binomial (which remains accepted today), he may not have employed clear descriptives in the pseudo-Latin, but he ensured that *Datura stramonium* would apply to a single species. A botanist, anywhere in the world, would know that *Datura* would mean any one of ten species in the Solanaceae ("Nightshades"), which have funnel-shaped flowers, prickly seedpods, and narcotic properties when prepared as drugs. The family Solanaceae (from the Latin *solanum*, the black nightshade of Pliny's *Natural History*, XXVII, 132 [*Solanum nigrum* L.]) has about seventeen hundred species and includes the genus *Capsicum* (the New World "red peppers" [derived from the Latin *capsa*, a "cylindrical case for storage of a rolled papyrus"]), the so-called Irish potato (*Solanum tuberosum* L.) native to the Andes Mountains of South America, the eggplant (*Solanum melongena* L., with the species name a Latinized form of the Italian *melanzana*, "mad apple"), the tomato (*Lycopersicon esculentum* Mill.) from Peru, Bolivia, and Ecuador (the neo-Latin coinage by Philip Miller [1691–1771] means "edible wolf-peach," and Renaissance Europe had believed the fruit to be the long-sought true aphrodisiac, hence the early name "love apple" after its introduction into Europe by 1554), the famous mandrake (*Mandragora officinarum* L.), and the ever popular and ever controversial tobacco (*Nicotiana tabacum* L.).

Linnaeus's nomenclature for tobacco takes account of both the origins and the native uses of the plant, as well as the name of the individual who presumably introduced tobacco into European culture: *tabacum* is derived from an Arawak or Guarani word (probably through Spanish) for the plant or for the pipe used by natives in northern South America to smoke the leaves; *Nicotiana* Latinizes the name of Jean Nicot, the French ambassador to Portugal, who took the seeds of this New World addiction to France in 1560.

Botanical terminologies and Latinate coinages are illustrative of the general principles of formation of modern scientific words, which presumably "use" Greek, Latin, or other languages for derivative terms: sometimes, the original meaning of the classical Latin or Greek is simply carried through into modern nomenclature (as in the case of the *Triticum* spp.), but frequently, ancient meanings have little connection with modern names, which display Latin-like endings but which are not Latin at all (*Nicotiana tabacum* L. as an example). Yet Latin itself was and is essential in almost all scientific coinages, and there are several reasons this has been so since the days of Linnaeus. In the first place, the ultimate origins of botanical Latin are in the terminologies of Pliny the Elder in his *Natural History* of A.D. 77; here is the fountainhead of Roman names for plants and animals, as well as numerous Latin adaptations of Greek plant names as they had appeared in the writings of Theophrastus of Eresus (*c.* 370–288 B.C.) and other, earlier Greek authors on agriculture and botanical lore. Those Latinized names passed into the tradition of botanical nomenclatures in the works of Isidore (A.D. 560–636), Albertus Magnus (1193–1280), Rufinus (*fl. c.* 1290), and thence into the writings on botany in Latin by Renaissance scholars, including Valerius Cordus (1515–44), whose *Historia plantarum* was one of the best of its kind. This long tradition, however, did not markedly improve the descriptive morphology of plants as set down by Theophrastus in his *Enquiry into Plants* (*c.* 300 B.C.). The concepts of botanical characters enunciated by Theophrastus—characteristics discerned by eye—remained essentially unchallenged for almost nineteen hundred years until technology produced good magnifying lenses and ultimately the microscope, which finally revealed the tiny structures within the flower (Greek *anthos;* Latin *flos*) as a collection of organs.

A second reason Latin has become the basic foundation ("with much plundering of ancient Greek," in the phrase of Stearn, *Botanical Latin,* 6) for botanical terms, as well as almost all other biological sciences, is also intertwined with historical matters. Renaissance Europeans used Latin, albeit a Latin somewhat distant from the Latin of Cicero and Vergil, in all learned subjects from law and theology to medicine and philosophy and literature. When one scholar wished to communicate with another scholar in a different country or in his own city, he almost always used Latin; his basic education often was in Latin literature, and if one aspired to high functions in the newly burgeoning nation-states of Renaissance Europe, one had to know Latin. Fewer knew Greek or Arabic or Hebrew, but an important aspect of the new scholarship in sixteenth-century Europe was the rediscovery of the classics in their original tongues, from the Greek of Aristotle and Galen, as well as the *koinē* Greek (this is the "common speech") of the New Testament, to the better readings gained by close perusal of actual manuscripts of ancient age. This "new philology" produced thousands of editions, spewed forth by the many printing presses that now dotted Europe, and those same printing houses made widely known (sometimes in Latin, sometimes in the vernacular tongues) the heady discoveries of lands and products, peoples and customs, which forcibly expanded the European world view. New plants, new animals, new drugs—all had to be described and catalogued in some way, and the base remained Latin, which soon became populated by many Latinized terms, coined from foreign words for which there were no near equivalents in Latin, or Greek, or any of the widely spoken vernaculars (English, French, German, Spanish, Portuguese, Italian, Dutch, Swedish, and so on). The adaptation of an Arawak word into the Latinized *tabacum* illustrates this process.

A third reason Latin became the basis for scientific coinages is perhaps the simplest and most practical: given the multiplicity of spoken languages at the various capital cities of the new nation-states, Latin provided an international tongue for scholars and scientists, a language also used by the Roman Catholic church as its international medium of communication. Much as priests and prelates could speak to one another in Latin, no matter what might have been their specific national origin, so also anatomists, botanists, physicians, legal experts, geographers, and so forth could communicate with one another on subjects of common interest and enthusiasm in Latin, no matter where one happened to be. Even today, when language barriers loom at international meetings of scientists and scholars, occasionally there will be a hasty brushing-off of one's rusty "school Latin," and a modicum of mutual understanding is often established. Yet one of the great strengths of using Latin (and to a lesser degree, Greek) as the language of labels is also simple: both are "dead languages," that is, neither classical Latin nor classical Greek remains as a spoken tongue anywhere in the world. There are, of course, the five Romance languages directly descended from Latin, and modern Greeks speak a form of Greek, which has the alphabet of ancient Greek but not the syntax, grammar, or vocabulary of the Greek of Plato's time. Latin and Greek as the substrata of scientific terminologies serve equally well for Russian biologists as they do for American chemists and botanists and as they will for Arabic-speaking or Chinese-speaking scientists. Latin and Latinate terms are the same to all these scientists of varying national origins or multiple linguistic contexts. Once established and accepted by the international community of specialists, scientific terms become specific: *Datura stramonium* L. may be "stinkweed" to the French and "Jimsonweed" or "thorn apple" to Americans but only *Datura stramonium* to the international world of the botanical sciences.

Classification of plants and animals remains rooted in the system established by Aristotle (384–322 B.C.), the brilliant philosopher and naturalist, who was the teacher of Theophrastus. Aristotle classed animals in a scale of nature that ascended to man (there is, however, no hint of an "evolution"), creating the "step-laddered" perception of nature wherein one still speaks of "higher" and "lower" animals and plants. If man (the animal) is the pinnacle of creation, how does man merit (in nature) that lofty status? Aristotle clearly understood the problems of classification, and his efforts to determine classes of animals led to the collection of "facts" in large numbers of "inquiries" (*historiai*, in Greek) on various subjects, which could then lead to a hypothesis (or a "law") by inductive logic; once a hypothesis was proposed, Aristotle and his students would apply the hypothesis to the collected data. Over many years and numerous observations of plants and animals (Aristotle dissected animals, and his comparative embryology was advanced enough to be appreciated well into the nineteenth century), Aristotle determined that nature (*physis*, in Greek) in its living forms existed and functioned in a teleology (*telos*, genitive *teleos* ["fulfillment," a "coming to pass," or "consummation" among several meanings]), which meant that animals and plants, and the parts of animals and plants, are what they are supposed to be, according to the *logos* (here "purpose") in nature. Living things thus followed development of their specific kinds through growth and change (*metabolē*), and higher animals by definition displayed movement (*kinēsis*), intelligence, a good deal of heat (*thermon*), and a soul (*psychē*) in terms of which all changes in the animal are expressed. Plants are simple by comparison with animals: plants take nourishment already prepared for them from the earth; they grow and reproduce themselves at a fixed season. To Aristotle, the most elementary *psychē* was assigned to the functions of growth, nourishment, and the production of offspring. Compared with animals, plants are devoid of life, but compared with other bodies, plants are endowed with life.

Classification of animals and plants, according to Aristotle, resulted from perception of higher functions beyond merely gaining food and reproducing according to one's own kind, and in a series of works, he set down this basic scheme of orderings in nature, each becoming enormously influential in the history of biology. In *On the Soul*, Aristotle treats the form of animals (that is, the soul) and its parts or functions; the *Inquiry into Animals* is a remarkable record of observations on numerous species; *Movement of Animals* explicates the functions common to the body and soul, excluding reproduction; *Generation of Animals* examines the parts used in reproduction and the reproductive functions common to the body and the soul; and the famous *Parts of Animals* treats the "causes" (*aitiai*) of why plants and animals are what they are (namely the teleology: nature with a purpose). One can illustrate in a streamlined manner Aristotle's notion of the causes by using an oak (*Quercus* spp. [Latin *quercus*, "oak"]) the parent tree is the "motive cause"; the seed (an acorn) is the "material cause"; the development into an oak tree is the "formal cause"; and the aim to produce a perfect oak tree is the "final cause." Aristotle's "causes" thereby explain differences among animals and plants and why some animals are "higher" on the scale of beings than others, with the highest animal of all being the male human.

Why male? In an infamous passage of *Generation of Animals*, Aristotle explains that "femaleness" is a natural "deformity" (that is, the aim in nature is to produce a male human) and that women are inferior to men due to women's lack of proportion (*symmetria*) of elementarty kinds of matter, especially the Hot (*thermon*), the Wet (*hygron*), the Cold (*psychron*), and the Dry (*xēron*). Women have less heat than men and are characterised by the Wet and the Cold (*Generation of Animals*, 767a–775a15 ["female deformity": *Generation*, 775a15]). If this long-term prejudice is puzzling to us today, then one may consult Aristotle's *Parts of Animals*, 650a2–8 and 652b8–11: here are the relationships between heat and the soul and the explanations of how the Hot is necessary for the soul and how nutrition is engendered by heat. The less heat, the less soul. Classification falls into place neatly enough, if one can determine the heat that reflects the soul. Aristotle's concepts of intelligence (he believed it emerged in the heart, the source of the body's heat) contrasted sharply with the teachings of *his* mentor, Plato (*c.* 429–347 B.C.), who taught that intelligence arose in the brain.

As Aristotle's student, Theophrastus inherited the constructs of a teleological classification system, but in the study of plants, the proportions of heat and the nature of the soul would not bulk too large. By definition, Theophrastus concentrated on the most basic functions of growth, nourishment, and reproduction in his *Enquiry into Plants;* morphology and taxonomy thereby reflected his recognition that the flower—whether leaflike or hairlike in such instances as the apple or the grape respectively—becomes the fruit or seed. Even in modern botanical classifications, there remain aspects of this ancient Greek notion of "higher" and "lower" plants, since "higher" plants generally are those that have flowers at some point in their life cycles. Modern botany, however, emphasizes the Linnaean "sexual parts" system, so that classification frequently turns on how one interprets either (1) the stamen (Latin's *stamen* is "the vertical threads in a loom, the warp"), with its upper anther (coined from the Greek *anthēros* ["flowery"]) and lower filament (Renaissance Latin's *filamentum* ["spun" or "wound thread"], drawn from Latin's *filum* ["thread"]), the anther being the pollen-bearing organ of the flower (Latin's *pollen* meant "dust" or "fine flour"), or (2) the pistil (*pistillum* in Latin meant "pestle"), with its upper style (from Latin *stylus* ["writing tool"]) and lower ovary (Renaissance Latin *ovarium,* from Latin *ovum* ["egg"]), the pistil being the seed-bearing, female organ of the flower. These are "higher" plants. "Lower" plants in today's botany include simple, unicellular organisms characterized by their chlorophyll (from the Greek *chloros* ["green" or "greenish yellow"] + *phyllon* ["leaf"], plural *phylla*) and phycocyanin (Greek *phykos* ["seaweed"] + *kyanos* ["dark blue"])—the blue-green algae, termed *Cyanophyceae* from the same Greek roots—as well as various mosses, mushrooms, ferns, yeasts, molds, bacteria, smuts, club mosses, horsetails, and many other genera and families of plants "below" those with flowers.

Plants and animals are called "kingdoms," in a semisubtle reflection of the division promulgated by Aristotle in the fourth century B.C. Within each "kingdom," there are subdivisions of animals and plants into phyla (Greek *phylon*, plural *phyla,* ["tribe" or "race"]), with a single "tribe" of plants known by the Latinized *phylum* and further subdivided into classes, subclasses, superorders, orders, families, genera (the plural of *genus,* the Latin for "race" or "kind"), and species (the plural is also species: Latin's *species* meant "visual appearance," "a thing of a particular kind," among about a dozen basic meanings in classical Latin; several species would be written "several spp." in most specialist works). The ancient stepladder survives in two forms: in the "higher" and "lower" notions, and in the taxonomic characteristics of all modern biological sciences. In botany, there are five phyla (or divisions) of plants, each with its subdivisions of classes, and the names ordinarily used show in vivid fashion their Latin or Greek origins:

> *Thallophyta:* a Late Latin coinage, based on the Greek *thallos* ("twig" or "young shoot") + *phyton* ("plant"), in which are—among several—the following classes:
>
> > *Algae* (Latin's *alga* meant "seaweed"), the algae, green scum, seaweeds, most microscopic, simple green plants
> >
> > *Fungi* (Latin *fungus* is "mushroom"), the yeasts, molds, mildews, blights, smuts, mushrooms, bacteria, most simple, nongreen plants
> >
> > *Lichens* (pronounced "lyekin") (the Greek *leichēn* usually meant "tree moss" or "scaly eruption on the skin"), the algae and fungi

that exist symbiotically (Greek *symbiōsis* ["living together" or "companionship"]) but with a common thallus (*thallos* as above)

Bryophyta (Greek *bryon* ["moss"] + *phyton* ["plant"]) has two classes:

Musci (Latin *muscus* is "moss"), mosses

Hepaticae (Greek *hēpatikos* ["one who suffers from a liver complaint"]), the liverworts (from the Middle English "lifer" + "wyrt" ["root"])

Pteridophyta (Greek *pteris* ["fern"] + *phyton* ["plant"]) includes

Filicales (Latin *filix,* pl. *filices,* ["fern"]), the ferns

Equisetales (Latin *equus,* pl. *equi,* ["horse"] + *saeta* ["bristle"]), the horsetails

Lycopodiales (Greek *lykos* ["wolf"] + *podion* ["little foot" or "footlike"]), the club mosses

Gymnospermae (Greek *gymno-* ["naked," "bare," or "exposed"] + *sperma* ["seed"]) incorporates

Coniferales (Late Latin *conus* ["cone"] + *-i-* + *-fer* [Latin suffix, "bearing," from *ferre,* meaning "to bear"]), the pine trees and cone-bearing plants with exposed seeds

Gnetales (a nineteenth-century Latinate coinage [*OED* gives 1886 as first use] of unknown derivation), the various spp. of Chinese Ma-huang (*Ephedra* spp.)

Cycadales (an early-nineteenth-century [*OED* suggests 1830s] fumbling pseudo-Latin adaptation of the Greek *koix* [gen. sing. *koikos,* nom. pl. *koikoi,* acc. pl. *koikas*—the modern genus is *Cycas*]), the "doum palm" in Theophrastus, *Enquiry into Plants,* I, 10.5, sago palms and others, "cycads"

Ginkgoales (from Japanese *ginkyo* = *gin* ["silver"] + *kyo* ["apricot"]), the maidenhair tree or ginkgo; only one species—*Gingko biloba* L. *Biloba* ("two lobes")—describes the shape of the leaf

Angiospermae (Greek *angio-* ["container" or "vessel"] + *sperma* ["seed"]) has two large classes:

Monocotyledons (Greek *mono-* ["alone," "one," "single"] + *kotylēdōn* ["navelwort" in Dioscorides, *Materia Medica,* IV, 91–92], derived from *kotylē* ["small cup"]), the flowering plants with seeds borne enclosed in a case; one cotyledon (the primary leaf of the embryo of seed plants)

Dicotyledons (Greek *di-* ["two"] + *kotylēdōn* [as above]), the flowering plants with seeds encased (as above) but with two cotyledons

This classification system (adapted from Brimble, *Intermediate Botany*) has five phyla (or divisions) and fourteen classes, each fitted according to characteristics of growth and reproduction. The botanical novitiate will quickly notice how professional botanists and botanical taxonomists quarrel about "what to name it" and "how to name it," as in the instance of Brimble's class of dicotyledons, which is a subclass" in Hickey and King, *100 Families*.

CHAPTER 3

INVERTEBRATES: PROTOZOA TO MOLLUSCS

Reference to zoological groups is by words (names), not by mathematical or other symbols, because the earlier taxonomists used the current Latin, Greek or vernacular names of particular groups of animals . . . Names are arbitrary. It would not matter in the least if all bears were always called men, and vice versa. There is no link between the words man, homo, hombre, *etc., and men except by custom. The choice of a name for a group is therefore in the last resort, entirely arbitrary.*
—A. J. CAIN, Animal Species and their Evolution

Scientists . . . tolerate uncertainty and frustration, because they must. The one thing that they do not and must not tolerate is disorder . . . the most basic postulate of science is that nature itself is orderly. In taxonomy as in other sciences the aim is that the ordering of science shall approximate or in some estimable way reflect the order of nature. All theoretical science is ordering . . . Taxonomy . . . is a science that is most explicitly and exclusively devoted to the ordering of complex data.
—GEORGE GAYLORD SIMPSON, Principles of Animal Taxonomy

THESE two apparently contradictory statements are not contradictory at all: Cain tells us that when we name something as we name it, the name we "choose" is the subject of whims of custom, history, habit, and just plain stubbornness; Simpson says that as we name things, we are seeking an order we assume in nature, even though we recognize that a complete understanding of nature is by definition impossible. The "ordering" is arbitrary, as all taxonomists acknowledge, and even in the new science that studies chaos and disorder in nature, there is an assumption that one *can* understand the mechanics of disorder and, moreover, that the study of unpredictables (for example, oscillations of the heart, random drippings from a water faucet, and the seemingly erratic swirling of smoke as it comes from my pipe) is an ordering of a new kind. "Where chaos begins, classical science stops . . . Chaos breaks across the lines that separate scientific disciplines . . . it is a science of the global nature of systems." (Gleick, *Chaos,* 3, 5). Association remains the intellectual key, analogy stands as a sturdy base for the new linking of subspecialties among the sciences, and randomness itself—so we are told—is subject to natural laws. Soon there will emerge a nomenclature for this fresh approach to physics and the world of nature, and the old struggles over "what shall we agree to call it" will be repeated. Essential will be the agreement among the international communities of scientists, or the science of chaos will certainly be chaotic.

Observing and naming animals is as old as humankind's observation and labelling of plants, perhaps older. Early humans lived and survived according to hunting skills, so that when one views the breathtaking Cro-Magnon cave art of *c.* 15,000 B.C., one also drinks in the vision of the large animals that sustained the clan. The Cro-Magnon sounds representing "mammoth," "bison," or "woolly rhinoceros" are totally lost to us, but the vivid colors breathe their own life and vibrancy after twenty millennia. Names here are irrelevant, but Cro-Magnons assuredly knew all these animals by some labels, and—important for the questions of nomenclatures in any society—everyone would know these names without reflection. Individuals would know more names of animals than names for plants, insects, or birds simply because many of the animals were larger and also because knowledge of plants, insects, and birds would demand careful and lengthy scrutiny, as contrasted to casual absorption through common words continually employed in ordinary speech. One would know a horse as different from an ox or a bison or a mammoth, as very different indeed from a bat or a mouse or a saber-toothed lion or tiger, but differences among hawks and eagles and falcons, or among daisy-like flowers, or among beetles or cockroaches or earwigs, would require a special interest or need, as found among the clan's food-gatherers (who knew the best berries, roots, seeds, and the like) or among those designated by the clan as medicine-persons (who distinguished herbs from merely edible plants). If prehistoric art shows what humankind early believed important, one perceives large animals, the rituals of stalking and slaughtering those animals, and the basics of sex and reproduction (the famous "Venuses" of Neanderthal and Cro-Magnon sites frequently display only oversized breasts, enormous buttocks, and sometimes an appropriately swollen belly). Prehistoric humans probably possessed more words in a technical vocabulary of religion and ritual than in the assumed basics of hunting or plant-gathering, and as one sees continuously throughout history, technical vocabularies almost always mirror those aspects and values most esteemed by particular societies and cultures.

Since animals are so "obvious" in their similarities and differences, one notices the paradox of how difficult it has been to "classify" animals. Citing Aristotle suggests how our ancestors sought that ordering among disparate forms, and the ancient Greek approaches to this problem of similarities and differences among animals have exercised an enormous influence in the history of biology, even as we still speak of "higher" and "lower" animals in a stepladdered blueprint of genera and species, in addition to orders and families that populate all versions of animal nomenclatures. Linnaeus's binomial system for naming entities in nature also has set patterns for animal nomenclatures, a binomial system laid out in his *Systema naturae* (10th ed., 1758), and pre-Linnaean systematics generally have been forgotten. Yet within binomial nomenclatures for animals, there lurks a curious series of internal paradoxes, since the Greco-Latinate descriptives presumably are based upon obvious features that will distinguish one kind of animal from another, features presumably embedded in the two-part name. Humankind's scientific name is *Homo sapiens* (Latin "wise" or "learned human being"), perhaps reflective of brain capacities as currently understood, but little else. Biologists commonly recognize the internal paradox as they half-humorously define *man* as an "unfeathered biped." Supposedly the "unfeathered" makes the distinction between man and bird, and the "biped" ("two-footed") provides the distinctive feature of human beings walking upright. But the difference from birds proves insignificant, and the distinctive feature is not, so that the Linnaean system of simply two linguistic markers for particular genera and species quite frequently leads to funny, if logical, results. Turgidly but succinctly, Crowson lays out the multiple problems faced by animal biologists as they seek clarity in nomenclatures:

> The words classification, systematics and taxonomy are now commonly treated as synonyms, an example of the confusion and carelessness in the use of words which is prevalent in so much modern scientific writing. Words, to quote a poet "decay with imprecision, will not stay in place," and however true this may be of his own art, it is at least equally so in science . . . [One must] distinguish between classifying things and naming them. The use of a name . . . implies the recognition of a group, the class of things referred to by that name, and such groups are the elements of which classification are composed. Classification . . . involves the incorporation of such groups into a rational, hierarchical system in which each group has a unique place. Classificatory groups (taxa) are of various grades, or categories . . . and for all categories except the lowest, each taxon will include one or more taxa of the next lower category. Crowson, *Classification and Biology*, 18–19.

Crowson remains impaled on the twin tines of similarity and difference, those opposites clearly defined in Aristotelian biology in the fourth century B.C. Similar things go together, runs the logic, while other things, which are different but are similar to one another, will be grouped accordingly. Put another way, the Aristotelian zoological systematics, which still wittingly or unwittingly has great weight among biologists, can be expressed Aristotelian-style as a syllogism (All—or some, or no—A is B) with zoological assumptions: all mammals have mammary glands among the females (the major premise); the extinct symmetrodonts and pantotheres of the Jurassic were mammals (minor premise); therefore, female symmetrodonts and pantotheres had mammary glands. Aristotle's methodology reveals something unverifiable through actual observation, important to paleontologists who must group animals from bones or bone-fragments in the fossils (a classic account of such specific problems is in Romer, *Vertebrate Paleontology*, chap. 16, "Primitive Mammals"). Thus as entomologists seek careful relationships among the thousands of newly discovered insects as published each year, or as parasitologists attempt to discern similarities and differences among the microscopic and submicrosopic creatures that may bedevil man and animals, there remains an often unspoken reliance on intellectual premises first enunciated in Greek biology by Aristotle and his students. Sometimes groupings are easy: beetles almost always look like beetles, elephants are unmistakable, and bats can only be bats. But shades between groups (recognized by Aristotle as animals "imperfectly formed," such as seals) frequently defy neat classification, a problem encountered particularly among protozoologists as they group the numerous genera and species of microscopic animals. Entomologists also fudge as they ponder "primitive" insects, even as they apply the Linnaean-style binomials.

SOME NUMBERS FOR PERSPECTIVE

Linnaeus's binomials, though very useful for labeling the fairly limited varieties among plants, sometimes cannot encompass the huge numbers of known and probable animals that have existed since the beginnings of life on earth. "It has been guessed that as many as 4,000,000,000 different species of animals and plants have evolved since the dawn of life" (Easton, *Invertebrate Paleontology*, 4). That number is 4 *billion,* and there are about 300,000 species of living plants currently catalogued, compared with roughly 1.4 million species of living animals. Among the animals, almost 75 percent, or about 1,050,000 species, are arthropods, with insects alone having 900,000 different species— or even more, according to some entomologists. Among the insects, beetles have the largest number of species. "One animal in every four is a beetle, and nearly 300,000 species have already been described" (Evans, *Life of Beetles,* 17). Among the insects, beetles roughly equal the number of species of *all* the plants, so that nomenclatures based on Linnaeus's binomials merely for the beetles will by necessity cause coleopterists to ask, "What shall we call it?" Moreover, zoologists of all stripes are constantly engaged in revisions of their classification systems, even up to the level of "kingdoms" (usually presumed as two, plant and animal, with the third—mineral—generally omitted in modern summaries), as illustrated by the kingdom *Protista* (a late-nineteenth-century coinage from the Greek *prōtistos* ["the very first"], the superlative of *prōtos* ["first"]), now occasionally split from the old animal kingdom into a kingdom of its own as listed (among several texts) by Buchsbaum, *Animals,* 2d ed. (the 3d ed., 1987, repeats this as well). *Protista* includes the *protozoa* (Greek *prōtos* + *zōon,* pl. *zōa* ["living animal"]), termed a "subkingdom" in an older edition of the standard handbook *The Invertebrata,* Borradaile and Potts, and merely a "phylum" in Mackinnon and Hawes, *Protozoa*.

Buchsbaum's *Protista* "include members that may be considered 'protozoans'" (*Animals,* 2d ed., 359), suggesting the behind-the-scenes debates and frequently heated arguments over revisions of nomenclatures. Enormous numbers, added to professional rethinking about what-goes-where in classification systems among animals, indicate that indeed any listing is arbitrary. The following is, therefore, quasi-traditional in its systematics, but any reader who looks up details in the current literature on taxonomies for almost any of the invertebrates will find differences and variations. That is assumed.

THE ANIMAL KINGDOM AND THE INVERTEBRATES

Linnaeus's hierarchy for animals in his *Systema naturae* of 1758 incorporated a basic sequence of seven levels: kingdom, phylum, class, order, family, genus, and species. But Simpson, in "The Principles of Classification," proposed twenty-one levels of hierarchy, often seen in the current literature (kingdom, phylum, subphylum, superclass, class, subclass, infraclass, cohort, superorder, order, suborder, infraorder, superfamily, family, subfamily, tribe, subtribe, genus, subgenus, species, subspecies). If this seems overcomplicated, one needs to remember that as zoologists study the relationships among animals, they repeatedly revise and change their views on both similarities and differences, almost as if they had gone back and pondered Aristotle's premises. Yet as shifting among kingdoms or orders into phyla and so on occurs, the Greco-Latinate terminologies are carried along as well, so that the names in themselves retain their original meanings, no matter where they may be placed in older or new taxonomies (sometimes, of course, entirely new names are proposed for newly classified animals, but more often, older labels are put into new slots).

Seeing how invertebrates receive accepted labels lucidly shows why the microscopic and larger creatures among the invertebrates are utterly fundamental in medicine. We are hosts to millions of animals, some harmless, some deadly, so that nomenclatures and relationships among creatures, ranging in size from the submicroscopic to the larger spiders, become basic for our understanding of precise treatments of numerous diseases. As is traditional, one considers animals beginning with "lower" forms and proceeding to "higher" animals. First on such a list is the phylum or subkingdom of *protozoa,* which includes about twenty-seven thousand living species and roughly nine thousand extinct species, subdivided into four classes:

> *Mastigophora* (Greek *mastigophoros* ["whip-bearing" or, in later Greek, "policeman"]) or *Flagellata* (derived from the Latin *flagellum* ["whip" or "lash"], here with the attachment of the Greek neuter plural [technically correct, since the Latin noun is neuter in gender]), has eleven orders, including:
>
>> *Euglenoidina* (an early-twentieth-century pseudo-Latin coinage from the Greek *eus,* neuter *ēu* ["good," "brave," "noble"] with adverb *eu* ["well," here in adaptation "true" or "genuine"] + *glēnē* ["eyeball" in Homer's Greek, and "shallow joint-socket" as used by Galen, *Bones for Beginners,* pref. (ed. Kühn, II, 736; Moore, *Galen,* 5 [Greek text] and 56 [English trans.])] + *-oidēs* ["having the form of"], here adapted as *-oid-* ["resembling" or "like"] + *-ina* [the transliteration of the neuter plural of *-inos* (Greek) and *-inus* (Latin), both emerging the same; here "of the nature of" or "made of"). Most famous in the order is *Euglena gracilis* Klebs, so familiar to beginning students in microbiology and protozoology. *Gracilis* is Latin for "slight" or "slender," perhaps in accounting for the extremely small size, about fifty to sixty microns in length (a micron is one-millionth of a meter, with the term *micron* pulled from the Greek *mikros* ["small"], which yields about two hundred *micro*-words in English including *microbiology* Greek *mikros* + *bios* + *logos,* thus "study of small lifeforms"). And *E. gracilis* is a freshwater organism, living "in standing water, such as duck-ponds, pools in meadows and pastures, especially those containing a certain amount of decaying weeds or other organic debris" (Mackinnon and Hawes, *Protozoa,* 76). The "brave eyeball" in the name records the "red eye-spot" of the protozoologists and appears on the anterior end of the animal, on the edge of the cavity that also gives rise to the flagellum that enables the organism to move in a screwlike manner, combining rotation with gyration.
>>
>> *Dinoflagellata* (Greek *deinos* ["fearful" or "terrible" or "powerful," or "clever," or as a noun, "round vessel"] + Latin *flagellum,* as above). An early-twentieth-century coinage perhaps with double meaning (the *di-* says "two" or "twice" [*duo* and *dis* respectively in Greek]), the word refers to tiny animals with two flagella and with rounded bodies of twenty-five to sixty microns quite like

the "rounded vessel" of alternative Greek meaning—and the aggressive eating habits suggest a "terrible" sense to other protozoans being consumed.

Sarcodina (Greek *sarkodēs* ["fleshy"] + *-ina*) or *Rhizopoda* (Greek *rhiza* ["root"] + *-pous*, gen. *podos* ["foot"]) includes the order *Amoebina* with the familiar *Amoeba proteus* (Greek *amoibē* ["change," "exchange," "transformation," "alteration" among several meanings] + Latin *Proteus* [a god of the sea who was the herder of Poseidon's seals and who was noted for his powers of changing his shape]); the order *Foraminifera* (Latin *foramen*, gen. *foraminis* ["hole" or "opening"] + *ferre* ["to bear"], whose name encapsulates the appearance of these shelled marine animals, pierced with holes through which extrude *pseudopodia* (Greek "false feet") that form feeding nets as they creep on seaweeds (most of the Foraminifera are about one millimeter in diameter, including the shells); and the order *Radiolaria* (a late-nineteenth-century Latinate coinage from Latin's *radius* ["rod" or "beam"] + *-olus* [variant of *-ulus* ("little")] + *-arium*, masc. *-arius* ["dealer in," which becomes "pertaining to" in modern scientific Latin]), many species of which display external skeletons of spicules.

Sporozoa (Greek *spora* ["sowing," "planting season," or simply "seed" or "offspring"] + *zōon*, pl. *zōa* ["living animal"]) is important in the history of humans and animals, since many species are parasites. The order *Coccidia* (Greek *kokkos* ["berry" or "seed" or "kernel of grain"] + *idion*, pl. *idia*, neuter forms of *idios* ["distinguishing feature" among many meanings in classical Greek, including "one's own," "private," "personal," etc.]) includes the genus *Eimeria* (the Latinized form of the German name Eimer, after Gustav Heinrich Theodor Eimer [1843–98], who made important discoveries in parasitic protozoology), which often infests the gastrointestinal tracts of such various animals as centipedes, chickens, geese, goats, donkeys, cows, rabbits, pigs, cats, and even mink, and the suborder *Haemosporidia* (Greek *haima*, gen. *haimatos* ["blood"] + *spora* + *idia*)—true blood parasites—with the notorious genus *Plasmodium* (Greek *plasma*, gen. *plasmatos* ["anything formed or molded"—"figure" or "image," sometimes "forgery" or "counterfeit"]), the cause of malaria (Italian *mala aria* ["bad air"]).

Ciliophora (Latin *cilium*, pl. *cilia* ["upper eyelid" or "eyelash"] + Greek *phoros* ["bearing"]) is so named to suggest the tiny cilia carried by many orders and genera. Imaginative names are common for orders in this class of unicellular animals, for example:

Order *Gymnostomatida* (Greek *gymnos* ["unclothed" or "naked"] + *stoma,* gen. *stomatos* ["mouth"]) includes the voracious *Holophyra nigricans* Lauterborn (Greek *holos* ["whole," "entire," "complete"] + *-phyra* of *porphyra* ["purple dye"] + Latin *nigricare* ["to shade into black" or "to verge on black"]), a freshwater protozoan that consumes large numbers of dinoflagellates and other Mastigophora. The binomial name indicates what R. Lauterborn observed and published on these creatures in 1894 and 1908, and *Holophyra* eat so many dinoflagellates that they become very obvious in the endoplasm, reminding one of "a fat gooseberry, broadly rounded behind and very slightly truncated in front" (Mackinnon and Hawes, *Protozoa,* 237). Everyone knows that gooseberries are purple, so . . .

Order *Suctorida* (Late Latin *suctorius,* derived from Latin *sugere* ["to suck"], participle *suctum*) has among its species *Discophyra piriformis* Guilcher (Greek *diskos* ["quoit" or "discus"] + *-phyra,* as above, + Latin *pirum* ["pear"] + *formare* ["to shape"] with Late Latin *formis* ["shaped"]), which bears from thirty to sixty tentacles that suck in favorite prey, various species of the genus *Paramecium* (immediately below).

Order *Hymenostomatida* (Greek *Hymēn* [god of marriage, addressed in wedding songs], which engenders many Greek terms beginning with *hymēno-* ["thin membrane"] + *stoma*) contains the famous genus of *Paramecium* (Greek *paramēkēs* ["oblong" or "oval"]), also favorites of beginning students in protozoology. Paramecia gobble up bacteria, making this single-celled animal beneficial in maintaining the balance of microscopic organisms in ordinary pond water.

In the phylum (or subkingdom) of the multicellular *Porifera* (Late Latin *porus* ["hole" or "pore"] + *ferre* ["to bear"]) are a comparatively small number of species (about twenty-five hundred living, and about eighteen hundred extinct), but everyone is familiar with them as the sponges. These animals have "skeletons" composed either of calcium or silicon, and zoologists number three classes within this phylum:

Calcarea (Latin *calcar,* gen. *calcaris* ["spur"], akin to Latin *calx,* gen. *calcis* ["pebble" or "lime" or "chalk"]), a name that captures the double sense of the structure of these sponges with skeletons formed from spicules of calcium carbonate (here, chalk).

Hexactinellida (Greek *hex* ["six"] + *aktis*, gen. *aktinos* ["ray" or "beam"] + *-ell-* [Latin *-ellus* or *ella*, variant of diminutive *-ulus*] + *-ida* [Late Latin from Greek *-idēs* ("offspring of"), with the coined Latin assumed as a neuter plural of a Latinate *-ides*]), which describes the sponges with siliceous (Latin *silex*, gen. *silicis* ["flint"], but in modern mineralology meaning "sandlike" [silicon dioxide, SiO_2]) skeletons with six-rayed spicules. These sponges are deep-sea species.

Demospongiae (Greek *dēmos* ["the common people"] but here derived most likely from *dēmos*—accented on the final omicron—["fat"] + *spongos* ["sponge"]). Since these are the most numerous of the sponges, the name may mean "the common sponges" or "the people's sponge," but among the Demospongiae, "the spicule skeleton can be supplemented or replaced by a spongin skeleton which is utilized either as a cementing element for the mineral skeleton, or to form fibres. Some genera have lost all specialized skeletal components" (Bergquist, *Sponges*, 153). Specialists have likened the looser structure in the class to something akin to fat in higher animals.

In the moderately numbered species (about ten-thousand living, five thousand or so extinct) of the phylum *Coelenterata* (Greek *koilos* ["hollow"] + *enteron*, pl. *entera* ["intestine" or "guts" or "bowels"] + *-ata* [Latin neuter plural of *-atus* ("wearing" or "possessing")]), there occurs a dualism of cellular layering, thought to be the evolutionary beginnings of how cells subdivide into varying functions in all of the "higher" animals. This phylum is made up of animals with body walls of two layers of cells, the inner enclosing an open and singly cavity (termed—from the Greek—an *enteron* by coelenterologists). There are three main classes within Coelenterata, and some of the creatures are quite familiar, some not.

Hydrozoa (Greek *hydra* ["water serpent"] +*zōon*, pl. *zōa* ["living animal"]) apparently reminded early microscopists of the Greek myth about Hercules (Heracles to the Greeks), who cleverly devised a way to kill a nasty water dragon with nine heads; if one cut off a single head, it grew back as two heads. Hercules killed the monster by burning shut each neck as he cut off each head. Among the six orders in this class is the *Hydra*, which indeed has the ability to regenerate lost parts, especially of its tentacles, numbering from five or six or twelve in common species to two hundred among some marine genera. The tentacles are equipped with stinging capsules that the animal uses to capture its prey, and these capsules are termed *nematocysts* (Greek *nēma,* gen. *nēmatos,* nom. pl. *nēmata* ["that which is spun," namely "thread" or "yarn" or sometimes "thread of a spider's web" or "silkworm's thread"] + *kystis,* gen. *kysteōs* ["bladder," or "pouch," or "bag"]), which serve as identity markers for classes and genera among the coelenterates. Large hydras can range up to twenty-five millimeters in length (1 inch), and they make up some of the few freshwater genera and species in Coelenterata.

Scyphozoa (Greek *skyphos,* gen. *skypheōs* ["cup"] + *zōon,* pl. *zōa*) are the common jellyfish, which live in moderately warm and colder oceans, and some are quite large. Infamous, due to their poisonous stingers that can inflict death even to humans, is the Portuguese man-of-war (genus *Physalia* [Greek *physallis,* gen. *physalidos* ("bubble" or "bladder"), from which comes *physalos* (a "toad which puffs itself up" or a "fish which puffs itself up")]), which can have a tangle of tenacles, lines of specialized polyps (Greek *polypous* ["many-footed"], which from medical writers [the Hippocratics, Galen] comes "abnormal growth in the nose" = Later Latin's *polypus,* thus our "polyp"), and what coelenterologists call *medusas* (from the Greek myth about the mortal Gorgon's snakelike locks of hair: Medusa was killed by Perseus), which can reach a length of twenty meters (about eighty feet). The trailing tentacles have particularly large stinging capsules, and although the vivid blue float of the Portuguese man-of-war is a beautiful sight, bathers on the shores of warmer seas know well the real dangers hidden below the translucent floating cup, which can attain a length of thirty-five centimeters (about fourteen inches). Enormous is what the British call "the Lion's Mane," the great pink jellyfish, *Cyanea capillata* L. (Greek *kyanos* ["deep" or "dark blue"] + Latin *capillus* ["hair"]): the lens-shaped disc can have a diameter of 2.5 meters (eight feet), and the tentacles (ranging up to eight hundred in number) can extend to over sixty meters (about two hundred feet). Given these extreme sizes, one is amused by an authority's understatement that normal lion's mane jellyfish are merely "3 feet in diameter, with tentacles of 75 feet when fully extended" (Miner, *Seashore Life,* 175). Most jellyfish are much smaller, as exemplified by the very common moon jelly or white sea jelly (*Aurelia aurita* Lamarck [Latin *aureus* ("gold" or "golden") + *aurus* ("ear")], which is ordinarily eight to twenty-three centimeters in diameter (about three to nine inches) and appears in large floating shoals as luminescent milky-pink or milky-orange. *Aurelia* is very common in the western Atlantic from Greenland to the West Indies.

Anthozoa (Greek *anthos* ["flower"] + *zōon*, pl. *zōa*) or *Actinozoa* (Greek *aktis*, gen. *aktinos* ["ray" or "beam"]) are the sea anemones, corals, sea fans, and similar animals. *Anemone* is a sixteenth-century borrowing from Greek's *anemōnē*, which designated various flowers, illustrated in Dioscorides' *Materia medica*, II, 176, as he writes of a "wild, wind-blown flower" (*anemōnē* in turn is akin to *anemos* ["wind"]). Sea anemones' hollow tentacles do seem to wave gently in the wind as they respond to minute currents in the surrounding waters of the shallow sea. Stony corals (Greek *korallion* ["coral," esp. "red coral"]) are somewhat like small anemones, but corals secrete a defensive cup of calcium carbonate (here, limestone) into which the fragile polyps can withdraw.

Sandwiched between the coelenterates and various "worms" (below) are the curious and remarkable animals in the phylum *Ctenophora* (Greek *kteis*, gen. *ktenos* ["comb," "rake," and sometimes "fingers," "ribs," and the "horn of a lyre"] + *phoros* ["bearing"]). Zoologists occasionally call these creatures "comb jellies" and, less frequently, what the Greek name would mean, "comb bearers." The resemblance to true jellyfish is striking, due to their transparency. Ctenophora, however, have no nematocysts, fundamentally distinguishing them from the Coelenterata. The name "comb bearers" was coined in the 1870s to suggest the eight rows of so-called comb-plates on the external surface of these skeletonless animals: the plates are hinged at one side and have toothy hairs projecting from the free edges; the plates beat the water back and forth, a motion that causes the tiny toothlike hairs to break up incoming light rays, so that the animal appears as if it were an inch-across, egg-shaped prism with continually changing rainbow colors at it moves across the surface of the sea. There are two classes in the small phylum:

> *Tentaculata* are those genra and species with tentacles (*tentaculum* is an eighteenth-century coinage from the Latin *tentare*, a variant of *temptare* ["to feel" or "to test by touching"], with the addition to the participle of the diminutive suffix *-culus*, neuter *-ulum* [this becomes "little feeler"]). Prominent among the Tentaculata are species in the genus *Pleurobrachia* (Greek *pleuron* ["rib" or "side"] + *brachiōn*, *brachionos* ["arm"]), which have two tentacles (thus the "ribbed

arms" of the scientific name). Known to many New Englanders as "sea gooseberries" and sometimes as "sea walnuts," many Pleurobrachia are swept to shore during storms where they are seen in death strewn on beaches. Some species of Pleurobrachia are striking even at night: when disturbed as they move slowly through the dark sea, they flash a cold light along the eight rows of their combs.

Nuda (Latin *nudus* ["naked" or "bare"]) lack tentacles but have the characteristic combed plates. There is only one genus in Nuda, represented by *Beroe cucumis* Fabricius (Greek *Beroē*, the name of a daughter of Ōkeanos [Latinized to Oceanus, whence our "ocean"] + Latin *cucumis* ["cucumber"]), which is about 1.25 inches long and resembles more an elongated helmet than a cucumber. Naming these creatures, as well as how and where to class the "Venus girdles" (genera *Cestum* and *Folia* among the Tentaculata, for example *Cestum veneris* [Latin *caestus* ("strip of leather"), with *Cestum veneris* ("Venus' strip of leather" or Victorianly "Venus' girdle"); *caestus* also means "weighted boxing-glove," a rather nasty ancestor of the twentieth-century version], which is long—up to about fifteen centimeters or six inches—and ribbonlike) engendered much heated controversy in mid-nineteenth-century zoology, arguments involving some of the great scientists of the day including Louis Agassiz, Thomas Henry Huxley, Alexander Agassiz (son of Louis), and several others. A good account of the "Ctenophore problem" is in Winsor, *Starfish, Jellyfish,* esp. 142–54; contextually, arguments reflected the sharp impact of Charles Darwin, whose *Origin of Species* appeared in 1859.

Collectively, the ten phyla that are "worms" and related animals are quite successful: there are about thirty-eight thousand living species (one thousand or so extinct). Some of the "worms" are parasitic, some are free-living, and the first phylum (the flatworms) suggest close links with the coelenterates.

In Linnaeus's day, all "worms" were simply *vermes* (Latin *vermis,* gen. *vermis,* pl. *vermes*), but as Borradaile and Potts, *Invertebrata,* 191–92, write, "Appearances have since been found to be deceptive and the collection has been broken up into separate phyla, one of which is the Platyhelminthes or flatworms . . . the name . . . of that heterogeneous collection of animals which in Linnaeus' times were called Vermes." The ancients were well aware of the problems in calling something a "worm," since Latin's *verminare* meant "to be affected with gripping or racking pain," as well as "to be infested with maggots or worms." Pliny, *Natural*

History, XVII, 220, uses *vermiculare* to mean (actively) "to infest with grubs" (perhaps those of beetles), and his noun for such an infestation is *vermiculatio,* gen. *vermiculationis,* with "swarming with maggots, worms, and the like" simply *verminosus.* Thus our "vermin" has a long and distinguished pedigree, even though we speak of vermin inclusive of flies, bedbugs, lice, fleas, mice, rats (and the American West includes the everadaptable coyote), as well as the Roman sense of slithery "wormy" critters. Swarming maggots (the larvae of flies, normally) on decaying tissue can rank as a digusting sight to many, and Linnaeus's *vermes* carried on a venerated tradition.

As is true for all phyla, classes, orders, and sometimes genera in the animal kingdom, specialists debate not merely the names for individual groups but also just how the parts of each animals shall be named. Consultation of modern texts of invertebrate anatomy will show that such nomenclatures vary, sometimes using analogies from the "body parts" of higher animals, sometimes with the zoologists inventing terminologies specific for the class or genus under particular consideration. When, for example, one reads that platyhelminthes differ from coelenterates in that the flatworms have a pair of cerebral ganglia, a student of human anatomy can say "A ha! I know what *that* is," and be more or less right. On the other hand, when an account of the flatworms relates how, on the outer layer of cells (the ectoderm—analogous to the term for humans and other animals), there are crystalline, rod-shaped bodies called rhabdites (Greek *rhabdos* ["wand" or "rod"]), unless one knew something of insect eyes, which have *rhabdoms,* or rod-shaped structures, or unless one chanced to recall from medical school such terms as *rhabdomyoma* and *rhabdomyosarcoma* (benign and malignant tumors, respectively, of striated muscle tissues), this special term would be meaningless. Thus the names for phyla, classes, orders, genera, and species overlay and frequently mask a separate and sometimes fulsome set of particular nomenclatures that apply *only* to the animals by those names. Modern zoology struggles with such terminologies, much as is expected, since duplication from subspecialty to subspecialty is fraught with the potential of misunderstanding or, worse, the potential of misinformation. At least international convention allows seeming duplication between botany and zoology, since (usually) botanists speak to other botanists, and zoologists to their own colleagues as contrasted to botanists. Scientific terminologies mirror that larger problem: how can various scientific subspecialties communicate with one another? From time to time, the Greco-Latinate words can help, yet often they can be confusing if one knows them only from the context, say, of medicine and wants to know about flatworms.

Considered the most primitive among the "worms," the classes making up the phylum *Platyhelminthes* (Greek *platys* ["flat," "wide," or "broad"] + *helmins,* gen. *helminthos* ["worm," esp. "intestinal worm," as in Aristotle, *HA,* 551a8, and in several Hippocratic writers]) display varying characteristics in both morphology and life-style. Traditionally, there are three main classes:

Turbellaria (a mid-nineteenth-century coinage from Latin's feminine plural noun, *turbellae,* gen. *turbellarum* ["stir" or "quarrel"], a diminutive of the Latin *turba,* gen. *turbae* ["disorder" or "riot"], to suggest the barely detectable vortical currents of water as generated by the cilia on the head of one of these small animals). In addition to a number of saltwater and terrestrial species, there are several freshwater species, including individuals in the genus *Planaria* (Latin *planus* ["level" or "flat"], with the mid-nineteenth-century word a borrowing from Late Latin's *planarius* [also "flat"]), "to which every zoology student is exposed in college" (Pennak, *Fresh-Water Invertebrates,* 1st ed., 114). "*Put a piece of raw meat into a small stream or spring and after a few hours you may find it covered with hundreds of black worms that are feeding upon it. These worms, each about half an inch long, are called planarias*" (Buchsbaum, *Animals,* 109).

Trematoda (Greek *trēma,* gen. *trēmatos* ["perforation," "aperture," or "hole"]) are parasitic flatworms with prominent suckers, which suggested the "creature of a hole or perforation" to parasitologists in the late nineteenth-century. In this class are a number of flukes, which have intermediate hosts among molluscs (usually snails) and are ultimately parasitic in man and cause schistosomiasis (genus *Schistosoma* [Greek *schistos* ["split"] + *sōma* ["body"]), or infestation by blood flukes. Various blood flukes produce endemic schistosomiases especially in tropical or semitropical parts of the world, and the life cycles of these nasty parasites have been thoroughly studied (see, for example, Wright, *Flukes and Snails,* as well as standard accounts in Wilcocks and Manson-Behr, *Manson's Tropical Diseases,* 285–336, and Faust and Russell, *Clinical Para-*

sitology, 519–627), but cures remain elusive. Typical are the comments under "Treatment" in Berkow et al., *Merck Manual*, 228: "Since the severity of schistosomiasis depends on the intensity of infection, the aim of therapy is to reduce the worm load. Prolonged or repeated courses of antischistosomal agents in an attempt to effect a cure are unwarranted. Praziquantel, a recently introduced antihelminthic, is the preferred treatment for all 3 types of schistosomiasis." A separate species of trematode, also with an intermediate snail host, is the Chinese liver fluke, genus *Clonorchis* (Greek *chlōn* ["branched"] + *orchis* ["testicle"]), which as *Merck*, 228, notes, "lives for 20 to 50 years in the biliary tree and passes operculated eggs into the feces."

Cestoda (Latin *caestus* as above under class *Nuda* among Ctenophora) are the tapeworms, including the most infamous human parasite of all, *Taenia solium* L. (Latin *taenia* ["ribbon"] + *solus*, gen. *solius* ["alone" or "lonely"], a name given by Linnaeus in 1758 and retained, in spite of its quaint meaning), the pork tapeworm. Thorough cooking of pork kills the parasite, yet infestations occur frequently in Latin America, Asia, Russia, and Eastern Europe. Famous too is the enormous length attained by the adult *T. solium* in the human gut: 2.5 to 3 meters (about eight to 10 feet) is about average, with lengths of 128 feet and 150 feet reported for extruded tapeworms by seventeenth- and eighteenth-century physicians in England and colonial America (quoted in Christianson, "Diagnostic and Therapeutic Authority," 66–67). Less well known, but still widely circulated in the popular scientific literature are the names for the "parts" of a tapeworm: the *scolex* (Greek *skōlex*, gen. *skōlēkos* ["worm," esp. "earthworm"] with pl. *skōlēkes* meaning "grubs" or larvae of insects), an odd, mid-nineteenth-century borrowing, since the scolex is the headlike segment of a tapeworm equipped with malevolent-looking hooks and suckers, not particularly analogous to an earthworm or even the grubs of insects; and the *proglottids* (Greek *proglōssis*, gen. *proglōssidos* [the "tip of the tongue," as one reads in Pollux, *Onomasticon*, II, 105]), a second, very curious mid-nineteenth-century coinage to describe one of the tapeworm's segments that contain complete male and female reproductive systems. Other tapeworms are also troublesome to humans, including the beef tapeworm and the fish tapeworm. Related are the far smaller tapeworms that cause hydatid cysts (Greek *hydatis*, gen. *hydatidos* ["watery vesicle" and especially a "disease of the liver with watery vesicles," as in Galen, *Use of Parts*, X, 7]) in intermediate hosts including sheep, moose, and human beings, with the primary hosts of the *Echinococcus* tapeworm (Greek *echinos* ["spine"] + *kokkos* ["berry"]) in dogs and wolves. In humans, hydatid cysts usually occur in the liver and occasionally in the lungs: "Surgical excision offers the only hope of cure" (Berkow et al., *Merck,* 231).

The phylum *Nemertea* (Greek *Nēmertes* [in Greek mythology, one of the Nereids or sea nymphs, in this case a daughter of Nēleus and Dōris]), sometimes termed ribbon worms, is a small group of about seven hundred species of animals that apparently have existed since the early eras of life-forms. It was Georges Cuvier (1769–1832), the great French zoologist and comparative anatomist, who first, in 1817, applied the "sea nymph" name to these worms, and it was Cuvier who was also first "to distinguish between planarians and nemerteans" (Gibson, *Nemerteans,* 13). Most nemerteans are long, soft-bodied, ribbonlike worms with abilities of extreme contraction and conversely extension. Species average a length of about twenty centimeters (about eight inches), but one of the heteronemerteans from the east coast of Scotland (appropriately labeled *Lineus longissimus* [Latin for "a very, very long line or string"]) reaches a length of thirty meters (somewhat less than one hundred feet). Even the longer ribbon worms are usually no more than a few millimeters wide, but "determination of nemertean sizes is . . . problematical in view of their great powers of extension and contraction" (Gibson, *Nemerteans,* 20). These animals, therefore, are not classified by length or colors (sometimes quite vivid, as in the mottled reddish-brown and white of the genus *Geonemertes* [derived from the Greek "earth nymph" if one assumes *Nemertēs* simply "nymph"]) but by the position of the longitudinal nerves relative to muscles as well as the structure of the *proboscis* (Greek *proboskis,* gen. *proboskidos* ["means for providing food," thus an "elephant's trunk or "the feeding-part of a fly" as in Aristotle, *PA,* 659a15, and *HA,* 528b29, respectively]), a term here meaning "feeding-part"; a nemertean's proboscis characterizes the phylum, and the organ is rather different from similar parts in other animals, like the arthropods. A ribbonworm's proboscis is within an internal cavity, shut off from the outside, and has muscular walls attached to the rear end of the sheath by a retractor muscle. "The proboscis may be compared with a finger of a glove with a string tied to the inside of the tip; when the proboscis is at rest the string, i.e., the retractor muscle, keeps it turned inside out within the sheath; when the muscles of the proboscis sheath contract . . . the proboscis is everted" (Borradaile and Potts, *Invertebrata*, 230). Nemertologists number two classes in the phylum:

> *Anopla* (Greek *anoplos* ["lacking the large shield, the *oplon*," thus in general "unarmed"]), a coinage to suggest those nemerteans lacking tiny (and probably poisonous) barbs on the proboscis. Prey is captured by species of Anopla with the proboscis coiled around the victim, and then the "feeding-part" retracts to bring it to the mouth, the entrance to the second cavity in these animals, a cavity just below that which houses the proboscis.
>
> *Enopla* (Greek *en* ["in" or "within"] + *oplon*, pl. *opla*), so named to indicate barbs on the proboscis, true for the species in the order *Hoplonemertini* ("armed nymphs," more or less) but not true for the order *Bdellonemertini* (Greek *bdella* ["leech"]), thus "leech-nymphs."

Among the several thousand species in the phylum *Nematoda* (Greek *nēma*, gen. *nēmatos* [here the meaning is "thread"] + *-odes* ["like," similar to Greek *-oidēs*]), usually called simply the roundworms, are a number of parasites causing untold suffering among humans and animals; nematodes are a major problem in agriculture. Extremely adaptable to a vast variety of environments, the nematodes are so plentiful that authorities are fond of quoting N. A. Cobb, whose long essay "Nematodes and their Relationships" appeared in 1914 and whose semipurple prose makes the point of enormous numbers:

If all the matter in the universe except the nematodes were swept away, our world would still be dimly recognizable, and, if as disembodied spirits, we would investigate it, we should find its mountains, hills, vales, rivers, lakes, and oceans represented by a film of nematodes. The location of towns would be decipherable, since for every massing of human beings there would be a corresponding massing of certain nematodes. Trees would still stand in ghostly rows representing our streets and highways. The location of the various plants and animals would still be decipherable, and, had we sufficient knowledge, in many cases, even their species could be determined by an examination of their erstwhile nematode parasites. N. A. Cobb, "Nematodes and their Relationships," in *United States Department of Agriculture Yearbook* (Washington, D.C., 1914), 457, as quoted in Buchsbaum et al., *Animals*, 214; selected sentences and phrases quoted by Thorne, *Principles of Nematology*, 1.)

Thorne concentrates on several dozen nematode genera that are specifically plant parasites, but most of the literature on these creatures is devoted to those genera and species parasitic in man. Far less is known about the one-thousand or so free-living species inhabiting freshwaters around the world, so that one assumes there are many species yet to be discovered and that, third after the arthropods and molluscs, the roundworms may turn out to be one of the most numerous kinds of animals on earth. In spite of their great variety, nematologists have only two classes in this great phylum:

> *Aphasmidia* (coined from Greek *a-* ["not"] + *phasma, phasmatos* ["apparition" or "phantom"]. Nematologists term caudal sensory organs in their animals *phasmids,* due to their faint appearance, and some specialists are uncertain about their function (Pennack, *Fresh-Water Invertebrates,* 3d ed., 226). Thorne, *Nematology,* 91, prefers *Adenophora* (Greek *adēn,* gen. *adenos* ["gland"] + *phoros* ["bearing"]) as the name for this class, perhaps knowing that *Phasmidia* is also the label of the insect order that includes walking sticks and other leaf insects. Among the Aphasmid roundworms are several genera parasitic in man, including *Trichinella,* or in older listings, *Trichina* (derived from the greek *thrix,* gen. *trichos* ["hair" or "bristle," and in later Greek "small vein"], especially *T. spiralis* (Greek *speira* ["something coiled"]) Railliet, a roundworm causing trichinosis, an endemic disease common in countries where "country sausage" remains a favored delicacy (not only can one become infested with the *Trichinella* worms from preparing or eating undercooked hog sausages, but there are recorded outbreaks of trichinosis among people who have eaten bear, walrus [Alaska, 1962; and Greenland, 1947], and sub-Saharan wild boar [Kenya, 1961]). Clinical parasitologists frequently cite analysis of wild animal infestation as reported by Zimmermann et al., "*Trichinella spiralis* in Iowa Wildlife." Slightly over seven thousand wild mammals were examined (forty-four species), and the trichina worm commonly occurred in fourteen species; expected was observation of worms in the Norway rat (a primary host), but the list includes mink, red fox, grey fox, opossum, racoon, striped skunk, spotted skunk, coyote, badger, beaver, least weasel, wolverine, and fox squirrel. Not only are arctic and temperate-zone meat-eating mammals commonly infested with the *T. spiralis,* but there is evidence that turtles are also subject to these tissue nematodes. One becomes infected by eating muscle (usually pork) containing the encysted (and usually calcified) worm, which is freed from its cyst by the stomach juices. Within a week

(after mating occurs between male and female worms inside the duodenal or jejunal mucosa), each female can produce over one thousand larvae, then carried by the bloodstream to various parts of the body. Larvae reaching skeletal muscle tissue survive; the rest do not. Commonly affected in humans are the diaphragm, the tongue, the pectoral muscles, the muscles of the eyes, and the intercostal muscles, and the worms can remain alive for many years. Nematodes are, one might say, careful parasites; should, for example, a larva come into myocardial or other nonskeletal muscles, it is killed by the body's natural defenses.

Some other nematodes among the genera in Aphasmidia, which engender long-term misery with their parasitic lives in human beings, are *Trichuris trichura* L. (Greek *thrix* + *oura* ["tail"]), the human whipworm first described by Linnaeus in 1771, a nematode of about fifty millimeters (about two inches), which burrows into the human intestinal mucosa and occasionally causes rectal prolapse, especially in children; *Capillaria hepatica* Bancroft (Latin *capillus* ["hair"] + Greek *hēpar,* gen. *hepatikos* ["liver"]), the capillary liver worm, a common parasite in monkeys, dogs, muskrats, and a number of other animals, which when contracted in humans mimics infectious hepatitis; and *Dioctophyma renale* (Goeze) Stiles (Greek *dionkōsis,* gen. *dionkoseōs* ["swelling" or "tumor"] + *phyma,* gen. *phymatos* ["growth"] + Latin *renes,* gen. *renium* [pl. noun "kidneys," sing. *ren*]), the giant kidney worm, blood-red as an adult attaining a length of twenty centimeters (8 inches), which is common in dogs, cats, racoons, and otters, which get the parasite from eating infected freshwater fish. The human form of the disease comes from eating undercooked freshwater fish infested with advanced larval stages of the worm.

Strongyloides stercoralis (Bavay) Stiles and Hassal (Greek *strongylos* ["round" or "spherical"] + *-oidēs* ["similar" or "like"] + Latin *stercus* ["dung," "excrement," more commonly "shit"]), the threadworm, is a very common parasite of humans in the tropics and is extraordinarily versatile in its life cycle, having both a free-living and a parasitic generation. The worm (female) is about one millimeter long, but it is the filariform larvae that enter the human system (usually through bare feet, thus imitating hookworms [see below]) to cause problems in the lungs and eventually in the intestinal tract. *Ancylostoma duodenale* (Dubini) Creplin (Greek *ankylos* ["crooked" or "curved"] akin to *ankylis,* gen. *ankylidos* ["hook" or "barb"] + *stoma,* gen. *stomatos* ["mouth"] + Medieval Latin *duodenum* = *intestinum duodenum digitorum* ["intestine of twelve fingerbreadths" as translated from the Greek—see *duodenum* in chap. 9

below]) is the old-world hookworm, which invades human beings through their bare feet to engender pulmonary lesions and infestation in the walls of the small intestine. *A. ceylanicum* Looss ("Ceylon" is the old name for Sri Lanka) and *A. braziliense* de Faria ("Brazil" as Latinized) are two other, geographically limited, hookworms, and *Necator americanus* Stiles (Latin *necare* ["to kill" or "to murder," part. *necatum*, thus "murderer" + Latinized "American"]) is the renowned, homegrown hookworm, often recalled by those children of the southern American states who repeatedly hear, "Wear your shoes!" *Enterobius vermicularis* (L.) Leach (Greek *enteron* ["intestine" or "gut"] + *bios* ["life"] + Latin *vermiculare* ["to infest with worms"]) is the very common pinworm or seatworm, entering the human system (particularly in children) through the mouth from licking fingers surfaced with embryonated eggs, and is one of the more annoying afflictions of childhood. Though almost never life-threatening, the migrating females of *E. vermicularis* cause an incredible itching at the anus, which leads to occasionally severe scratching and infection of the perianal tissues.

Aristotle, *HA*, 551a8–10, records that the ancient Greeks were well aware of large roundworms (as well as flatworms and probably also the tinier roundworms) as he speaks of *helminthes strongylai* ("roundworms"), most likely the giant intestinal roundworm *Ascaris lumbricoides* L. (Greek [corrupted] *askaris* ["intestinal worm"] + Latin *lumbricus* ["earthworm," sometimes "intestinal worm"] + Greek *-oidēs* ["like" or "similar"]). Linnaeus gave the binomial name in 1758 and this has remained the preferred label, even though the giant roundworm does not resemble an earthworm except in size (a female *Ascaris* can be fifty centimeters long [about twenty inches]). Horrific complications can occur, from blockage of the appendix and the lumen of the intestine, to pulmonary gangrene and rare cases of invasion of the heart. *Ascaris* spp. are the most widespread parasites in humans in many parts of the world: mankind is the primary host. And among other phasmid nematodes that live in man, two species have long been recognized, if until recently poorly understood. *Wuchereria bancrofti* (Cobbold) Seurat is a filarial worm (Latin *filum* ["thread"] that causes severe problems in human blood and lymph glands in a disease often called *elephantiasis* (straight Greek, *elephas*, gen. *elephantos* ["elephant"]); common clinical symptoms are enormously swollen legs and scrota in men (so large that one parasitologist commented that victims "had to haul their balls about in wheelbarrows"). *Wuchereria* is the Latinized form of Otto Wucherer (1820–73), a German physician who worked in Brazil for many years and became famous for his pioneering findings in parasitology. *Bancrofti* is likewise a Latinized form of a name, Joseph Bancroft (1836–94), an English physician who spent some years in Australia. At least seventy species of mosquitoes serve as vectors of the parasite, so that elephantiasis is endemic throughout the tropics. The second species of phasmid nematodes prominent in the descriptions from antiquity is *Dracunculus medinensis* L., the unhappily famous guinea worm of the tropics (Latin *dracunculus* ["little snake"] + *medinensis* ["of Medina," one of the two important cities in northwestern Arabia, revered by Muslims]), which in its adult form (the females are larger, as usual) grows into a length of one hundred centimeters on average (about forty inches). Linnaeus's nomenclature of 1758 reflected that this gruesome-looking worm, which in its final stages of development ruptures through the skin to release motile first-stage larvae, was known to be common in the Middle East in the eighteenth-century. The intermediate host is a minute crustacean in the genus *Cyclops* (Greek *Kyklōps* ["round-eye," in mythology one of the giants with a single eye centered in the forehead]), easily and frequently ingested by people who engage in religious bathing (as is common in India) or who swim in or drink infested water (as is common in Africa and the Middle East). The evidence for ancient knowledge of both elephantiasis and the guinea worm is assembled and discussed by Hoeppli, *Parasites and Parasitic Infections,* 33–38, and 8, 19, 32, 213, 242–45. One is fascinated to read how guinea worms were slowly twisted out of the erupted lesions, following ancient directions for treatment, and one is even more fascinated to read: "Treatment consists of slow extraction of the adult worm by gradual traction on its head over a period of 10 days" (Berkow et al., *Merck,* 226).

Humans are a small percentage of the animals serving as hosts of nematodes. Veterinarians commonly encounter similar worms that weaken cats, dogs, and almost all pets and domestic animals, but the greatest number of nematode parasites are in the most numerous of the animals: insects. Most insects harbor parasites, and of the thousands of species of animals, many are nematodes specific to equally numerous species of arthropods. The genus *Spherularia* (Greek *sphaira* ["globe" or "ball"] + Latin diminutive *-ulus* ["little"]) inhabits the gut of the common bumblebee, and the large-sized, sausage-shaped nematode somehow does not kill its host. Among the beetles, there teems a veritable universe of nematode parasites, varying from a species in the genus *Tylenchus* (Greek *tylos* ["knot" or "knob"] + *enchos,* gen. *encheos* ["spear" or "lance"]) that lives inside a pine-borer bark beetle (the beetle's genus is *Ips* [Byzantine

Greek *ips,* gen. *ipos* ("worm")], in reference to its wormlike burrowings under pine bark) during the winter, to another species in *Allantonema* (Greek *allas,* gen. *allantos* ["sausage"] + *nēma,* gen. *nēmatos* ["thread"]) that winters inside pine weevils among *Hylobius* (Greek *hylē* [here, "wood"] + *bios* ["life"]). The list seems infinite.

After the countless genera among the nematodes, many other phyla are rather smaller collections of animals, with the phylum *Nematophora* (again Greek *nēma,* gen. *nēmatos* ["thread"] + *phoros* ["bearing"]) having about eighty species, almost all of these threadworms (sometimes called horsehair worms) living in freshwater. If amateur zoologists chance to know any species among the horsehair worms, most likely they would recognize the fairly long (up to seventy centimeters [about twenty-seven inches]) and inextricably tangled species in the genus *Gordius* (named, naturally enough, after the famous Gordian Knot of classical antiquity). Freshwater nematophores are parasitic in insects, with *Gordius* parasitizing crickets that live near the water. Marine species are parasitic in crustaceans. The occasional *Gordius* that appears in humans is considered a pseudoparasite; that is, if accidentally ingested, it is passed out of the body in the urine or feces without consequences.

The spiny-headed or thorny-headed worms (phylum *Acanthocephala* [Greek *akanthos* ("thorn") + *kephalos* ("head")]) is an even smaller group of parasitic animals, which are fairly large as worms go (females can measure up to sixty-five centimeters [about twenty-six inches]), especially the giant, leechlike acanthocephalan labeled *Macracanthorhynchus hirudinaceus* (Pallas) Travassos (that multisyllabic binomial consists of Greek *makros,* fem. *makra* ["large" or "long"] + *akanthos* [as above] + *rhynchos* ["snout" or "muzzle"] + Latin *hirudo,* gen. *hirudinis* ["leech"] + *-aceus* [suffix meaning "resembling" or "made of"]). Hogs are normal hosts for this wicked-looking and ominous-sounding parasite, with intermediate hosts among the arthropods, especially cockroaches. Rats also are ordinary hosts for other species among the acanthocephalids.

Phylum *Rotifera* (Latin *rota* ["wheel"] + *ferre* ["to bear" or "to carry"]) has about eighteen hundred species, and the phylum consists of microscopic animals ranging from forty microns to 2.5 millimeters. First described by the pioneering Dutch microscopist Antony van Leeuwenhoek (1632–1723), in letters to the Royal Society in London, as animals with "revolving toothed wheelwork" (letter of 28 June 1713, quoted in translation by Dobell, *Anthony van Leeuwenhoek,* 292, 294), the "toothed wheelwork" remains as a part of the official nomenclature. What Leeuwenhoek saw is now explained as a beating of cilia (Latin's *cilium* ["eyelash"]) around the edges of the two, disc-shaped lobes at the head end of the animal, and they *do* look like rotating wheels, spokes and all. These creatures have a variety of fascinating shapes, ranging from tulip-forms, what looks like a profile of a legless tarsier (genus *Pedalion* [Greek *pēdalion* ("steering oar" or "steering paddle," one of the two used from the stern of Greek ships)]), and the profile of a spoon, to a folded-up toad (genus *Gastropus* [Greek *gastēr,* gen. *gastros* ("paunch," "belly," or "stomach")]), an armored seedpod (genus *Distyla* [from the Greek *dis* ("two") + *stylos* ("a pointed stick for writing in wax" = Latin *stylus*]), and plain old worms. It is not surprising that Leeuwenhoek found an abundance of these animals in the pools and drainpipes around his home, since "the rotifers are one of the few groups that have unquestionably originated in fresh waters . . . and here . . . they have attained their greatest abundance and diversity" (Pennak, *Fresh-Water Invertebrates,* 1st ed., 159). There are two classes in Rotifera:

> Digononta (Greek *dis* ["two"] + *gonos* ["seed" or "genitals" or "procreation"]), a classification based on the paired ovaries in the females.
>
> Monogonata (Greek *monos* ["alone," "only," "single"]), which are those rotifers whose females have a single ovary—over 90 percent of known species. Males of both classes are poorly known: they are far smaller than females and apparently live at most for two or three days.

The phylum *Gastrotrichia* (Greek *gastēr,* gen. *gastros* ["paunch," "belly," or "stomach"] + *thrix,* gen. *trichos* ["hair"]) encompasses about four hundred species of small, semitransparent animals (average length about 250 microns) that resemble both rotifers and ciliated protozoans. Gastrotrichs are sometimes *hermaphroditic* (Greek *Hermaphroditos,* in Greek mythology the bisexual offspring of Hermēs and Aphroditē [whence the combined name], thus a being with both sets of sexual organs) and sometimes reproduce through *parthenogenesis* (Greek *Parthenos* [an epithet of the goddess Athena meaning "virgin," which is the origin of the name of the famous Parthenon at Athens] + *genesis,* gen. *geneseōs* ["origin," "source," "generation," "production," among several meanings]). "No males have ever been seen" (Buchsbaum et al., *Animals,* 237).

The phylum *Kinorhynchia* (Greek *kinein* ["to move"] + *rhynchos* ["snout" or "muzzle"]—named to describe the animals' retractile heads) consists of half a dozen genera of minute animals that live in marine slime or mud and are related to nematodes, as well as to gastrotrichs and rotifers. The phylum *Priapulida* (Greek *Priapos* [the god of male procreative power, a son of Aphrodite and Dionysos], hence simply "penis" from his continual erection [thus too the modern *priapism* for the unfortunate man with this affliction]) has two genera and a dozen or so marine species, which are cylindrical, brown-fleshy wormy animals growing up to fifteen centimeters long (about six inches). Priapulids appear to be related to nematodes, rotifers, and gastrotrichs, but the priapulids' heavily spined proboscis (see above under phylum Nemertea) suggests a relationship with echiuroids, a minor class in annelida.

Phylum *Endoprocta* (Greek *endon* ["within"] + *proktos* ["anus"]) is a small collection of species of wormy-like, anchored animals (only one kind lives in freshwater) grouped into three genera and often classed together with bryozoans; the name suggests the anus in these creatures, which occurs inside a circle of tentacles, contrasted with the structure of bryozoans. Buchsbaum, *Animals,* 2d ed., 176, has a short paragraph on these animals, small and hydralike, but in *Animals,* 3d ed., even this terse account is omitted, with endoprocts renamed as phylum *Kamptozoa* (Greek *kamptos* ["flexible"] + *zōon,* pl. *zōa*) on page 561. "Arrow worms" are three or four genera in the phylum *Chaetognatha* (Greek *chaitē* ["flowing hair"] + *gnathos* ["jaw"]), which some zoologists link with echinoderms, while others place these transparent sea animals (about ten centimeters long [about four inches]) between brachiopods and bryozoans. *Sagitta* (Latin for "arrow") is a representative genus, and these creatures form an important part of the *plankton* (a late-nineteenth-century borrowing from Greek *plazein* ["to go astray"] with adj. *plankton* or *planktos* ["wandering" or "roaming"]), which make up the diet of so many sea animals. The name for the phylum originates from the sight of the huge numbers of arrow worms as they drift and flow on the surface of the sea like gigantic tresses of long flowing hair (Buchsbaum et al., *Animals*, 3d ed., 247, however, "translates" *Chaetognatha* as "bristle-jawed," certainly not what the Greek says). Perhaps the original namers in the late nineteenth century had in mind both the "long hair" and the adapted Latinate term of the day, *chaeta*, which did mean "bristle" in zoological nomenclatures.

Creatures in the phylum *Bryozoa* (Greek *bryon* ["tree moss," or "liverwort," but most commonly "catkin"] + *zōon*, pl. *zōa*) are often called "moss animals." Consisting of about three thousand living species and the same number of extinct varieties, some bryozoans in the shallow marine estuaries appear at first glance like very delicate seaweeds, but on closer examination, the seaweeds turn out to be branched colonies of encased animals, each with a set of tentacles that make currents around the top of the creature, allowing it to feed. Bryozoans also grow as flat sheets on seaweeds and boulders, and among the fifty or so freshwater species, enormous colonies occur (measuring up to forty centimeters long [about fifteen inches] and fifteen centimeters thick [about six inches] by the fall, in globuolous masses investing submerged twigs) in the class *Phylactolaemata* (Greek *phylaktos* ["capable of being preserved"] + *laimos* ["throat"] + *-ata* [Greek nom. pl. ending])—so named from the boxlike casing occupied by each member of the colony, the top of which opens for extension of the feeding tentacles, which rest on a circular ridge that specialists term a *lophophore* (Greek *lophos* ["mane," "crest," or "tuft" of hair, or sometimes the "comb" of a rooster] + *phoreus*, gen. *phoreōs* ["bearer" or "carrier"]). Among the *Phylactolaemata* and formerly quite common in unpolluted streams of the eastern United States (bryozoans are signals of a stream's purity) is the remarkable *Pectinatella magnifica* Leidy (Latin *pectinatus* ["resembling the form of a comb"], from *pecten*, gen. *pectinis* ["comb"], which may have more than eighty tentacles; the colonies encircling sticks and twigs now favor public water systems, where they clog various screens. Americans who reflect on the loss of pristine freshwaters may wince when they read a 1933 report stating that colonies of genus *Plumatella* (Latin *plumare* ["to cover with feathers" with part. *plumatum*, "feathered"] + *-ellum*, diminutive variety of

-*ulum*) were observed "exceeding 1 meter (= a little over 3 feet] in width extending along half a mile of shore of Douglas Lake, Michigan" (Ryland, *Bryozoans*, 151).

The phylum *Brachiopoda* (Greek *brachion,* gen. *brachionos* ["arm"] + *pous,* gen. *podos* ["foot"] are shelled animals (called *bivalves* from Latin *bis* ["two"] + *valva* ["a leaf of a folding door"]) that resemble clams. Brachiopods are similar to free-living bryozoans and are about fifty times larger than the small moss-animals. Zoologists who coined *brachiopod* in the 1840s were apparently struck by the two coiled ridges inside the shells and made the (mistaken) analogy to the "foot" of a clam; thus "armed-footed" is not a good label for this phylum, and likely a new name will appear in the literature within a few years. There are slightly more than two hundred living species of brachiopods, with at least fifteen thousand known extinct species, suggesting that the heyday of these animals has long past. Living brachiopods are divided into two classes:

> *Ecardines* (Latin *e* or *ex* ["from" or "out of"] + *cardo,* gen. *cardinis* ["hinge"]) are brachiopods lacking a hinge between the shells. Buchsbaum et al., *Animals,* 246, prefers "inarticulates" as the name. Representatives of this class are very common, including the Far Eastern genus *Lingula* (Latin *lingulatus* ["tongue-shaped"]), which describes the extended muscular stalk. The Japanese gobble up these creatures in huge numbers.
>
> *Testicardines* (Latin *testa* ["brick," "tile," or "shell"] + *cardo,* as above) are the brachiopods with hinges between the two shells. Fairly common in the sea-bottom mud in deep waters off the Atlantic coasts of Europe is the genus *Terebratula* (Latin *terebrare* ["to drill a hole"], part. *terebratum* + diminutive suffix *-ulum*). This genus provided common parlance with the name "lamp-shell," since the animals are oval-shaped and resemble ancient oil lamps, with the "wick" the extended muscular stalk.

Invertebrate paleontologists, with their thousands of species of brachiopods, have shown that all prehistoric forms were also members of these two classes, and some of the oldest survive into the present with little change (for example, *Lingula,* known from Cambrian rocks, five hundred million years old [Rudwick, *Living and Fossil Brachiopods,* 14, 164–65]).

At least there is little argument that the phylum *Annelida* (French

INVERTEBRATES: PROTOZOA TO MOLLUSCS 57

annelés ["ringed ones"], ultimately derived from the Latin *anellus* ["little ring," usually "a ring for a finger"], are indeed "worms." These animals include the common earthworms, "perhaps the most familiar annelids" (Dales, *Annelids,* 11). Not all the species in Annelida look like earthworms (the phylum groups animals having segments generally repeating one another), and the three major classes and roughly nine thousand species display some intriguing variations on the basic structure. The three classes are

Polychaeta (Greek *polys* ["many"] + *chaitē* ["flowing hair," here taken to mean "bristle"]), so named from the multiple bristles that protrude from each segment of the worm; these bristles both anchor the worm in its burrow and provide the basic means of locomotion for the animal. Each segment is equipped with longitudinal and circular muscles, which expand and contract in a front-to-back rhythm through the segments, yielding a forward motion distantly analogous to peristalsis (see chap. 9 below) in the human intestine. Polychaeta include most of the marine worms, many of which are active and swimming species, sometimes with exotic shapes: the coral worm or Christmas-tree worm (genus *Spirobranchus* [Greek *speira* ("coiled," "wreathed," or "twisted") + *branchos* ("hoarseness"), but in Aristotle's zoological Greek, the plural diminutive *branchia* means "gills," and learned Greek in the Roman Empire had the singular *branchion* ("gill"), as one reads in Aelian, *On Animals,* XVI, 12—and modern *gill* words frequently borrow this *branch-* root from the Greek, which must be carefully distinguished from *brach-* words, usually meaning "arm" and the like) is a tropical genus that lives in a tube fashioned within a coral reef, with the animal's feeding and respiratory crown protruding as a miniature and spiraled evergreen. Familiar are the clam worms (United States) or rag worms (England) used as bait by fishermen; these worms are also called "nereids" from the name of the genus, *Nereis* (Greek *Nēreis,* gen. *Nēridos,* a sea nymph, a daughter of Nēreus in Greek mythology). The American name comes from the worm's habit of sheltering in empty clam shells, whereas the British name reflects the generally ragged profile presented by the large and flapping *parapods* (Greek *para* ["from beside," "near," "along"] + *pous, podos* ["foot"]), the technical term for the protrusions that carry the worm's bristles.

Oligochaeta (Greek *oligos* ["few"] + *chaitē* as above) receive their label from the fewer bristles on the parapods than among the Polychaeta. Here are the earthworms, with *Lumbricus terrestris* L. (Latin *lum-*

bricus ["earthworm" or "intestinal worm"] + *terrestris* ["earthly," "on earth" and similar meanings, adj. from *terra* ("dry land," "earth," "ground," or "soil")]) the most familiar of all earthworms. A large *Lumbricus* in temperate climates can measure about thirty centimeters (about a foot) and have around 180 segments, but some tropical South American species of *Lumbricus* can be as long as 2.5 meters (that translates into eight feet or so) and have as many as 600 segments. Long recognized by farmers as extremely beneficial, *Lumbricus* species in normal abundance (before the wide use of pesticides) enormously enhance production of *humus* (another Latin word for "earth" or "ground"), the dark organic soil matter made from the decomposition of animal or vegetable matter. Earthworms pull leaves and other plant parts into the soil as they burrow along but leave the parts only partially digested in what agriculturalists call "castings," the semidigested remnants of the earthworm's eating of seeds, insect eggs, plant matter, and ground soil-particles, which pass through *Lumbricus'* long digestive tract. A soil's fertility is often dependent on earthworms. The freshwater species *Tubifex tubifex* (O.F.M.) (Latin *tubus* ["pipe" or "tube"] + *-fec-* from *facere* ["to make"], thus "pipe-maker") is a negative measure of pollution: *Tubifex* thrives on sewerage.

Hirudinea (Latin *hirudo*, gen. *hirudinis* ["leech"]) are indeed the leeches, once the main instruments of a venerated part of medical therapeutics of "bloodletting," sometimes simply called "leeching." In contemporary American English, calling someone a "leech" is understood as describing a person who "sucks" others "dry" of something important (usually money), a neat historical recollection of the "bloodsuckers" once very common in medical practice. Medicinal leeches usually are *Hirudo medicinalis* L. in Europe (the Latinate Linnaean binomial is self-explanatory), and the corollary species in North America is *Macrobdella decora* Say (Greek *makros* ["large"] + *bdella* ["leech," sometimes "lamprey"] + Latin *decorus* ["becoming" or "beautiful"]), a rather showy animal (green, bright orange, red, and the expected black in living specimens; only the red and black survive in preservative fluids). Wilderness fans of the lakes in northern Wisconson and northern Minnesota are all too familiar with freshwater leeches, especially the common *Philobdella gracile* Moore (Greek *philos* ["beloved," "dear," "pleasant," and similar meanings] + *bdella* + Latin *gracilis* ["slender"]), and the binomial seems to be some kind of grim joke. Almost all leeches are parasitic on animals other than man, and fish, frogs, salamanders, turtles, and snails are usual hosts.

Leeches secrete one of the finest known anticoagulants (named, naturally enough, *hirudin*), a substance that has been widely studied by medical chemists and physiologists. Hirudin is a specific inhibitor of *thrombin* (Greek *thrombos* [ordinarily "lump" but also a "clot of blood" and sometimes "curd of milk"]), defined as the enzyme derived from prothrombin, which changes *fibrinogen* to *fibrin* (Latin *fibra* ["fiber" or "lung- or liver-part," and sometimes "entrails"] + French -gène, from Greek -genēs ["born" or "produced"]; fibrin is the insoluble protein product of bloodclotting, formed from fibrinogen by the action of thrombin in the presence of calcium ions. Hirudin is a *polypeptide* (Greek *polys* ["many"] + *pepsis*, gen. *pepseōs* ["cooking" or "digestion" with adj. *peptikos*]), based on amino acid composition but lacking *tryptophan* (Greek *tripsis*, gen. *tripseos* ["rubbing" or."friction"—for the enzyme *trypsin*, see chap. 9 below] + *phainein* ["to appear"]), *arginine* (Latin *argentum* ["silver"] + Latin -*inus*), ["pertaining to" but in chemistry "with nitrogen-containing compounds"]), and *methionine* (Greek *methy*, gen. *methuos* ["wine" esp. "honey-wine" = "mead"] + *theion* [sulfur"] + -*inus*), which, added to hirudin's high concentration of dicarboxylic acids, suggest the chemical reasons why a leech's secretion would be so effective. The same biochemistry operates while the leech digests its blood meal.

Greek and Roman physicians knew what we call the "anticoagulant properties" of applying leeches, and Galen's little tract *Leeches, Reaction [to them], Cupping Instruments, Scarring and Incision* (ed. Kühn, Vol. XI, 317–22) is a summary of second-century bloodletting techniques. Antyllus (*fl.* sometime in the late second century) was the master of leech-lore, and as a surgeon of high repute, he provides the best details we have about Greco-Roman employment of leeches in medical treatments (we have quoted a text of Antyllus's *On Leeches* in Oribasius, *Medical Collection*,, VII, 21 [ed. Raeder, Vol. I, 219–20]: Oribasius was friend and physician of Julian the emperor A.D. 361–63). Roman physicians used the "medicinal leech" (*H. medicinalis* L.) and were familiar with other species not as useful in bloodletting (Beavis, *Insects* 8–10). In recent practice, employment of leeches has been revived as a means of removing blood from inflammations and congested areas of skin, particularly if physicians desire meticulous freeing of clotted capillaries.

Phylum *Mollusca* (Latin *molluscum* ["a protuberance which grows on maple trees," so Pliny, *NH*, XVI, 68] or *nux mollusca* ["a nut with a soft shell," also Pliny, *NH*, XV, 90], akin to Latin *mollis* ["soft"]—the modern Latin term is the assumed neuter plural of *molluscum*, taken to mean "soft-bodied") has about one-hundred thousand living species, roughly forty-two thousand extinct, and includes the following classes (sometimes listed as orders):

Polyplacophora (Greek polys ["many"] + *plax*, gen. *plakos* [anything "flat" or "broad," namely "slab," "plate," "tablet," and similar meanings, with a special "flap" or "tail fin" in crustacea as in Aristotle, HA, 526b9] + *phoros* ["bearing"]), a name describing soft-bodied animals whose upper surfaces are protected by overlapping plates of shell; the underparts are often called a "foot," which clamps down on rocks when the creature is disturbed in its seashore habitat. Off the coast of California occurs the largest of these animals in the genus *Chiton* (Greek *chitōn* ["garment worn next to the skin" or "tunic"]), commonly called gumboot chitons, which average about thirty-five centimeters (about fourteen inches) in length. *Chiton* is pronounced "kyeton," almost identical to *chitin* pronounced "kye-tin" (*chitin*—also derived from Greek's *chitōn*—is the usual name for the exoskeleton casing of insects), so there is understandable confusion when entomologists and malacologists converse. And instead of the expected "molluscology," specialists who study molluscs call themselves malacologists (Greek *malakos* ["soft"] + *logos*).

Monoplacophora (Greek *monos* ["alone," only," "solitary," and similar meanings], + *plax, plakos,* + *phoros,* as above) were well known only from the fossil finds of limpetlike animals from the Cambrian and Devonian eras (about five hundred million to about two hundred million years ago) until malacologists were electrified in 1957 by discoveries made on the Danish Galathea Expedition: "Dr Henning Lemche . . . announced the most exciting discovery in the history of malacology: a living mollusc of the highly primitive class Monoplacophora . . . Dredged from 5000 meters off the Pacific coast of Mexico and named *Neopilina galatheae,* this new mollusc has a flat, saucer-shaped shell up to 4 cm long, and a ventral foot, a mouth in front and the anus behind" (Morton, *Molluscs,* 18). The discovery indicated that the "primitive" forms of prehistoric molluscs were quite complex in their own right, with five pairs of gills and a fairly complicated system of muscles and nerves. The name *Neopilina* derives from Greek *neos* ("new" or "fresh") fused with Latin's *pilus ("hair"),* a cognate of Greek's *pilos* ("hair"), which engenders *pilinos* ("made of felt"), so that this Greco-Latinate coinage means "a new felt cap"; the *galatheae* commemorates the Danish expedition, in turn named for Galateia, one of the sea nymphs in Greek mythology.

Aplacophora (Greek *a-* ["not" or "without"] + *plax, plakos* + *phoros,* as above) are small and wormlike, lacking a shell as suggested by the name of the class. Malacologists occasionally call them *solenogasters* (Greek *sōlēn,* gen. *sōlēnos* ["pipe"] + *gastēr,* gen. *gastros* ["belly" or "paunch"]), which also suggests their appearance.

Familiar are genera and species among the *Gastropoda* (Greek *gastēr,* gen. *gastros,* as above, + *pous, podos* ["foot"]), about seventy thousand species of snails, slugs, limpets, abalones, sea slugs, oyster drills, sea hares, and similar animals. French cuisine features "escargot" (French for "snail"), with the favored genus for the table being *Helix* (Greek *helix,* gen. *helikos* ["anything which is spiral-shaped"]), some of the larger European (and now American) land snails, often with brilliantly colored shells. Snails are very common in temperate climates, where they are sometimes serious pests to gardeners, but are even more common in saltwater and freshwater. "Every conceivable type of fresh-water environment, from the smallest ponds and streams to the largest lakes and rivers, has its characteristic population of snails, or univalve mollusks" (Pennack, *Fresh-Water Invertebrates,* 1st ed., 667). Some freshwater snails are intermediate hosts for trematodes and are important to humans not for their gastronomic value but for their role in schistosomasis. Slugs are essentially land snails that have lost their external shells. "[There is] economy in calcium [and] the slug habit has many structural advantages: these molluscs can glide through narrow spaces, or—like *Testacella*—burrow actively for animal prey which can then be swallowed into a distensible body" (Morton, *Molluscs,* 50). *Testacella* (a mid-nineteenth-century coinage from *testaceus* [Latin for "having a hard outer covering," here taken as a diminutive, since slugs have only a thin, oval plate covering a small part of the back]) is a European genus of carnivorous slugs, favoring earthworms as their primary diet. Slugs' sliminess is legendary, as demonstrated by malacologists, who enjoy showing how these animals can slither at right angles over a razor with no harm.

Limpets (the common name ultimately stems from the Greek *lepas,* gen. *lepados* ["limpet"], illustrated by the passage in Aristotle, *HA,* 528b1) are marine gastropods that subsist on algae scraped from rocks and seaweeds or that are omnivorous, as in the case of the keyhole limpets, genus *Diodora* (from the Greek *diodos* ["passageway"]). They grow to seventy millimeters (a little less than three inches) and range from Alaska to lower California. Abalones are large molluscs (mature specimens can measure twelve centimeters [over five inches]) in the genus *Haliotis* (Greek *halios* ["of the sea"] + *ous*, gen. *ōtos* ["ear"] = "ears of the sea," so named from their seeming resemblance to human ears) whose shells have a row of respiratory holes. Those shells are a primary source of mother-of-pearl.

Sea slugs or, more properly, *nudibranches* (the order or suborder is named *Nudibranchiata,* which translates from the Greco-Latinate as "naked gills") are frequently brightly colored, nature's way of signaling fish and other marine predators that many species of sea slugs are poisonous; nudibranches lack both a shell and a mantle cavity but make up for these with copious mucous secretions and reuse of the nematocysts (above, under phylum Coelenterata) of their otherwise digested prey, usually anemones, hydroids, and algae. Representative species include the common Atlantic plumed sea slug, *Aeolis papillosa* L. (in Greek mythology, *Aiolos* was god of the winds, and in ordinary Greek, *aiolos* came to mean "wriggling," "color-changing," "slippery," or simply "subject to change," and Linnaeus's added Latinate *papillosa* [Latin *papilla* can mean a "nipple-like protuberance" as well as the usual "nipple"] provides a rather vivid mental picture of an animal that changes color and is full of "little nipples," quite appropriate for the plumed sea slug, whose length can reach ten centimeters [about four inches] and is covered with long, tapering papillae [malacologists term these "little nipples" *cerata,* coined from the Greek *keras,* gen. *keratos,* usually "horn," but Aristotle, *HA,* 526a31, has *kerata* as "antennae of crustaceans," leading to this specialized, modern meaning.]). "Sting cells (nematocysts) often occur in the cerata. These sting-cells have been swallowed alive by the nudibranchs, along with the coelenterates to which they belong, and are then incorporated into the cell-structure of the nudibranchs themselves, where they function as in the coelenterates that produced them originally" (Miner, *Seashore Life,* 670). Related to the sea slugs are the sea hares, which have curled earlike tentacles; since they feed on algae, the sea hares have reminded malacologists of "rabbits on the sea bottom." A soft rounded back may appear to invite petting from divers, but the animal exudes a slimy purple ink when annoyed. Sea hares can grow large, with the genus *Aplysia* (Greek *aplysia* [either "filth" or "an uncleanable sponge," the latter in Aristotle, *HA,* 549a4]—malacologists recall the nasty and inky defense ejected by sea hares) sometimes reaching a length of seventy-five centimeters (about 2.5 feet) and weighing in at about sixteen kilograms (about thirty-five pounds) in species off the coast of California. *Aplysia* is the largest gastropod in the world.

Gastropods also include marine species in the genus *Cypraea*

INVERTEBRATES: PROTOZOA TO MOLLUSCS   63

(Greek *Kypros,* the island now called Cyprus, the birthplace of Aphrodite), famous as cowrie shells (*cowrie* is a seventeenth-century Anglicization of the Hindi word *kauri*), especially the "money cowrie" (appropriately named *Cypraea moneta*), used as such in sections of Asia and Africa.

Scaphopoda (Greek *skaphē* [usually "trough," "tub," "baker's tray," or "skiff," but here "digging"] + *pous,* gen. *podos* ["foot"]) has about 250 species, collectively known as "tooth shells," which occur in great numbers along both coasts of North America (they are cosmopolitan, in all seas and almost all depths). The early-twentieth-century nomenclature for this class of molluscs apparently was chosen to delineate scaphopods' ability to bury themselves in the mud of sea floors, foot down and shell straight up (hence the "digging foot" label). Many species superficially resemble the shapes of elephants' tusks and thereby are sometimes called "tusk shells," and one common genus, *Dentalium* (Latin *dentale,* gen. *dentalis,* with neuter plural *dentalia,* gen. pl. *dentalium* ["the sole or share beam of a plow"]) bears a name reflective of both the "tooth-shape" (Latin *dens,* gen. *dentis* ["tooth," "ivory," or "prong"]) and Roman agriculture's common "toothed plow," quite in keeping with a scaphopod's digging habits. *Dentalium entale* L. (*Dentalium* + Greek *entos* ["within"], which evolved into Renaissance Latin's *entalis* [medieval Latin's *entare* meant "to insert"]) is the common tooth shell of our eastern coasts from North Carolina up to Arctic latitudes, and it has a shell about five centimeters long (two inches). Larger species can attain a length of thirteen centimeters (about five inches) and were favored as parts of necklaces among Indians in the Pacific Northwest.

Authorities differ over what to call molluscs with two shells (clams and oysters and similar animals). Buchsbaum likes *Bivalvia* (Buchsbaum et al., *Animals,* 266), which he translates as "two valves" (not correct, since Latin's *valva* is a "leaf of a folding door"), and Miner, (*Seashore Life,* 555), gives *Pelecypoda* (Greek *pelekys,* gen. *pelekeōs* ["double-bladed axe"] + *pous,* gen. *podos,* as above with the tooth shells). Borradaile and Potts, (*Invertebrata,* 622), prefer *Lamellibranchiata* (Latin *lamella* ["thin metal plate"] + Greek *branchion* ["gill"] + neuter plural ending *-ata*). Most current texts have dropped Lamellibranchiata in favor of either Pelecypoda or Bivalvia; both are adequately descriptive of animals in the class, with the Latinate "two-leaves-of-a-folding-door" reasonably good, and the Greco-Latinate "double-bladed-axe-footed" a nice mental picture if one thinks of the two shells of the animal flattened out while still connected by the hinge. Unlike the air-and-water division among gastropods, Pelecypoda (or Bivalvia) are all aquatic and are abundant in both fresh and salt waters. There are about twelve thousand extant and sixteen thousand extinct species in the class, most familiar as clams, oysters, cockles, mussels, scallops, and the famous shipworms.

Venus mercenaria L. (Latin *Venus* [the Roman goddess of erotic love and beauty] + *mercennarius* ["working for pay"]) is a very common marine clam, and Linnaeus knew that North American Indians used the shells to make wampum, cutting and piercing small beads of white and purple and stringing these beads for ease of transport; thus the nomenclature for this widely consumed seafood preserves an aspect of early North American economic history from colonial days. *V. mercemaria* carries a number of vernacular names (depending on regions of the United States), including quahog, little neck clam, cherry stone clam, round clam, and hardshell clam. Before 1960 or so, when pollution and damming of river drastically reduced the populations of freshwater clams and mussels, there was a flourishing "pearl button" industry in the Ohio and Mississippi river valleys, which harvested millions of *Fusconaia* (Latin *fuscare* ["to blacken" or "to darken"]), *Quadrula* (Latin *quadrus* ["square"], with diminutive *quadrula* ["little square"]), and other genera, mostly from the Kentucky, Tennessee, and Arkansas rivers. Most buttons are now made from plastic. Famous too are the marine horsehoof clams in the genus *Hippopus* (Greek *hippos* [horse"] + Latin *opus* l"work"]—thus "workhorse clams") which grow to thirty centimeters (about twelve inches) in length, quite large for clams, which generally average about eight centimeters long (about three inches). The "giant clam" of the divers' horror stories are species in the genus *Tridacna* (Greek *tridaknos* ["requiring three bites," as Pliny the Elder records this Greek word in the Latin transliteration *tridacnus* to describe how long it took to eat a large oyster in *NH*, XXXII, 63]), which can reach lengths of 150 centimeters (about five feet) and weigh close to 250 kilograms (about 550 pounds). Readers of sea stories know that *Tridacna* live off the coasts of Australia, and therefore divers fearing giant clams off the coast of North Carolina have got their geography wrong.

Oysters have one genus, *Ostrea* (Greek *ostreon* ["oyster"), with the *O. virginica* L. (the Latinate "Virginian," named for Elizabeth I of England, the "Virgin Queen") being the succulent species so favored by aficionados of seafoods. Cockles have two shells of equal size, and looking at the animal edgewise shows a modified heart shape, engendering the genus name *Cardium* (Greek *kardia* ["heart"] with diminutive *kardion* ["heart-shaped"]), a widely dispersed marine bivalve. Representative species include *C. muricatum* L. (Latin *muricatus* ("armed with spines like the shell of a murex"—the shellfish that yielded the famous Phoenician purple—as one reads in Pliny, *NH*, XX, 262; Linnaeus was reminded of the famous murex of antiquity]), sometimes called the Florida cockle or the Southern spiny cockle, abundant off the Atlantic coast of Florida. Scallops are *the* seashell shape, figuring frequently in ancient art as well as modern depictions, familiar as the logo of Shell Oil Company. Common scallops on both sides of the Atlantic are in the genus *Pecten* (Latin *pecten, gen. pectinis*]"comb" but also simply "the scallop," apparently by analogy to the comblike ribbing of the shell]), with representative species including *P. irradians* Lamarck (Latin *irradiare* ["to shed rays of light upon" or "to illumine"]), the common scallop that gives seafood fanciers its tender adductor muscle as a marine delicacy; as *P. nodosus* L. (Latin *nodosus* ["full of knots" or "gnarled" or "full of nodes" and similar meanings]), the appropriately named knobbed scallop; and the largest American scallop, *P. magellanicus* Gmelin = *P. grandis* Solander (*magellanicus* is the Latinized form of Ferdinand Magellan [*c.* 1480–1521], whose fleet—actually, only a single ship survived—was the first to circumnavigate the world [1522], and *grandis* is Latin for "large," "great," "noble, and magnificent"), the giant scallop or deep-sea scallop, which can measure up to fifteen centimeters (about six inches).

"Shipworms" are greatly elongated clams and are the most notorious of the boring bivalve molluscs. Highly destructive to wooden ships, wharf pilings, and the like, this animal was named *Teredo navalis* by Linnaeus (Greek *terēdōn, gen. terēdonos* ["wood-boring worm," as commonly in classical Greek, but also "larva of the wax moth," which infests beehives] + Latin *navalis* ("of ships," the adj. from *navis, gen. navis*("ship")], perhaps recalling Theophrastus, *HP*, V, 4.4–5, and the vivid description of troubles suffered by ancient Greeks and resulting from the habits of these animals: "The woods which deteriorate in the sea are eaten by a *terēdōn* . . . and a *teredon* lives only in the sea. The *terēdōn* is quite small but has a large head and teeth . . . and the damage done by the *terēdōn* cannot be corrected" (trans. Scarborough). This account is quite like what one reads in a modern handbook, which concludes, "Eventually the timber becomes so weakened it falls apart" (Miner, *Seashore Life,* 607). Theophrastus suggests pitch to coat the ships' hulls before they are launched, and modern authorities say to use creosote to impregnate the wood to be submerged. *Kreosote* was coined in German (1832) to describe the distillation products of coal and wood tars, an oily liquid found to have preservative properites—thus our *creosote* from the German, created from two Greek words "*kreas,* gen. *kreōs* ["flesh" or "meat"] + *sōtēr,* gen. *sōtēros* ["savior" or "deliverer"]).

Teredo has developed enzymes that digest "90 per cent of the cellulose contained in the ingested wood" (Thorson, *Life in the Sea,* 164), "enzymes which are almost unique in the Animal Kingdom, which digest cellulose and hemicellulose" (Borradaile and Potts, *Invertebrata,* 635). *Teredo* can be as long as fifteen centimeters (about six inches) with a whitish-yellow wormlike body, and only the most anterior centimeter has the covering of two very short white shells. Even in its tiny, pinhead-sized larval form, *Teredo* can make its initial hole, since the larva already possesses the major enzyme *cellulase* (Latin *cellula* ("small room" and other meanings, for which see chap. 9 below under "salivary glands: ptyalin and carbohydrates"] + biochemical coinage *-ase,* the suffix to designate enzymes [Greek *asis,* gen. *aseōs* meant "slime" or "mud," and *enzyme* comes from a Byzantine Greek word—earlier Greek's *zymē* meant "leaven" or "beer yeast"—that denoted simply "leaven," so that when biochemists discovered how the process of fermentation worked in the presence of necessary substances that took no part in the chemical changes, they sought terms that combined some of the multiple actions involved and came up with *leaven* from Greek fused with the appearance of yeasty, fermenting stuff, thus *slime* and the *-ase* suffix still used today]).

Whereas *Teredo* and another genus called *Xylophaga* (Greek *xylon* ["wood"] + *phagein* ["to eat"]; *phagos* or *phagas* as a derivative noun usually means "glutton") are wood borers, causing enormous damage to shipyards, docks, and piers, there are other genera that thrive as they bore into inorganic matter. Representative are *Pholas* (Greek *phōlas, phōlados* [any animal—a spider or a bear—that lurks in a hole"], and in the Greek of the Roman Empire, *hai phōlades* are "the shellfish which bore into rocks," as one reads in Athenaeus, *Deipnosophistae,* III, 88a), which lives in the holes it bores into sandstone or chalk, and *Saxicava* (Latin *saxum* ["rock" or "boulder"] + *cavus* ["hollow" or "cavity" or "hole"], which makes its home in the burrows it excavates in hard limestones.

Cephalopoda (Greek *kephalē* ["head"] + *pous,* gen. *podos* ["foot"]) or *Siphonopoda* (Greek *siphōn,* gen. *siphonos* [usually "pipe" or "tube"] + *pous,* gen. *podos*) are thus "head-footed" of "footed-head" animals (or pipe-footed) and include some of the most amazing creatures that live in the sea. Octopuses and squids have shells, but

INVERTEBRATES: PROTOZOA TO MOLLUSCS

they are internalized, so that the casual observer assumes these animals are soft-bodied, a rather reasonable assumption from appearances alone. The third group of animals prominent among the cephalopods is the beautifully shelled nautilus, one of the most ancient members of this class (paleontologists have fossil examples from the late Cambrian of about four hundred million years ago) yet one of the most sophisticated and successful: the coiled, multichambered shell allows the nautilus to swim in varying depths of the sea, since the small compartments can be filled and emptied with different levels of gas or liquid in a continual adjustment of buoyancy.

Squids, cuttlefish, and similar animals are among the *Decapoda* (Greek *deka* ["ten"] + *pous*, gen. *podos*), so named for their ten arm-tentacles, each supplied with numerous suction-cups (the "suckers") with which these creatures grasp their prey. Quite common are the cuttlefish, usually genus *Sepia* (Greek *sepia* ["cuttlefish"]); the "cuttlebone" is the animal's shell, embedded in its fleshy mantle, frequently given to caged birds as a source of calcium. In English, *sepia* is dark brown," a name derived from the pigment in the cuttlefish's ink sac, expelled as the creature swims away from danger (nature's underwater "smoke screen"); real sepia (that is, the cuttlefish pigment) remains favored by artists, and the best brown inks still contain some cuttlefish. Squids vary in size from the gigantic *Architeuthis* (Greek *archi-* ["chief"] + *teuthis*, gen. *teuthidos* ["squid"], which can grow up to eighteen meters long (about sixty feet) and weigh about one thousand kilograms (close to a ton), making it by far the largest invertebrate in the world, to the common eight-inch-long (about twenty centimeters) *Loligo* (Latin *lolligo*, gen. *lolliginis* ["squid"] or "cuttlefish"]).

Octopoda (Greek *oktō* ["eight"] + *pous*, gen. *podos*) include the well-known octopus, most of which are moderately sized, similar to species in the genus *Octopus*, which range in the north Atlantic from Newfoundland to the Carolinas, having lengths up to seventeen centimeters (about 6.5 inches). There are giants among the octopuses (sometimes the plural is written as octopi): some species off the coasts of Oregon, Washington, and British Columbia can attain weights up to fifty kilograms (about 110 pounds).

Tetrabranchia (Greek *tettares* ["four"] with *tetras*, gen. *tetrados* ["the number four"] + *branchion* ["gill"], thus "four-gilled") are cephalopods with well-developed shells and with two pairs of kidneys and two pairs of gills. These animals are occasionally called living fossils, since *Nautilus pompilius* L. (Greek *nautilos* ["sailor" or "seaman"], with the more common word for "sailor" [*nautēs*] +

pompilos ["a fish that follows ships"]), and other species of *Nautilus* are sole survivors from a number of similar genera that flourished in large numbers until a mysterious extinction about seventy million years ago (at the end of the Cretaceous era [Latin *creta* is "chalk"]). *Nautilus* resembles a squid living inside a coiled and chambered shell, which gives its common name of pearly nautilus. *Nautilus* has about ninety small tentacular arms to seize fish and crabs.

The coinage of the modern nomenclature is an illustration of twisting from ancient to modern: in addition to its ordinary meaning of "sailor" in Greek, *nautilos* in Greek zoology (for example in Aristotle, *HA*, 525a21) is a name for a curious member of the Octopoda called either the paper nautilus or the argonaut (in modern nomenclature, labeled *Argonauta argo* L.), which secretes a thin, paperlike shell from the expanded ends of its two upper arms (only the female does this, anticipating deposition of eggs). Greek seamen believed that the creature was making sails and that it could perform like a ship by spreading its presumably membranous arms and "sail away." Linnaeus's name for the paper nautilus simply means "an individual who sailed with Jason on the ship Argo in search of the Golden Fleece."

Modern medicine has appropriated many Greek and Latin terms, not only in naming anatomical parts but also in attempting to define precisely the *aetiology* (Greek *aitios* ["cause" among several related meanings] + *logos*) of parasitic diseases. The termininologies employed by protozoologists, malacologists, and other specialists in invertebrate zoology continually interweave with the descriptions used by physicians as they seek therapies and cures for illnesses engendered by human populations of invertebrate parasites. Zoologists frequently collaborate in medical research, and there is an increasing appreciation by physicians for the basic data uncovered in "pure" invertebrate physiology and zoology: life cycles among plasmodia, for example, are as important in combating malaria as are pharmaceutical approaches; and how these facts are recorded—the words used—becomes the basis for a tomorrow when malaria will take its place among those ailments banished into history. The study of such animals as cuttlefish, or sea slugs, or scallops, also reveals unexpected mechanisms of natural defenses against parasites or ailments afflicting sea creatures, and the basics of physiology among marine invertebrates occasionally suggest new insights into mammalian biochemistry.

The huge natural laboratory of living animals without backbones links more and more in medical research to what humankind can comprehend of the nature of disease and the essentials of survival. Nomenclatures become the tools of communication, and clarity in those names (generally derived in some fashion from Latin and Greek) becomes even more important as the numbers of species-variations increase. This is especially true when one considers the huge variables among the arthropods, taken up in the next chapter.

CHAPTER 4

ARTHROPODS

Little Miss Muffet
Sat on a tuffet
Eating her curds and whey
Along came a spider
And sat down beside her
And frightened Miss Muffet away.
—Traditional Nursery Rhyme

There was a young lady from Ryder
Who screamed when sight of her outsider
Revealed through a glass
Showed the orange ass
Of a barbed and carnivorous spider.
—Anonymous Student Limerick (1989), University of Wisconsin

INSECTS, spiders, scorpions, and related invertebrates are those "lower animals" generally known by sight. Most kinds receive disgust or revulsion, suggested by the often repeated lines about Miss Muffet (and its updated version). If movie producers wish to induce a mood of basic horror or deep gloom, standard props almost always include spider webs (to suggest "old" or "spooky" settings) and large, nastily hairy spiders. It rarely occurs to the typical horror buff that the presence of cobwebs in large, drooping quantities (especially if there are no insects *in* the webs) indicates few spiders are about and that the American tarantulas set to crawling on the hero's clothes are some of the least dangerous arachnids.

Yet no matter how many entomologists (Greek *entomon* ["an animal that is incised"] + *logos*) wax eloquently about the beauty of beetles, or about the incredible engineering feats that are the webs constructed each night by our common black-and-yellow garden spiders, there is usually resistance by the general public to any rationalization of this deep-seated fear of "the bugs." Newspapers enjoy detailing the frightening stories of killer bees, advancing inexorably from Brazil into Texas, and familiar are scenes of army ants eating paths through tropical jungles. The image projected is always of enormous numbers "flooding" an area, and in essential respects, this evocation is partially true: insects and their kin generally do exist in huge numbers, as one will remember from those motion pictures of the thousands of ants in a traveling tropical colony, or as we note with annoyance the millions of mosquitoes attacking in squadrons anywhere in temperate North America (in Wisconsin, we with some sarcasm call the mosquito our "state bird"). Arthropods literally are everywhere on the earth (the extreme Arctic and Antarctic excepted), in the air, and in and on the fresh and salt waters girdling the globe. It is little wonder that biologists say that if humankind indulges in self-destruction, the dominant species afterwards would be cockroaches on the land and related cousins in the seas. Arthropods compete with humans everywhere, even within and on our bodies, and the annals of parisitology bulge with grim tales of the continual struggle.

Popular natural history and television nature programs often emphasize humankind's natural rivalries with the larger land animals (elephants, lions, bears, etc.), many now approaching extinction. It is often said that man and bear occupy similar "biological niches" and that man's encroachments, settlements, and agriculture will doom such animals. Perhaps so, but our major rivals for dominance on the earth are not the larger carnivores or plant-eaters like bison or elephants, but the arthropods. Nature has fashioned these creatures with some dazzling technologies of their own, ranging from the purely mechanical wizardry that enables a large dung roller beetle or an even larger stag beetle to fly ("a tank with wings," as one entomologist says), to the remarkable and specific chemical defenses and attractants ordinary among the arthropods and their botanical hosts. We are all familiar with how bees are attracted to flowers, but we may not know how millipedes exude a form of hydrogen cyanide as a defense against ants—a very exact chemical weapon that prevents ants from devouring a millipede on the spot but that does not save it from other millipede-loving creatures. Natural history and medicine in the twenty-first century will doubtlessly focus on these matters and the myriads of similar particulars, especially as human populations expand and as human health and food supplies are constantly challenged by the anthropods. The new natural history and medical toxicology of tomorrow not only will provide computer models (for example) of molecular chains characteristic of spider venoms but also will seek understanding of the multiple chemical and mechanical relationships that exist over the earth among the millions of species of arthropods and of their survival techniques in the presence of giants like humans, bears, and whales.

The phylum *Arthropoda* (Greek *arthro-* ["jointed"] + *pous,* gen. *podos* ["foot"], thus animals "with jointed feet") includes spiders and the huge class of insects, as well as centipedes and millipedes, lobsters and crabs, and the famous if extinct trilobites. One million or more species of animals are arthropods. Molluscs have one hundred thousand species, an impressive number until compared with the arthropods, with their ten-times-greater tally. Moreover, entomologists continually discover new species in this phylum (especially insects), so that the phenomenal bulk of animals living on our small globe becomes even more amazing. Yet more astonishing are arthropods' enormous aggregates of offspring: one hundred thousand from a single individual is commonplace.

Nature's carefully honed balances reflect how thousands of fish, amphibians, reptiles, birds, mammals—not to mention fellow arthropods and many other phyla—consume literally billions of these joined animals. Survival among insects and their kin depends on numbers, illustrated in a small way by the seasonal life cycles among American praying mantises (which devour huge numbers of other insects, to the great delight of farmers and gardeners). Each mantis egg-case usually yields about two hundred miniature mantises in June, but only one or two mature to mate in October (the female does, indeed, eat the male immediately after copulation, and sometimes she indulges in her final feast even while he performs his last act). Once she produces her egg-case, the female dies, and the following June, two hundred more mantises emerge.

Entomology is a direct coinage from the Greek of Aristotle, who wrote, "I call *entoma* those creatures which have incisions (*entoma*) on their bodies, either on their undersides alone or on both their undersides and backs: (*HA,* 487a33), and the modern term frequently assumes an incorporation of not only insects but also spiders and myriapods (Greek *myrios* ["a thousand" or "numberless" or "countless"] + *pous,* gen. *podos* ["foot"]), yet not other "incised" creatures like lobsters and the prehistoric trilobites. Purists use *entomology* to designate the study of insects only, an enormous collection of animals that seems sometimes to defy the neat binomial system of Linnaean nomenclature, since there are so many creatures encompased within the basic and relatively simple morphology of what an insect should be: six-footed or six-legged, thereby the traditional *hexapoda* (Greek *hex* ["six"] + *pous,* gen. *podos*) as the label for this class of animals subsumed under the phylum Arthropoda. The English word *insect* emerges from a classical Latin translation of Aristotle's *entomon,* as in Pliny, *NH,* XI, 1, 108, and XVI, 90, where the Latin *insectum* or the participle *insectus* (*insecare* meant "to make an incision in" or "to cut") became adapted to describe these numerous animals important in Roman folklore, medical entomology, and agriculture. Pliny, like Aristotle before him, included all sorts of "incised animals" among the *insecta,* so that one can discern in Aristotle's descriptions (often borrowed directly by Pliny) spiders, centipedes, millipedes, and some worms along with flies, beetles, wasps, moths and butterflies, grasshoppers, cicadas, bees, ants, and a few other insects. And even though Aristotle's studies of animals were the first to incorporate insects, it is surprising that he designated only about fifty different kinds among his *entoma.* Among the many classes within Arthropoda—even before one takes up the insects—are the following:

> *Onychophora* (Greek *onyx,* gen. *onychos* ["talon" or "claw"] + *phoros* ["bearing"]) is occasionally made into a phylum, since these widely distributed caterpillar-like animals (species in the genus *Peripatus* [from the Greek *peripatein* ("to walk around")] attain a length of about twelve centimeters [a little less than five inches] and live in southeast Asia and Australia, as well as Central and South America and tropical Africa) seem to form a missing link between arthropods and annelids. Much sought after by students and scholars of invertebrate natural history, these creatures are rather rare in spite of their frequent notices in the literature. The seventy or so species in this class carry the name "claw-bearers" or "talon-bearers" because the short legs (the non-Australian species can have up to

forty-three pairs) end in tiny claws or nails, which resemble those of insects. Psychiatrists have also borrowed Greek's *onyx* to create *onychophagia* (*onyx* + *phagos* ["eating"]), the oddly bothersome habit of "biting one's fingernails," an act perhaps characteristic of those frustrated as they seek the elusive *Peripatus*.

Trilobita (the early-nineteenth-century Latin *trilobites* was coined from the Greek *trilobos* ["three-lobed"] + *-itēs* [a suffix suggesting a "component" of something]) includes several prehistoric and extinct animals that are the most familiar—next to the dinosaurs and mammoths, perhaps—to the general public. Paleontologists (Greek *palaios* ["old" or "ancient"] + *onto-* ["being," a participial form of the verb *einai* ("to be")] + *logos*—the term coming into English from the early-nineteenth-century French coinage *paléontologie*) consider these extinct arthropods extremely important in analyzing life-forms from the Cambrian period (some 500 million years ago) through the Permian period (to about 250 million years ago [*Cambria* is medieval Latin for "Wales," in turn a Latinization of the Welsh *Cymry,* so that this geologic period bears the Latin name for Wales, where fossils were discovered from this earliest time of life in the sea; *Permian* emerges from the Russian *Perm* or *permskii,* the first a city on the Kama River in eastern European Russia, the second a name for a subfamily in the Finnic languages]) In his lovely photographic atlas and commentary on these animals, Riccardo Levi-Setti lists nine orders as determined by paleontologists (*Trilobites,* 58), suggesting a great variety of form among these creatures, which ranged in size from a short 2.5 centimeters (one inch) to sixty centimeters (about two feet) in length. Although many species bear pseudo-Latin terms coined either from the place of discovery or after the discoverer, most of the orders and a number of the species have nomenclatures in the sturdy tradition of mining Latin or Greek for descriptives. For example, the order *Ptychopariida* (Greek *ptyx,* gen. *ptychos* ["fold" or "layer" or "plate"] + late Latin *pari-* ["equal" from Latin's *par*] + zoological Latin's suffix *-ida* [from Latin's *-ides* ("offspring of"), but here specifically the suffix designating orders and classes of animals], thus this order of trilobites means "equal folds" or "equal plates") includes the genus *Trimerus* (Greek *treis, tria* ["three"] + *meros,* gen. *mereos* ["part"]), among which is the species *T. delphinocephalus* Green (Greek *delphis,* gen. *delphinos* ["dolphin"] + *kephalē* ["head"]), a rather fancified label for a small creature as illustrated by Levi-Setti (*Trilobytes,* 179 plate 138). Yet even this "dolphin-headed, three-part and equal-plated" trilobite is a handsome specimen, and indeed, "trilobites are the hallmark of paleontology" (Easton, *Invertebrate Paleontology*, 489).

Crustacea (the nineteenth-century Latinate term is taken to be a fictional neuter plural of *crustaceum* ["a hard-shelled animal"], pulled from classical Latin's *crustare* ["to cover with a layer or coating"], with its participle *crustatum;* in fact, Pliny, *NH,* XI, 165, uses the neuter plural *crustata,* gen. *crustatorum,* to mean "animals with a hard shell," that is, our "crustacea") includes most of the familiar marine arthropoda: lobsters, crabs, and shrimps. Numbering about thirty-five thousand species, the crustacea also take in the barnacles, the parasitic rhizocephalans, the tiny water fleas, fresh- and saltwater ostracods and copepods, the frequently observed freshwater crayfish of the American South, and the tropical land crabs as well as the extremely common land-living sowbugs.

Zoological specialists who study crustacea call themselves *carcinologists* (Greek *karkinos* is "crab" as well as "ulcerous sore"), and they are careful to distinguish their insectlike inamorata from the similar objects of ardor among the entomologists: "Unlike insects, Crustacea typically have two pairs of feelers, or antennae, whereas the insects and their nearer relatives have but a single pair" (Schmitt, *Crustaceans,* 13). Schmitt could have added that insects *always* have six legs, whereas some members of the crustacea can have ten limbs, and others are equipped with from four to twenty-seven pairs of trunk limbs.

Under the subclass or division called *Branchiopoda* (Greek *branchion* ["gill"] + *pous,* gen. *podos,* thus "gill-footed") appear three or four orders of crustaceans, and many are freshwater genera. The *Anostraca* (Greek *an-* ["without" or "lacking"] + *ostrakon* [here, "shell"]) are the "fairy shrimps." American species have eleven pairs of legs, exemplified by *Streptocephalus texanus* Packard (Greek *strephein* ["to twist"] with adj. *streptos* ["twisted" or "turned"] + *kephalē* ["head"] + Latinization of "Texas"), whose genus name nicely describes the shape of the head and appendages in the male. The *Notostraca* (Greek *nōton* ["back"] + *ostrakon*) or "tadpole shrimps" or "shell-backed shrimps" are minute, with a large animal ranging to fifty-eight millimeters long (a little more than two inches), and these animals can have from thirty-five to seventy-one pairs of legs, but "the number of legs [is not] constant within a species" (Pennack, *Fresh-Water Invertebrates,* 1st ed., 326). The genus *Apus* (Latin *apus,* gen. *apodis* [a "swallow" or "swift"]—from the doubled tail) = *Triops* (Greek *treis, tria* ["three"] + *ops,* gen. *opos* ["eye" or "face"]) is famous among carcinologists, since *Apus* (*Tri-*

ops) *longicaudatus* LeConte ("lengthy tail," renders the Latin) produces eggs that are incredibly hardy: the eggs of an English species of *Apus* are recorded to have survived 132 years in the dried mud of a Hampshire pool. Appearing like a miniature horseshoe crab, *A. longicaudatus* is a serious pest in American rice paddies. "Clam shrimps" are grouped in the order *Conchotraca* (Greek *konchē* ["mollusc" or "seashell"] + *ostrakon*), and the order *Cladocera* (Greek *klados* ["branch"] + Latin *cera* ["wax"]) are creatures called "water fleas."

Ostracoda (Greek *ostrakōdēs* ["like a potsherd," describing crabs, turtles, oysters, and eggs]) is the subclass of Crustacea commonly called "seed shrimps" or "mussel shrimps," generally small creatures of marine habitat reaching a length of two millimeters (not quite .08 inch); their appearance has a vague resemblance to seeds with shrimp-like appendages. The modern name (which entered biological nomenclatures in the 1860s) is taken directly from the Greek adjective and fashioned into a neo-Latin noun, appropriately since Aristotle had used the term to designate the shells of crabs (*HA*, 525b12), a turtle's shell (*HA*, 600b20), an oyster shell (*HA*, 531a17), and sometimes eggshells (558a28).

The copepods (subclass *Copepoda* [Greek *kōpē* ("handle of an oar" or simply "oar") + πους, ποδος ("foot")]) are some of the most numerous animals on earth, with "a rough estimate of the number of individuals produced annually in a mere ten cubic meters of Baltic sea water [at] nine billion" (Schmitt, *Crustaceans,* 55). These "oar-feet" are tiny creatures, large specimens reaching less than 1.5 centimeters (.5 inch) in length. Copepods are consumed by enormous tallies of aquatic animals, from whales to freshwater whitefish, and the copepods in company with the ostracods form the base of the pyramid of marine life, "transforming . . . the microscopic vegetable life of the sea and inland waters into food which can be utilized by animals larger than themselves" (Schmitt, *Crustaceans,* 55). In turn, however, copepods parasitize almost every other sea creature, so that carcinologists subdivide this subclass into free-swimming and parasitic animals. Careful study of the copepods shows a remarkable development of mechanisms for "moving exoskeletal parts" (Manton, *Arthropoda,* 174), and many genera are equally remarkable for the beauty of their form, as in the case of the "butterfly copepods" (*Notopterophorus* spp. [Greek *nōton* ("back") + *pteron* ("feather" or "wing") + *phoros* ("bearing," from *pherein,* meaning "to bear" or "to carry")]), which display a miniature splendor in the four "wings" of the female.

Goldfish aficionados are grumpily familiar with the subclass

Branchiura (Greek *branchion* ["gill"] + *oura* ["tail"]), "gill-tails" known as "fish-lice," which are parasitic on almost all species of aquarium fish, from the common varieties of goldfish to the exotic tropicals so favored in the colorful homebound aquatic tanks. Usually in the genus *Argulus* (from the Greek *argos,* with diminutive neo-Latin coinage as *argulus* ["idler" or "lazy one"]), the fish-lice (normally about one centimeter [about .5 inch]) feed on the blood of their hosts, and those argulids that are parasitic on fish migrating from saltwater to freshwater to lay eggs can shift with their hosts from saltwater to freshwater (or the reverse).

The subclass name for the barnacles is *Cirripedia* (Latin *cirrus,* gen. *cirri,* nom. pl. *cirri* ["a lock of curly hair" or "a tuft on the head of a bird" or "a tuft on a plant"] + *pes,* gen. *pedis* ["foot"]), animals synonymous with anything (person or otherwise) that clings tenaciously to something. And cling the barnacles do, fastening themselves to hard and softer surfaces by means of a cementlike glue exuded from a gland next to the last joints of the exterior antennae; another set of glands on the animal's back secretes the shell. The barnacles were formerly classed among the molluscs, but careful observation of the larval stages proved them to be true crustaceans. Barnacles develop from a free-swimming stage beginning with the newly hatched *nauplius* (Greek *nauplios* ["the paper nautilus" or "argonaut," for which see *Tetrabranchia* in chap. 3]) into an adult that latches onto surfaces particular to its species. Familiar are the stalked and sessile barnacles in the order *Thoracia* (Greek *thorax,* gen. *thorakos* ["breastplate" or the area covered, that is, "chest"]), grouped by carcinologists into two major suborders. The *Lepadomorpha* (Greek *lepas,* gen. *lepados* ["limpet"] + *morphe* ["shape" or "form"]) are stalked barnacles or "goose barnacles," so-called from their necklike attachments (the *penduncle* [Latin *pes,* gen. *pedis* ("foot") + *-unculus,* a diminutive suffix, or *unculus* ("single")—the mid-eighteenth-century coinage enfolds the double-meaning, and thus "single, little foot" is an accurate translation]); this suborder includes the worldwide genus *Lepas* (Greek *lepas* ["limpet," suggestive of the shell's shape]) averaging about twelve centimeters (about 4.5 inches) inclusive of the shell. The second major suborder is *Balanomorpha* (Greek *balanos* ["acorn," but due to its lookalike appearance, already "barnacle" in Aristotle, *HA,* 535a24, and elsewhere in medical Greek] + *morphē*), which are the "acorn barnacles" or "stone barnacles" or what carcinologists term "sessile" barnacles (Latin *sedere,* part. *sessus* ["to sit"] with *sessilis* ["fit for sitting on"], the early eighteenth-century zoological Latin taken to mean "permanently attached" [but in botanical Latin, "sessile" means "attached by the base"]), the most common barnacles scraped from the hulls of ships in dry dock. Zoologists enjoy citing Agassiz and Thomas H. Huxley, who are supposed to have said that barnacles are little more than shrimps that stand on their heads inside an encased limestone house and kick food into their mouths with their feet (Miner, *Seashore Life,* 420; Schmitt, *Crustaceans,* 67–68; Buchsbaum, et al., *Animals,* 342), but the humorous summary disguises the striking physiology of feeding among the Cirripedia: "The barnacles form a casting net from their long setose thoracic endo- and exopods (cirri) and the net cleans itself as it curls up after each cast, passing food material to the mouth . . . From a position with curled up or retracted limbs, the body and limbs are projected outwards through the opened valves of the carapace (shell). The force causing extrusion of the body and limbs is largely hydrostatic . . . a special blood pump forcing blood into the cirri, so extending them. There are no extensor muscles to the hinge joint on each cirrus, but a long flexor muscle passes along the whole length of each exopod and endopod. The vascular system is canalized . . . there is no heart as in a normal arthropod" (Manton, *Arthropoda,* 157). And among the barnacles, the order *Rhizocephala* (Greek *rhiza* ["root"] + *kephalē* ["head"]) preys as killer-parasites exclusively on crabs.

The subclass *Malacostraca* (Greek *malakos* ["soft"] + *ostrakon* [here, "shell"]) embraces the numerous crustacea with compound eyes, usually stalked, and normally a *carapace* (Spanish *carapacho* ["the dorsal shell of a turtle, or crab, etc."]) covers the thorax (the dorsal section of the animal immediately behind the head). Here are the shrimps, sow bugs, sand hoppers, whale lice, crayfish, lobsters, and crabs. Grouped in the order *Stomatopoda* (Greek *stoma,* gen. *stomatos,* nom. pl. *stomata* ["mouth"] + *pous,* gen. *podos* ["foot"]) are the "foot-breathers," often called "mantis shrimps" thanks to their jackknife claws, so similar to those of the praying mantis; also among the Stomatopoda are the shrimp mammies, nurse shrimps, and split thumbs. Opossum shrimps are in the order *Mysidacea* (Greek *mysis,* gen. *myseos* [a "closing up"—of pores, the uterus, etc.]), gaining their popular name from the brood pouch of the female, and these enormously numerous pseudo-shrimps (several species are prominent in North American freshwater lakes) can grow as long as thirty millimeters (slightly more than one inch). *Isopoda* (Greek *isos* ["equal"] + *pous,* gen. *podos*) include the common land-dwelling sow bugs, pill bugs, trichoniscids, and rock slaters. The genus *Oniscus* (Greek *oniskos* ["wood louse"], diminutive of *onos* ["ass" or "donkey" but "wood louse" in

Aristotle, *HA*, 557a23]) are common sow bugs occurring frequently in eastern North America after introduction from Europe. These small land-crustaceans (average length 1.6 centimeters [about .6 inch]) cannot roll up into a ball, unlike their cousins among the cosmopolitan pill bugs (genus *Armadillidum* [diminutive of Spanish *armadillo*, in turn a diminutive of *armado* ("armed one"), derived from Latin *armare*, part. *armatus* ("armed")], so named from their ability to "roll up like an armadillo"). The vernacular "pill bug" has a history of its own, since Greco-Roman pharmacy indeed used these creatures as actual "pills" (the rolled-up state), and "the range of ailments against which they were said to be efficacious is not inconsiderable" (Beavis, *Insects*, 18). Rock slaters (*Ligia* spp. [Greek *Ligeia* ("water nymph")] are also isopods, which inhabit creviced and stony seashores, feeding on seaweed at low tide, and which are slightly larger than either sow bugs or pill bugs (rock slaters—also called rocklice or sea slaters—are about thirty-five millimeters long [about 1.25 inches]), and *Trichoniscus* spp. (Greek *thrix*, gen. *trichos* ["hair"] + *ischas*, gen. *ischados* ["thistle"]) are small (four millimeters [.2 inch]) isopods common in damp spots in the northeastern states (the genus name suggests the "brushy" or "tufted" appearance of both the second pair of antennae and the doubled tail). *Amphipoda* (Greek *amphi* ["around" or "on both sides" or "double"] + *pous*, gen. *podos*) is the order incorporating sand hoppers or beach fleas in Isopoda. In spite of their common name, these small animals are totally harmless to beach lovers; in fact, sand hoppers are the most efficient scavengers that live on the world's shores. *Cyamus* (Greek *kyamos* ["bean"]) is the genus in Amphipoda parasitic on whales (thus "whale lice"), and each of the eighteen species of whale lice is parasitic on one—and only one—species of whale.

Almost everyone knows the animals of Malacostraca in the order *Decapoda* (Greek *deka* ["ten"] + *pous*, gen. *podos*), which carcinologists break down into two suborders: *Natantia* (Latin *natare* ["to swim"], with neuter pl. present part. *natantia* ["swimmers"]); and *Reptantia* (Latin *reptare* ["to creep" or "to crawl"], with neuter pl. present part. *reptantia* ["creepers" or "crawlers"]). Natantia are the true shrimps and prawns (the larger specimens among commercial shrimp are known as "prawns"), and *Peneus setifera* L. (Greek *Pēneios* [a Thessalian river god], perhaps muddled with Greek *pēnion* [the "chrysalis" or "pupa" or "cocoon" of a moth, as in Aristotle, *HA*, 551b6] + Latin *seta* ["bristle"] + *ferre* ["to bear"]) is harvested from the sea in millions of tons for human consumption (*Peneus* can grow as large as twenty centimeters [about eight inches]). The genus *Crangon* (Greek *krangōn*, gen. *krangonos* ["small crustacean," as in Aristotle, *HA*, 525b2]) are "snapping shrimps," so termed from the snapping noise they make when disturbed; and the dozens of other genera among the shrimps include freshwater species (genus *Macrobrachium* [Greek *makros* (here, "long") + *branchion* ("arm")]), the gulfweed shrimps (genus *Latreutes* [Greek *latreus*, gen. *latreōs* ("hired servant")]), and several other distinctive varieties.

The "creepers" and "crawlers" in Reptantia are crayfish, lobsters, and crabs, numbering in thousands of species as some of the more successful forms among the arthropods. One muses on the binomial nomenclatures for a few of these creatures, since some are whimsical at best, as in the example of the large spiny lobsters (the West Indian "sea crayfish" can reach forty-five centimeters [about sixteen inches] in length), which have received the genus-name of *Palinurus*. In Roman myth, Palinurus was a pilot of Aeneas, but as helmsman, Palinurus fell asleep at his tiller and tumbled into the sea (Virgil, *Aeneid*, V, 833 and following lines). Many of the names for these well-known "creepers" have been the subject of long-term controversy, as in the instance of the genus *Astacura*. Even though Huxley assures us, in his classic 1880 *The Crayfish*, that *astakos* (Greek for "lobster") is the firmly accepted genus name for the crayfish—"as this nomenclature is generally received, it is desirable that it should not be altered; though it is attended by the inconvenience, that *Astacus* . . . does not denote that which the Greeks, ancient and modern, signify, by its original, *astakos*" (*Crayfish*, 13–14)—one notes that Schmitt uses *Astacura* to designate the "tribe" of "true lobsters and crayfish" (*Crustaceans*, 198). Nowadays crayfish are *Cambarus* spp. (another Greek word for lobster was *kammaros*, Latinized as *cammarus* [Pliny, *NH*, XXXII, 148] or *gammarus* [Varro, *Agriculture*, III, 11.3] and re-Latinized in zoological terminologies as *Cambarus*); and although Huxley's discussion of lobster names (*Crayfish*, 13) remains current, since modern authorities list *Homarus* (a Latinization of the old French *omar* or *homar* ["lobster"]) as the genus that encompasses lobsters (*H. americanus* Milne-Edwards is the usual lobster of restaurant and supermarket, the "New England" lobster, dark greenish-gold-brown while alive, bright pinkish-red after cooking), there is some initial confusion at first glance at the literature. *Procambarus* (Latin *pro* ["before"] + *Cambarus*) is the common genus of North American freshwater crayfish, whose burrows (those mucky "chimneys" of the American South) appear in marshes and wet pastures where there is no open water.

The suborder *Anomura* (greek *anomos* ["erratic" or "irregular"]

+ *oura* ["tail"]) are the genera of hermit crabs, mud shrimps, the large coconut or robber crabs of the southern Pacific, king crabs, and a number of similar animals. Hermit crabs are famous for borrowing the empty shells of marine snails, and as the crabs molt and increase in size, they must "move house," sometimes by ejecting another hermit crab from a larger shell. The large Australian hermit crabs in the genus *Dardanus* (Latin *Dardanus* ["Trojan" or "descendant of a Trojan" = "Roman"—but third-century legal Latin's *dardanarius* meant "speculator" (Ulpian in Justianian's *Digest*, XLVII, 11.6), which is the connotation of the modern zoological Latin]) can be thirty centimeters (one foot) long, but the cosmopolitan *Pagurus* spp. (Greek *pagouros* ["crab"]) normally are about half this size. Mud shrimps include the genera *Callianassa* (Greek *kallion* ["more beautiful"] + Latin *nassa* ["wicker-basket fishtrap" or "weel"]) and *Calocaris* (Greek *kalos* ["beautiful"] + *karis* ["shrimp"]). *Birgus* spp. (a Latinization of *Birges,* an older spelling of *Bruges* [Flemish *brugge* ("bridge")], with "Bruges satin," simply "satin," the meaning intended here) are the subject of many tales from the South Pacific, where these large coconut-drilling and -feeding climbing crabs (forty-five centimeters [about eighteen inches] long) are hunted for their sweet flesh and rich oil—a single robber crab can yield as much as a quart of oil (see Schmitt, *Crustaceans,* 113–18, for a collection of yarns about these animals, the only creatures known to have "strength and ability to open the tough-husked coconut unaided" [117]). King crabs (the North American genus is *Lithodes* [Greek *lithos* ("stone")], and the genus of the northern Pacific is *Paralithodes* [Greek *para* ("beside," here "beyond") + *lithos*]) have become frequent choices of seafood fanciers, and one occasionally hears these goodly sized edible crabs called "stone crabs" to avoid confusion with horseshoe crabs (not crustaceans at all, but an arachnid), traditionally known as "king crabs." Especially prized are large specimens of *Paralithodes camtschatica* (a Latinization of Russian Siberia's Kamchatka peninsula), the so-called Alaskan king crab, which ranges from the Gulf of Alaska to the Kamchatkan side of the Bering Sea.

Finally among the Reptantia, carcinologists place "true crabs" (either the tribe or suborder *Brachyura* [Greek *brachys* ("short") + *oura* ("tail")]). Among the fifty or so major genera is *Macrocheira* (Greek *makros* ["long"] + *cheir* ["hand"]), the Japanese giant spider crab, whose long clawed appendages can reach 3.65 meters (twelve feet) across, and the genus *Cancer* (Latin *cancer,* gen. *cancri* ["crab"]), which forms one of the most important items in the profits of fisheries on both East and West coasts of the United States.

THE MYRIAPODS

As the name indicates, these are creatures with "countless feet" (the Greek *myrioi* as a definite numeral, written ,ι, is "10,000," but the common adjective *myrios* in classical Greek usually means "numberless" or "countless" and sometimes "infinite"; when a writer wanted to express something "immense" or "measureless" in size, he often used *myrios*). "Countless" may express a superficial observation of these animals, but the literal "10,000 feet" does not, so that this former class name among the Arthropods is generally discarded in favor of class names for particular groups of creatures: the millipedes, the centipedes, the pauropods, the garden centipedes (the symphilids). All are land-living, and zoologists sometimes argue that the myriapods represent a kind of evolution from crustacea on the analogy of sow bugs and wood lice, which are crustaceans. As classes of animals, the myriapods are kin to both the crustaceans and the arachnids (spiders, scorpions) and are related to the insects.

> Class *Diplopoda* (Greek *diploos* or *diplous* ["twofold" or "double"] + *pous*, gen. *podos* ["foot"]) are wormlike, multilegged creatures commonly called *millipedes* (Latin *mille* ["a thousand"] + pes, gen. *pedis* ["foot"]), found frequently in houses and in moist settings of southern forests. There are about seven thousand species in the class Diplopoda, with about six hundred occurring north of the Rio Grande River in North America. Some American species attain remarkable lengths: heavy rains in the Ohio Valley during the spring and summer of 1982 engendered heavy arthropod populations in the upper southern states, and a specimen of *Narceus americanus* (Greek *narkē* ["numbness" or "stiffness"] + Latinized "American") in the order Spirobolida (Greek *speira* ["coil" or "twist"] + *bolis*, gen. *bolidos* ["missile"]) that I collected in Montgomery County, Kentucky, measured twenty centimeters (eight inches) in length. Greco-Roman toxicologists viewed the larger millipedes with unease, assuming these animals could give poisonous stings or bites (for example, Nicander, *Theriaca*, 811), but "harm to humans from any millipedes . . . has not been verified in the modern literature" (Scarborough, "Nicander's Toxicology," 18). Yet large millipedes do secrete defensive acids "in the form of a fine jet or spray" (Cloudsley-Thompson, *Spiders*, 36), and the spray causes chemical burns on human skin, turning it black. Modern research has determined

that millipedes in a number of orders exude hydrogen cyanide, polyzonimines, bezoquinones, along with chlorine and iodine, "as natural defensive agents against their enemies, especially ants" (Scarborough, "Nicander Toxicology," 32 n. 197). Hellenistic physicians and naturalists may not have been so wrong after all. Most millipedes are cylindrical, and the name *Diplopoda* suggests how each fused segment of the animal bears two pairs of limbs, but these "rings" are variable in number, even in particular species; for example, the common eastern North American *Chordeumida* spp. (Greek *chordeuma,* gen. *chordeumatos* ["sausage"]), averaging four centimeters (about 1.5 inches) in length, can have from twenty-eight to fifty-nine rings. Millipedes are easily distinguished from their land-crustacean cousins: millipedes have a single pair of antennae, crustaceans have two pairs.

Class *Chilopoda* (Greek *chilioi* ["a thousand"] + *pous,* gen. *podos*) are the *centipedes* (Latin *centum* ["a hundred"] + *pes,* gen. *pedis*). The scientific name for centipedes is deliberately artificial as a label, and the common name is closer to appearance. Widely feared by homeowners, centipedes are very beneficial predators of household pests, from silverfish (the bane of book lovers) to gnats and flies, and the speedy, very common *Scutigera* spp. (Latin *scutum,* gen. *scuti* ["shield"] + *gerere* ["to carry" or "to wear"])—often found trapped in slippery washbasins—have fifteen pairs of long legs (among centipedes, "the fewer the legs, the faster they can go"). Here in Wisconsin, *S. coleoptrata* L. (Greek *koleon* ["sheath"] + *-pt-* [an abbreviated form of *pteros* (here, "feather")], suggesting the plated back and "feathery" look while in motion) averages three centimeters (1.2 inches) and is a welcome help in mosquito control inside houses. Gardeners know well the stone centipedes (*Lithobius* spp [Greek *lithos* ("stone") + *bios* ("life")], up to 4.5 centimeters [about 1.7 inches], with fifteen pairs of legs. The eyeless soil centipedes in the order *Geophilomorpha* (Greek *gē,* gen. *gēon* ["earth"] + *philos* ["fondness"] + *morphē* ["form" or "shape"], thus rendered as "formed to love the earth"), which are the long, wormlike centipedes (*Strigamia* spp. [Latin *striga* ("a strip"—here, "a strip of bristles")] have fifty-seven pairs of legs, and our reddish-brown specimens may reach five centimeters [about two inches] in length). Some tropical Geophilomorphids have 177 pairs of legs, and "the largest species, like the North African *Orya barbarica,* measure about six or seven inches in length" (Cloudsley-Thompson, *Spiders,* 51). The largest centipedes, however, are in the order *Sclopendromorpha* (Greek *skolopendra* ["centipede"—wrongly given as "millipede" in LSJ] + *morphē*), with some tropical American *Scolopendra* spp. reaching thirty centimeters (twelve inches) in length. Greco-Roman toxicologists believed such large and nasty-looking *entoma* were dangerous, and "though not actually poisonous, the bites of these Scolopendromorphs can produce painful swelling of the affected area, so that the fear they evoked in classical times is quite understandable" (Beavis, *Insects,* 10). Nicander's *Theriaca,* 812, recorded the belief that both "heads" of the large centipede could inflict a painful bite, and "viewing the gross aspects of the larger centipedes . . . may also help explain why Nicander (or his source) might believe that the animal had two heads, and that both could bite. A ventral view of the postcephalic segment reveals a very prominent pair of venom jaws, while the last pair of legs are modified into lengthened prehensile limbs, which can deliver a firm pinch" (Scarborough, "Nicander's Toxicology," 19–20).

Discovered in 1886, the minute arthropods in the class *Pauropoda* (Greek *pauros* ["little"] + *pous,* gen. *podos*) are widely distributed in decaying and dampish leaves, sticks, and almost any deteriorating organic matter. Usually two millimeters (about .1 of an inch) or less in length, these creatures are soft-bodied, with twelve segments and normally nine pairs of legs. Cloudsley-Thompson *Spiders,* 75–76) quotes a study by a North Carolina student of Pauropods who gives an amazing estimate of the density of the "little-footed" myriapods: "an annual average of 1,672,704 per acre (to a depth of five inches) in oak stands on clay soil, and 2,178,000 in pine stands on sandy loam in the Duke Forest, North Carolina." Specialists have described about 350 species in this small class.

An even smaller class are the 120 species in *Symphyla* (Greek *syn* ["with" or "along with": *m* replaces *n* before *b, m,* and *p*] + *phylum,* pl. *phyla* [Greek *phylon,* Latinized into *phylum* ("tribe," but in modern biology, "a primary subdivision of animals or plants, grouping together those with the same body plan")]. Considered serious pests in greenhouses, these "garden centipedes" are from two to eight millimeters long (.1 inch to .3 inch), with twelve pairs of legs; unlike true centipedes or millipedes, symphilids walk by moving all legs on one side together and survive by the unusual "ability to change direction of running very suddenly and often, to turn in a hairpin bend or run off in a different direction" (Manton, *Arthropoda,* 372). Common are *Scutigerella* spp. (Latin *scutum* ["shield"] + *gerere* ["to carry"] + diminutive suffix *-ellum,* thus "little shield carriers"), equipped with fifteen segmented dorsal plates; Scutigerellids will feed on both living and dead plant matter.

THE INSECTS

These arthropods almost defeat the Linnaean binomial system of nomenclature, simply through sheer numbers. The basic morphology is very straightforward: all insects have six legs (hence the formal Class name *Hexapoda* [Greek *hex* ("six") + *pous,* gen. *podos* ("foot")]) and have bodies divided into three parts (from front to back: head, thorax, abdomen). Defining an insect, illustrated by the following from Richards and Davies, *Imms' General Textbook,* 10th ed., Vol. I, 3, shows how entomologists separate their animals from all the rest:

The insects are tracheate arthropods in which the body is divided into head, thorax, and abdomen. A single pair of antennae (homologous with the antennules of the Crustacea) is present and the head also bears a pair of mandibles and two pairs of maxillae, the second pair fused medially to form the labium. The thorax carries three pairs of legs and usually one or two pairs of wings. The abdomen is devoid of ambulatory appendages, and the genital opening is situated near the posterior end of the body. Postembryonic development is rarely direct and a metamorphosis usually occurs.

If one were to "translate" this paragraph into "ordinary" English, it might read:

The insects are air-breathing, jointed-limbed animals in which the body is divided into a head, a middle section, and a rear-ended portion. Two sensory frontal appendages (similar in function and structure to the smaller, double pair of sensory appendages of the Crustacea) are present, and the head also has two hard jaws and four (in two pairs) segmented mouthpart structures furnished with sensory appendages, with the second pair joined in the middle to form what is called the "labium." The middle section of the insect carries three pairs of legs and usually one or two pairs of wings. The rear-ended portion of the insect lacks appendages with which the animal walks, and the sexual organ is close to the rear of the creature. The form of the insect emerging from the egg is rarely the same as an adult, and usually a complete alteration occurs in structure from hatchling to mature insect.

A perceptive reader immediately notes how terms derived from Greek and Latin lend precision and why the presumably "ordinary" English emerges as occasionally vague. As in the accepted vocabulary of medicine, the particular adaptations of classical words by entomologists to designate and describe body parts of insects say exactly what they need to say, no more or no less. The "translation" of Imms' "antennae," for example, into "two sensory frontal appendages" not only violates the rules of clear writing but also uses four words in place of one. To be sure, Latin's *antenna,* gen. *antennae,* nom. pl. *antennae,* does not in entomology carry the meaning of the word as used by Cicero, Ovid, Horace, Catullus, or even Pliny the Elder (*antenna*—usually spelled *antemna*—meant "sail yard" or "yardarm" or simply "sail" in classical Latin), but television and radio people know exactly what *they* mean by *antenna,* and so do entomologists and carcinologists know *their* meaning as they employ the neo-Latin in modern, technical English. And the muddled "ordinary English" account of an insect's mouthparts (feeding antennae, jaws) fails to suggest the beautifully complex mechanisms summarized by *mandibles* and *maxillae;* and the "translation" must employ *labium* (Latin *labium* ["lip"]) to avoid the specialized and multiword definition of the term as employed by entomologists: "the posterior, unpaired member of the mouthparts of an insect, formed by the united second maxillae." These sixteen words mean *labium* for the entomologist, but *labium* for the botanist has another meaning, and yet a third meaning for an anatomist. In all three, the original *lip* survives from the classical Latin, but in each of the three, *labium* acquires a precise meaning according to the particular science. "Rear-ended portion" is certainly less elegant than "abdomen," but the greatest violation to clarity occurs when the "translation" of *metamorphosis* becomes "complete alteration . . . in structure from hatchling to mature insect."

Metamorphōsis, gen. *metamorphōseōs,* is Greek for "transformation," a word borrowed directly into Latin, where its basic meaning summarized Ovid's famous "transformation myths" Latinized as the *Metamorphoses* of about A.D. 8. In modern entomology, the metamorphosis of an insect is either "complete" (butterflies, moths, beetles, flies, mosquitoes) or "incomplete" (grasshoppers, mantises, crickets), and when an entomologist uses *metamorphosis* in its fullest sense, four stages of an insect's growth are assumed: the egg, the larva, the pupa, and the adult.

Larva (Latin *larva*, gen. *larvae*, nom. pl. *larvae* ["evil spirit" or "demon," akin to *Lar*—an Etruscan word—"a Roman god associated with the protection of a particular place"]). Seventeenth-century Latin reused *larva* in its special sense of "mask—usually horrible" to suggest how what came out of a butterfly egg was but a "ghost" of the beautiful adult, thus *larva* frequently means "caterpillar" in ordinary English.

Pupa (Latin *pupa*, gen. *pupae*, nom. pl. *pupae* ["girl" or "doll"]) is the stage of metamorphosis in which the insect larva has fashioned for itself a protective *cocoon* (French *cocon* ["egg-shell"] from the Latin *coccum* ["scarlet dye" or the insect that yielded the dye]) or a *chrysalis* (Greek *chrysalis*, gen. *chrysallidos*: Aristotle, HA, 551a19, uses the word as it is used today), a term employed by entomologists to designate the hard-shelled pupa of a butterfly or moth.

Entomologists call the "adult" an *imago* (Latin *imago*, gen. *imaginis* ["picture," "likeness," "image," "shape," "form," or "species," among a number of meanings]), that is, the "mature form" of the insect that emerges from its cocoon.

One cannot "translate" metamorphosis without explicating the phases of an insect's life, so that any "translation" of this term is inadequate and hopelessly vague, unless accompanied with some details of the wonder-provoking "transformations" common among the insects.

Entomologists debate how to classify and what to call the over one million species of insects, and that rounded-off million is a conservative estimate, since new species turn up and are published each year; over twenty years ago, a commonly cited taxonomy of insects had thirty-five orders and not quite eight hundred thousand species (W. Henning, *Stammegeschichte der insekten* [Frankfurt, 1969]), with an actual count of 781,226 species—two hundred thousand new species discovered in merely twenty years. And to the question "What constitutes an order of insects?" entomologists give a standard definition with an enormous loophole, exemplified in Borror and DeLong, *Study of Insects*, 56: "The class Insecta is divided into orders on the basis of the structure of the wings and mouthparts, the metamorphosis, and on various other characters. There are differences of opinion among entomologists as to the limits of some of the orders." (Borror, Triplehorn, and Johnson, *Study of Insects*, 146, has very minor changes in this definition: substituting "Hexapoda" for "Insecta," adding "primarily" before "into orders," and ending the first sentence with "metamorphosis," omitting "and on various other characters.") That loophole of "differences of opinion" leads to varying enumerations of insect orders: Henning, *Stammegeschichte,* lists thirty-five orders; Borror and DeLong, *Study of Insects,* has twenty-six; Borror, Triplehorn, and Johnson, *Study of Insects,* gives thirty-one; Imms, *General Textbook,* 10th ed., names twenty-nine; and Essig, in his widely used, post–World War II text *College Entomology,* has thirty-three orders.

The debate continues, but nomenclatures of insect orders are easy and simple compared with labeling problems for genera and species, especially among the beetles, the most numerous of the insects (Hennig has 350,000 species of beetles, Borror and DeLong 276,700, Borror, Triplehorn, and Johnson 300,000, Imms 10th ed. 330,000 [but Imms 9th ed. has 220,000—110,000 new species in twenty years], and Essig's text counts "no less than 250,000 described species" [518]). Typical is the proposed nomenclature for a newly discovered beetle from Borneo, as published by Bright, "Two New Species of *Phloeosinus* Chapuis." The genus *Phloeosinus,* so Bright informs us, is controversial in its own right, even though it is "well-known" (Essig, *College Entomology,* 605, has thirty-one species in the genus; forty years later, Bright tells us it now has "more than 90 species"). But unless one happened to know about Mount Kinabalu in Malaysian Borneo, would one be able to comprehend Bright's species name of *kinabaluensis?* The genus *Phloeosinus* (Greek *phloios* ["bark"] + Latin *sinus,* gen. *sinus* ["cavity"], thus "bark-cavity" beetles) in the family *Scolytidae* (Greek *skolyptein* ["to cut short"]—suggesting the short snout and truncated bodies of these common bark beetles) thus has an addition named *P. kinabaluensis* Bright. The genus name too bears the name of its nomenclator: M. F. Chapuis was a famous Belgian entomologist of the mid-nineteenth century, and in beetle listings, Scolytidae will carry "Kirby" as giving the name to this family. William Kirby (1759–1850) was one of the greatest British entomologists, and his "cut short barkbeetles" appeared in the literature of entomology in 1836. And *Coleoptera* (Greek *koleos* ["sheath"] + *pteron,* nom. pl. *ptera* [here, "wing"], thus "sheath winged") is the name provided for the beetles by Linnaeus in 1758.

Extended to fossil species, nomenclatures of the about fifty thousand known species of prehistoric beetles in the order *Protocoleoptera* (Greek *prōtos* + *koleos* + *ptera* ["first sheath wings"]) engender problems in nomenclature as paleontologists and entomologists continue to mine Greco-Latinate terms, and one encounters Latin-like geographic names (Bright's *kinabaluensis* is illustrative) with great frequency, or Latinizations of personal names, usually the discoverer or a relative of the discoverer. Geographical names aim for precision, but as students of modern political geography well know, names get changed according to shifting regimes, and names that mirrored precise geography in decades or centuries past become instantly obscure with changes in culture or politics (British Ceylon became Sri Lanka, to take one example). Shifts in historical or cultural assumptions may also serve to bury the meanings originally intended in the binomial nomenclatures with their Greek and Latin foundations. Anyone who collects insects sooner or later learns about the destructive labors of the small beetles in the family *Dermestidae* Gyllenhall (Greek *derma* ["skin"] + *esthein* ["to eat" or "to devour"]), which will consume a painstakingly assembled and mounted collection unguarded by paradichlorobenzene crystals (usually called "mothballs") or a similar chemical defense. Incomprehensible is the entomological nomenclature unless one knows that the name was given in 1808 by Leonhard Gyllenhall (1752–1840), an eminent Swedish coleopterist who presumed "everyone would know" (and they would in the early nineteenth century) that "skin-eaters" were obviously those little beetles that wrought such destruction on the leathers ("skins") in the tanneries of the day. Within Dermestidae, the genus *Dermestes* has about seventy species, and museums occasionally use *D. vulpinus* Fabr. (Latin *vulpinus* ["of a fox" or "belonging to a fox," thus "cunning"]) to clean dried flesh from bones: the beetles do the job far better than any chemical, leaving museum osteology with perfectly scoured bones, totally cleaned yet completely undamaged. Johann Christian Fabricius (1745–1808), the great Danish entomologist, gave this name presumably from the beetles' preference for fox pelts, or perhaps from the "cunning" way in which they cleaned dried flesh from bones.

In the 10th edition (1758) of his *Systema naturae,* Linnaeus gave the name of this class as *Insecta* and established seven orders within the class. Yet almost immediately scientific colleagues wondered if there might be a better descriptive than this simple Latin term, derived from Pliny the Elder's *Natural History*. In 1825, the French naturalist P. A. Latreille (1762–1833) proposed *Hexapoda* as the name for the class, and Insecta and Hexapoda occasionally appear side by side. Linnaeus used wings (or the lack of them) to classify insects, but this alary system (Latin *ala*, gen. *alae*, nom. pl. *alae* ["wing"]) failed to account for many particular structures distinguishing various insects; among the seven orders set down by Linnaeus, only four remain in modern listings: *Coleoptera* (the beetles); *Lepidoptera* (Greek *lepis*, gen. *lepidos* ["scale"] + *ptera*, thus "scaled-wings" [the butterflies and moths]); *Diptera* (Greek *dis* ["twice"] + *ptera*, thus "paired wings" [flies, gnats, midges, mosquitoes]); and *Hymenoptera* (Greek *hymēn* [here, "thin skin" or "membrane"] + *ptera* [bees, wasps, and ants]). The Linnaean instinct in using wings (simply *aptera* ["without wings"] and *pterygota* ["winged ones"], from the Greek adjective *pterygōtos* ["winged"] as used by Aristotle, *PA,* 659b7) seems to have been accurate, since modern entomologists favor the alary system as opposed to other insect body parts for taxonomical clarity. Imms, *General Textbook*, II, 121–31, gives a survey of the controversies over classifications (the seventy-seven-item bibliography—English, French, German, Russian—under "Literature on Classification and Phylogeny" mirrors the continual arguments conducted on an international scale).

GREEK AND LATIN FOR INSECT NAMES

Repeatedly, common names obscure exact species, and entomology is replete with modern adaptations of the two classical languages. Often there are borrowings familiar to students of medicine in another context, and this interconnectedness of Greco-Latinate coinages among the biological sciences should be kept in mind as one learns the special nuances chosen by each science. The following entomological nomenclatures are merely illustrative, with some orders providing basic groupings of merely a fraction of the million or more species involved:

> Order *Thysanura* (Greek *thysanos* ["tassel" or "fringe"] + *oura* ["tail"]) includes the wingless insects called bristletails, silverfish, and fire-

brats. Latreille established the name of the order in 1796, and genera rarely exceed three centimeters in length (about 1.25 inches), although one sometimes sees skittering silverfish a bit longer. Thysanurids bear a characteristic three-tined tail that appears fuzzy or hairy (thereby, "bristletail"). Silverfish (Family *Lepismidae* [Greek *lepis* ("scale")]) are destructive feeders on the starches and sugars in the glues of bookbindings, but a goodly population of household centipedes keeps one's library free of these pests. There are about fifty species in Thysanura in North America, and seven hundred or so worldwide.

Order *Collembola* (Greek *kolla* ["glue"] + *embolon* [here, "wedge," "peg," or "stopper"], so named from gummy ventral tubes or collophores) has about twenty-five hundred, widely distributed species, normally not longer than .1 centimeter to .2 centimeter (.25 to .5 inch). Known as springtails and snow fleas, these wingless insects are dependent on a ready suppy of moisture, and several species exist on seashores daily submerged by tides. The snow fleas (Family *Poduridae* [Greek *pous,* gen. *podos* ("foot") + *oura* ("tail")]) are minute creatures appearing in large numbers on the surface of snow, revealing themselves as dark insects equipped with a double-pronged "jumping tail."

Order *Ephemeroptera* (Greek *ephēmeros* ["short-lived" or "living only a day"] + *pteron,* nom. pl. *ptera* ["wing"]) are about two thousand species of the very familiar mayflies. In spite of the oddly incomplete description in Aristotle, HA, 552b18–23 (where the insect called *ephēmeron* inhabits Crimean Russia), the numerous allusions to *ephemera* by Greek and Roman authors show familiarity with the swarmings of the larger mayflies—and with their extremely short life-span in the adult form (some larvae, however, live for three years before emerging for their single day on the wing). Using the thumb and index finger, collectors can easily grasp mayflies by their wings before inserting them into a killing jar, since at rest the insect holds its two wings together above the body. Depending on species, these delicate creatures have either two or three hairlike tails, and the common European mayfly (*Ephemera vulgata* L. [*vulgus* is Latin for "common"]) is abundant from May through August (length up to twenty-four millimeters [not quite an inch]). Aristotle's southern Russian mayfly is *E. longicauda* Olivier (the Latinate *longicauda* means "long tail"), also abundant and about twice as large as its western European cousin.

Long admired for their dazzling aerial abilities, matched by their elegance in color and grace, are members of the order *Odonata* (Greek *odous,* gen. *odontos* ["tooth"]), the dragonflies and damselflies (other common names include darning needles, snake doctors, and the exactly appropriate mosquito hawks). Fabricius gave the name for this order in 1793, perceiving the fundamental role of these insects' formidable mouthparts, perfectly suited for their predatory feeding habits. The aquatic nymphs (Greek *nymphē* ["young wife" or "bride," sometimes "young girl"]), which emerge from dragonfly or damselfly eggs, are as endowed with slicing and chopping mouthparts as are the adults (the *imago,* as above under "metamorphosis") that come forth from the last stage of nymph growth (these stages are *instars* to entomologists [Latin *instar* ("the equivalent in measure," or "counterpart," or "equal"), with *ad instar* meaning "according to the pattern of"]). Nymphs feed voraciously on mosquito and gnat larvae and are the natural control mechanism of mosquitoes where dragonflies flourish. There are more than five thousand species in Odonata around the world, with about five hundred in North America, and they range in size from the South American genus *Megaloprepus* (Greek *megas* ["great"] + Latin *praepes,* gen. *praepetis* ["bird" or simply "something that flies"]) with a wingspan of twenty centimeters (about 7.5 inches) to the Australian damselflies in the genus *Agriocnemis* (Greek *agrios* ["living in the fields" or "wild"] + *knēmis,* gen. *knēmidos* ["spoke," but more commonly "greave" or "legging"]) with wings measuring across 2.5 centimeters (one inch). Prehistoric dragonflies were far larger: *Meganeura* spp. (Greek *megas* ["great"] + *neuron* ["cord," "sinew," or "tendon"]) from the Upper Carboniferous had a wingspan of over sixty centimeters (slightly over two feet) about three hundred million years ago. The remarkable helicopter-like hovering, darting, and diving movements in flight by dragonflies and damselflies come from complex musculatures controlling the two pairs of wings.

The Tropics are not the only parts of the world in which new insects turn up to puzzle entomologists. In 1914, E. M. Walker published an article in which he described some odd insects, from the Canadian Rockies, that seemed to combine the features of both cockroaches and crickets, but were wingless. By the 1930s, a new order of insects, *Grylloblattodea* (Latin *gryllus* ["cricket"] + *blatta* ["cockroach"]) had appeared in the entomological listings. These small creatures (the largest among the twenty known species is three centimeters long [1.25 inches]) live in mountains from four thousand to seven thousand feet above sea level in moss or under stones or in alpine soils.

Order *Orthoptera* (Greek *orthos* ["straight"] + *pteron,* nom. pl. *ptera* ["wing"]) includes the locusts, grasshoppers, katydids, common crickets, mole crickets, and kindred insects. Next to the terror evoked by plagues and pestilences in human history, nothing quite matches the dismay and fear produced from nature's whims when the daylight becomes smothered from swarms of locusts. Usually numbering in the hundreds of millions, such a "plague of locusts" guarantees famine for man and animal, and Saharan Africa, western North America, and other areas suffer occasional orthopteran invasions even in our era of widespread use of insecticides and sophisticated understanding of life cycles—especially of the desert locust (*Schistocera gregaria* Forskal = *S. tatarica* L. [Greek *schistos* ("split" or "divided") + *keros* ("beeswax" or "wax," here "wax-colored") + Latin *gregarius* ("pertaining to a flock or herd")]; the Linnaean *tatarica* is a variant of *Tartaros* from the Greek, namely "the infernal regions" or, in the eighteenth century, "hell," which is where these creatures seemed to come from). *S. gregaria* is in the family *Locustidae* (Latin *locusta* ["locust," but *locusta marina* meant "lobster"]), in turn one of the families in the suborder *Acridodea* (Greek *akris,* gen. *akridos* ["a locust, grasshopper, or cricket conspicuous by reason of its song," in Beavis, *Insects,* 62]). The adult desert locust can grow to eight centimeters long (a little more than three inches), and a swarm of a couple of million can literally darken the sky and eclipse the sun. The ancients knew that swarming locusts could fly long distances, and modern accounts confirm the ancient ones in terms of the huge masses of drowned locusts washing up on shores to putrify as a forecast of yet another kind of plague. During a hopeful eradication campaign on the island of Cyprus in 1881, thirteen hundred tons of eggs were destroyed (that would be about 1.6 billion egg cases). The female inserts about one hundred eggs per case (called a pod) down into the sand, and a single female can deposit ten to twenty pods, with at least one thousand first instars emerging with the first rains.

Fortunately not all members of the Locustidae are this destructive, and everyone in temperate climates recalls the rasping, clicking, and chirping by locusts, grasshoppers, and crickets as a pleasant sound of summer. The Greek *tettix,* gen. *tettigos* (usually "cicada") misleadingly provides the family name for the katydids, long-horned grasshoppers, and bush crickets: *Tettigoniidae.* Childhood memories of something that chirped in the dark "katy did, katy didn't" are the sounds of a common, green katydid of eastern North America, *Pterophylla camellifolia* Fabricius (Greek *pteron* ["wing"] + *phyllon* ["leaf" or "plant"] + eighteenth-century Latin *camellia* [the genus of several Asian trees and bushes, the most famous of which is *Camellia sinensis* (L.) Kuntze, "tea"] + Latin *folium* ["leaf"]), which translates as "winged leaf," that is, "the leaf of a tea-tree." In Fabricius's day, the actual shape and size of tea leaves as shipped from the Far East would have been familiar to natural historians, and the botanical name shows Linnaeus originally provided the genus name. The coinage of *camellia* itself indicates the intertwining of entomology, botany, and herbal lore in the eighteenth and nineteenth centuries—suggesting why our common katydid bears the Latinate name for Chinese tea: *Camellia* is the Latinized form of Georg Josef Kamel (1661–1706), who was born in Brünn (Moravia) and who became a Jesuit in 1683. The Latinized form of his name is properly Camellus; the Jesuits sent him to the South Seas and then to the Philippines, where he opened a pharmacist's shop in Manila for the distribution of remedies to the poor. Kamel became an expert on herbal botany and sent specimens and drawings to European scientists, including the influential English botanist, John Ray (1627–1705). Kamel's corruption of a Chinese term, heard among speakers of the Xiamen dialect in Spanish Manila, gave Europe—and especially England—"tea." One cannot hear "katy did, katy didn't" and not reflect on why our beautiful, sometimes gray-emerald katydid carries the name of a Jesuit who gave his name to tea. Many names, however, among the insects mirror this fusion of botany, medicine, and pharmacy, since these sciences were followed by students of what was called "natural history" well into the twentieth century.

Order *Phasmida* (Greek *phasma*, gen. *phasmatos* ["apparition," "phantom," "strange phenomenon," and similar meanings]) are the leaf insects and walkingsticks as grouped by Imms (*General Textbook*, 10th ed.). This order contains some of the most extraordinary known insects, which have almost perfected their mimicry of leaves and sticks around the world. Unless one looks very carefully indeed, one will miss the common American walkingstick, *Diapheromera femorata* Say (Greek *dia* ["through"] + *pherein* ["to bear" or "to bring"] + *mēros* ["part"] + Latin *femur*, gen. *femoris* ["thigh," but here the "thigh-bone" known as the femur]), which—until touched—remains motionless among the twigs of the tree on which it is perched, even mimicking the swaying of nearby limbs if a breeze should come along. I observed specimens in Kentucky about ten centimeters long (almost four inches) while walkingsticks here in the Old Northwest reach five to eight centimeters (two to three inches). Most of the leaf insects are tropical and carry the logical family name *Phyllidae* (Greek *phyllon* ["leaf"]). These creatures not only mimic almost perfectly the colors and shapes of leaves but also display the veins of those leaves; many species have leaflike attachments on the first two pairs of legs to add to the illusion. Many of the oriental Phyllidae attain lengths of ten centimeters (about four inches), but the giants in the order Phasmida are in the family Phasmatidae (walkingsticks): the genus *Eurycantha* (Greek *eurys* ["wide"] + Latin *cantus* ["rim" or "iron tire"]) of New Guinea is a twenty-five-centimeter long spiny stick (about ten inches), and an example of a Malaysian *Podocanthus* (Greek *pous*, gen. *podos* ["foot"] + Latin *cantus*) in my collection is a bulky sixteen centimeters in length (slightly over six inches), celery-green except for its curiously pink pair of wings. Most of the two thousand five hundred species in Phasmida are East Asian.

Order *Dictyoptera* (Greek *diktyon* ["net," but specifically "fishing net" in Homer, *Odyssey*, XXII, 386, and "hunting net" in Pollux, V, 26.27; other common meanings in Greek were "lattice work" and "the bottom of a sieve"] + *pteron* ["wing"]) are the common cockroaches and praying mantises, and the order has two suborders (Imms, *General Textbook*) carrying the names of former orders: *Blattaria* (the cockroaches) and *Mantodea* (the mantids). Latin's *blatta* included various insects: cockroach, clothes moth, and bookworm, among several, but the adjective *blattarius* meant particularly "connected with or suitable for moths." *Blattaria* are the loathed cockroaches, common throughout the world within the dwellings of humankind. Among the four thousand or so species of cockroaches, the usual ones we see at midnight, scattering from a suddenly switched-on light, are *Blatella germanica* L. (*Blatta* + diminutive suffix *-ella* [thus "little roach"] + Latinized "German"), the smallest of the domesticated cockroaches (*B. germanica* can reach a length of twelve millimeters [a little less than .5 inch])— and in the strictest sense of association and dependence on human beings and their food supplies, cockroaches are among the most "domesticated" of animals. Often placed in the family *Phyllodromiidae* (Greek *phyllon* ["leaf"] + *dromomeus* ["that which runs"], thus "running leaves"), *B. germanica* is closely related to the largest American cockroach, *Blaberus cranifer* Burmeister (Greek *blaberos* ["noxious" or "harmful"] + *kranion* ["skull"] + Latin *ferre* ["to carry" or "to bear"]) of Florida (up to sixty millimeters [a little less than 2.5 inches]). The nomenclature "noxious skull-bearer" reflects the common name of this species, the "giant death's head roach," a fanciful epithet suggesting some light markings on the dark-brown thorax, thought to resemble a skull. Common too are cockroaches called "waterbugs" or "kitchen roaches" or "black beetles" (*Blatta* *orientalis* L. [Latin *oriens*, gen. *orientis* is "morning" and therefore "east"]), the Asiatic cockroach that infests garbage dumps, seedy hotels, and unhygienic slaughterhouses throughout the world (normal length about 2.5 centimeters [one inch]), as well as the so-called American cockroach (*Periplaneta americana* L. [Greek *peri* ("around") + *planēs*, gen. *planētos* ("wanderer" or "vagabond")]), reddish-brown with well-developed wings (adults usually are 3.5 centimeters long [slightly less than 1.5 inches]). Frequently suspected of being disease vectors, cockroaches do carry pathogenic viruses, including that for poliomyelitis (Greek *polios* ["grey or "grizzled"] + *myelos* ["marrow"] + neo-Latin suffix *-itis* ["inflammation of"]), several protozoans, and bacteria troublesome to man (for example, *Escherichia* spp. [named after T. Escherich, a German physician (1857–1911) who described these anaerobic, rod-shaped bacteria often found in mammals' large intestines], *Staphylococcus* spp. [Greek *staphylē* ("bunch of grapes") + *kokkos* ("berry") or "grape")], and *Salmonella* spp. [named for Daniel E. Salmon (1850–1914), an American pathologist]). But medical entomologists generally believe that although cockroaches contribute to the spread of diseases, "mainly intestinal" (Service, *Medical Entomology,* 152), these insects are not primary vectors, especially since the illnesses engendered by cockroach-carried organisms are spread in many other easier ways. Yet cockroaches' feeding habits—and they eat anything organic, from fresh to fecal—include vomiting up of partially digested food onto their nutritional swill, causing a manure-like odor if the insects are numerous, so that keeping one's kitchen and dining areas free of them makes good sense. Still recommended for cockroach control is borax (medieval Latin *borax,* gen. *boracis* [from Persian *būrag,* in turn from Arabic *būraq* ("golden halter"), from its tincture produced in the manufacture of glass, porcelain, or enamel]) or boric acid powder, which occurs in nature as hydrated sodium borate and is a contact insecticide as well as a stomach poison.

Suborder *Mantodea* (Greek *mantis*, gen. *manteōs* ["prophet," "seer," or "a kind of grasshopper," here "praying mantis," as one reads in Theocritus, *Idylls,* X, 18] + *eidos* ["form," "shape," or "kind"]) are the famous praying mantids, and common names in many languages echo long-standing veneration or wonderment. In English, these insects are sometimes known as mule killers, rearhorses, and devil horses, as well as the expected praying flowers, preachers, and mendicants. In German, praying crickets (*Fangheuschrecken*) and god-worshippers (*Gottesanbeterinnen*) are traditional labels, and early settlers in Australia called mantids "the Hottentot's god," due to their importance in aboriginal mythologies. Mantids, like their cousins among the walkingsticks, are mostly tropical, and many of the eighteen hundred or so species occur in eastern Africa. Native to the United States is *Stagmomantis carolina* (L.) Johannsen (Greek *stagmos* or more commonly *stagma*, gen. *stagmatos* ["that which drips," that is, "perfume" or "aromatic oil"] + *mantis* + medieval Latin *Carolinus*—Latin *Carolus* ["Charles," in this instance Charles I of England (1625–49), for whom North and South Carolina are named]), a grayish-brown mantis that inhabits the American southern states north to New Jersey and west through southern Indiana and southern Utah and Arizona (average length of the female adult is six centimeters [about 2.25 inches]). Most familiar are two introduced species: *Mantis religiosa* L. (Greek *mantis* + Latin *religiosus* ["sacred" or "marked by awe"]), the so-called European mantis (common in southern Europe, northern Africa, India, China, and Japan), which arrived in America on nursery stock and was first recorded in New York State in 1899; and *Paratenodera sinensis* Saussure (Greek *para* ["beside" or "near"] + *tenōn*, gen. *tenontos* ["sinew" or "tendon"] + *deirē* or *derē* ["neck" or "collar"] + Byzantine Greek *sinai* ["the Chinese"]), the Chinese mantis first observed in Philadelphia in 1896. Both the European and the Chinese mantises are common in the eastern United States, and by far the largest is *P. sinensis*, which grows to eleven centimeters (about four inches long) and is distinctive with its bright-green or yellowish-green color. The pale-green European mantis reaches a length of five centimeters (two inches). The eminent Swiss entomologist Henry Louis Frederic de Saussure (1829–1905) was reminded of the sternocleidomastoid (see chap. 7 below ["Muscles"]) by the length and striated wings of the Chinese mantis.

About twelve hundred species are in the order *Dermaptera* (Greek *derma* ["skin"] + *pteron* ["wing"]), the earwigs, famed in folklore for crawling into the ears of sleepers to enter the brain. The vernacular *earwig* owes its origin to the shape of the insect's wings (when expanded), vaguely resembling a human ear, but the early-nineteenth-century coinage *Dermaptera* suggested the skinlike wing bases. Earwigs carry a distinctive double-pronged "tail," a pair of curved pincers markedly like curved shears (entomologists call the rear pincers of an earwig *forceps* [Latin *forceps*, gen. *forcipis* = *forfex*, gen. *forficis* ("tongs," "pincers," "shears," and "scissors"), with a special sense of *forceps* as a "claw" of a crab, so Pliny, *NH*, IX, 97]). Earwigs have nocturnal habits comparable to cockroaches, and in temperate regions earwigs can become serious pests in garbage dumps. In the wild, however, their favorite diet is fly maggots, so that they are beneficial—even as one observes their horrific cannibalism as they devour each other with startling ferocity. Species in the suborder *Arixenina* (Greek *Areios* [the Greek god of war, hence "warlike"] + *xenos* ["foreigner" or "stranger"]), first recorded in the Dutch East Indies (now Indonesia) in the early twentieth-century, frequently occur in huge numbers associated with bats in their caves: the insects swarm over the bat droppings, larvae feeding on the dung and each other, while adults devour smaller specimens, both adults and larvae. The common European earwig is *Forficula auricularia* L. (Latin *forfex,* as above, + *auris,* gen. *auris* ["ear"] and *auricula,* gen. *auriculae* ["external ear" or "earlobe," and as diminutive, "little ear"]), a cosmopolitan species attaining a length of fifteen millimeters (slightly more than .5 inch), normally shiny and brownish-black. Longer by ten millimeters is the Asian black earwig, *Chelisoches morio* Fabricius (Greek *clēlē* ["cloven hoof" but also "claw" of a crab, as in Aristotle, *HA,* 527b5] + *isos* ["equal"] + Latin *morio,* gen. *morionis* ["idiot" or "fool"]), common in Hawaii and California, where it feeds on sugarcane leafhoppers and similar insects. "Equal-clawed fool" suggests that Fabricius was thinking of the earwigs' self-destructive cannibalism.

A rare word in classical Latin is *tarmes,* gen. *tarmitis,* pl. *tarmites,* which meant "maggot" or "wood-eating worm," whereas the more common *termes,* gen. *termitis,* pl. *termites,* was the name of a specific kind of tree, most likely the wild olive (in a general sense, *termes* was "a bough of a tree"). Yet when Linnaeus invented a neo-Latin word for what are frequently known as "white ants" in temperate America, he returned to the literally correct Latin and Greek verbs (Latin *terrere,* derived from Greek *teirein,* both "to bore" or "to rub") to gain his term for these "maggots" that ate wood. Half a century earlier, English writers were employing *termes* to mean "maggot" or "a little worm, call'd a Death Watch" (in 1706, so *OED* s.v.), and by the end of the century, *termite* had entered the language as the name of these usually tropical insects so incredibly destructive of wooden dwellings. Even though termites do occur in southern Europe, Greek and Latin writers did not classify them as such, and the sole description of termites in classical literature is in Aelian's *Characteristics of Animals,* XVI, 15—and this is an accurate account of the termites and their raised hillock nests in India. Linnaeus's coinage did not stand up to further observations and studies of taxonomies by entomologists, so that by the late nineteenth century, the name *Isoptera* (Greek *isos* ["equal"] + *ptera* ["wings"]) became the accepted name for the order of social insects called termites. Not all of the two thousand or so species in Isoptera are capable of digesting *cellulose* (the mid-eighteenth-century coinage of the Latinate *cellularis* was taken as equivalent to *cellula* ["live cell"], in classical Latin literally "little room" + Latin's suffix *-osus* ["full of" or "abounding in"]), the inert carbohydrate making up the main portions of cell walls in wood, cotton, most plants, paper, and all wood products. But careful scrutiny of those species that do have cellulose-digesting protozoans in the rectal pouch illuminates the repeatedly observed process in nature called *symbiosis* (Greek meaning "living with," "companionship," sometimes "good fellowship" and even "club" or "society"): two very dissimilar organisms—here the insect and the protozoan—are essential for each other's survival. As one author puts it, "Termites by themselves cannot digest cellulose" (Howse, *Termites,* 17–18). Howse also emphasizes that other insects have this kind of symbiosis (an American cockroach, for example), and on reflection, one realizes how dependent even humans are upon the gut bacteria for proper digestion. About sixty species of termites live in North America; the workers and soldier termites are about .6 centimeters long (about .25 inch), and the queens reach lengths up to nine centimeters (3.5 inches). Once a colony is established, the queen can live fifteen years and produce a million eggs (there is, to be sure, a termite king, but he remains of minute size compared with his royal wife; entomologists call the queen and her king "reproductive castes," and they are the parents of *all* members of the colony).

Among smaller orders of insects are the *Zoraptera* (Greek *zōros* ["pure"] + *aptera* ["without wings"]), twenty-two species of tiny creatures normally three millimeters long (.125 inch), existing gregariously under tree bark and in rotting leaves throughout the tropics. The first species described in 1913 was wingless (and blind), and the nomenclature then suggested remains, although some species since narrated have wings that are sometimes shed in the manner of termites, which zorapterans resemble.

Order *Embioptera* (Greek *embios* ["lively"] + *pteron,* pl. *ptera* ["wing"]) are about three hundred species of tropical insects often called web spinners from their self-spun silken galleries and tunnels, in which they live in quasi-colonies (web spinners do not display the social interactions characteristic of termites, bees, ants, and wasps—true social insects). Web spinners are small (a large specimen is seven millimeters long [about .25 inch]) and feed on moss, lichens, bark, and dead grasses and leaves; some species reproduce by *parthenogenesis* (above in chap. 3 under phylum Gastrotrichia).

Order *Psocoptera* (Greek *psōchein* ["to powder" or "to rub small or fine"] + *pteron*) has about two thousand species of minute insects variously known as book lice, dust lice, bark lice, or simply psocids. The order formerly had the name *Corrodentia* (Latin *corrodere* ["to gnaw" or "to chew up"], with present participle *corrodens* ["gnawing" or "chewing up"]), describing what happened to books or museum specimens of birds, insects, and other mounted animals after these "powder-makers" finished their meal; they seek out dessicated organic matter including glue, paste, beeswax, fungi, and insects long dead. Psocids are very small (some species are five millimeters long [a little less than .25 inch]), but the cosmopolitan book louse or cereal psocid (*Liposcelis divinatorius* Müller [Greek *leipein* ("to lack") + *skelis*, gen. *skelidos* ("rib of beef" or "side of bacon") + Latin *divinatio*, gen. *divinationis* ("prophecy," but here a Late Latin adj. coined to mean "foretold")] is even smaller and at one millimeter is one of the smallest insects known. The Greco-Latinate name suggests a sense of humor: "a forecasted lack of a side of bacon" remains funny, recalling how these tiny insects infested old houses in the nineteenth century, feeding happily on the glues behind layers of wallpaper or, when they ventured forth, consuming slabs of ham or beef hanging in kitchens or cooking rooms. The vernacular parlance of "lice" for the psocids reflects their appearance, barely visible to the naked eye, much as Greek and Roman authors termed such as insect *sēs*, "a creature too small to be readily identified with any group of larger invertebrates . . . [even as they] attacked books and papers" (Beavis, *Insects*, 136–37).

About three thousand species are in the order *Mallophaga* (Greek *mallos* ["lock of wool"] + *phagein* ["to eat"]), the bird-fanciers' bane known as "bird lice." The German entomologist C. L. Nitzsch (1782–1837) coined this name in 1818 from observation that these minute insects (a big specimen will be ten millimeters long [about .4 inch]) feed on wool and hair. Most of the Mallophaga, however, live on birds, with fewer species infesting mammals, on which they can be as irritating as on their avian brethren. Bird lice live on feather fragments, epidermal flakings, and blood as available from wounds and lacerations. Ornithologists believe that when birds roll in dry dirt or take "dust baths," they are attempting to remove these parasites, which can occur in large numbers on both wild and domestic fowl. Chicken farmers know too well the cosmopolitan chicken or hen louse, a very small (one millimeter [about .04 inch]) pale-yellow insect, which received from Linnaeus the curiously appropriate name *Menopon gallinae* (Greek *menein* ["to lodge" or "to remain"] + *ponos* ["work" or "toil"] + Latin *gallina*, gen. *gallinae* ["hen"]), although Nitzsch's alternative *Menopon pallidum* (Latin *pallidus* ["pale," "wan," or "colorless"]) sometimes appears in modern accounts of bird lice. Heavy numbers of *M. gallinae* L. reduce egg production, so that chicken farmers usually dust their birds with sodium fluoride every ten days or so. Many species of Mallophaga are specific to their hosts (pigeons, turkeys, ducks, flamingoes, guinea pigs, storks, pigs, kangaroos, cats, dogs, horses, goats, and peacocks, as examples). On the death of a host, the Mallophaga populations usually perish after a few hours, suggesting a very recent evolution (there are no known fossil species).

Smaller in number but of enormous importance in human history are the three hundred species in the order *Anoplura* (Greek *anoplos* ["without a shield," thus "unarmed"] + *oura* ["tail"], thus "naked tail," so named from the absence of a tail), sometimes labeled *Siphunculata* (Latin *siphunculus* ["a small tube through which water is forced"], a rare word in classical Latin but used by Pliny the Younger, *Letters*, V, 6.23, 36, to indicate the "jets" of a fountain). The Anoplura are the sucking lice, true bloodsuckers of mammals, causing untold misery and death from frantic itching and as vectors of various human diseases, including *typhus* (Greek *typhos* ["fever" of four kinds, one accompanied by stupor]). Species of Anoplura are host-specific as ectoparasites on most mammals, including humans and domesticated animals; entomologists have classified sucking lice peculiar to rabbits, seals, elephants, mice, etc.). Humankind has the distinction of having two species, each living particularly on one of the two heavily haired parts of our bodies: the common head louse is *Pediculus humanus* L. (Latin *pediculus* ["louse" but literally "little foot"] + *humanus* ["human being"]), which inhabits the hair on the human head; and the crab louse, *Phthirus pubis* L. (Greek *phtheir*, gen. *phtheiros* ["louse" of animals and plants] + Latin *pubes*, gen. *pubis* ["pubic hair," as technical meaning in Celsus, VII, 19.1; generally "genitals" or "age of puberty" and most commonly "adult population"]), which lives in the stiff hairs of the groin (as well as the equally stiff hairs of beards and mustaches). Subspecies appear in the literature of medical entomology, and one reads of a "body louse" with the label *Pediculus humanus* var. *corporis* (Latin *corpus*, gen. *corporis*, nom. pl. *corpora* ["body"]) and a "head louse" called *P. humanus* var. *capitis* (Latin *caput*, gen. *capitis* ["head"]), as set forth in Busvine, "*Pediculus humanus* L." Busvine summarizes some of his research in his *Insects, Hygiene, and History*, where he notes, "Body lice were obtained from naturally infested tramps, who assisted us in our researches for a small financial reward" (43). Whatever these small ectoparasites are called (the crab louse averages about two millimeters in length and width [about .08 inch], and the head louse or body louse is one millimeter wide and four millimeters long [about .2 inch]), they rank among the insects next to honeybees and silkworms in their influence on human beings since the beginnings of our species.

In conditions of continuous filth (as in war, when troops wear the same clothing for days on end), human lice multiply first, causing severe itching and *eczema* (Greek *ekzema,* gen. *ekzematos* ["cutaneous eruption," in Dioscorides (Wellmann, ed.), I, 43; the technical term in the Greek of the first century A.D. was derived from *ekzesis,* gen. *ekzeseōs,* which meant "a boiling out" or "boiling over" and thus—in medical matters—a "breaking out" of sores]), which physicians often label *pediculosis* (from the Linnaean name for the genus). Soap and hot water remove adult lice from the hair, but not the eggs (termed "nits"), and insecticidal cleansers are necessary for total elimination of the parasites. Sometimes a very fine toothed comb must be used to remove the eggs, which are "oval and white, and have distinct opercula," with small holes giving the nits "the appearance of minuscule pepper pots" (Service, *Medical Entomology,* 138). Sometimes simply shaving off the hair is the best treatment (followed by a hot, soapy shower), depending on conditions. *Pediculus* spp. are transmitters of epidemic typhus and the feared wartime trench fever; causative organisms are *rickettsiae,* sing. *rickettsia* (the Latinized name from Howard T. Ricketts [1871–1910], an American pathologist), with the genus *Rickettsia* comprising species of microorganisms that resemble rod-shaped or round bacteria but that behave like viruses and are as small as a large virus, reproducing only inside a living cell. Before the advent of vaccines and modern antibiotics, fatality rates could reach 60 percent of adult populations, and Hans Zinsser (1878–1940) suggested that even in the early twentieth century, three million deaths occurred between 1917 and 1923 in eastern Europe from louse-transmitted typhus (Zinsser's comments carry weighty authority, since he was a central figure in the development of the typhus vaccine; his sprightly *Rats, Lice and History* remains a model account among histories of epidemiology).

There are five thousand species of *Thysanoptera* (Greek *thysanos* ["fringe" or "tassel"] + *pteron*), commonly called "thrips" (the Greek *thrips,* gen. *thripos* ["wood-boring worm," in Theophrastus, *HP,* V, 4.4] is "the most usual Greek term for the smaller timber pests" [Beavis, *Insects,* 181]) from their knack of poking holes in and sucking sap from the leaves and stems of various plants. Some species are serious pests on onions, citrus fruit leaves, cotton, and certain grains, so that there is a large literature on their control. Thysanoptera are rather small insects, ranging from the .9-millimeter-long "very small thrip" (thus *Thrips minutissima* L., of about .02 inch) to the giant thrips of Australia, which attain lengths of fourteen millimeters (a little more than .5 inch). First introduced into the nomenclature in 1836, *Thysanoptera* as a name suggested the odd fringe-edged four wings of these insects, which sometimes swarmed in large numbers and appeared to "suck" on human beings (in dry weather, sweaty laborers were "bitten" by swarming thrips that sought moisture, not blood).

Even more damaging are the sucking and piercing mouthparts of the thirty-five thousand species in the order *Hemiptera* (Greek *hēmi* ["half"] + *pteron*), the only insects entomologists call "bugs." Linnaeus's 1758 label encapsulated the structure of wings particular to these insects: the anterior pair of four wings displays a hardened basal ⅔, with the apical ⅓ membranous (*anterior* is Renaissance Latin's comparative form of *ante* ["before"] and here would mean "toward the head"; *apical* here describes the "outer edge" or "outer surface" and derives from the Latin *apex*, gen. *apicis* ["summit"], with nom. pl. *apices* [usually *apex* in modern English means "tip" or "point," with "summit" and "peak" as occasional connotations]). Bugs are very familiar, since this order includes stinkbugs and shield bugs (large numbers of species grouped in the families *Pentatomidae* [Greek *pente* ("five") + *tomos* ("cut" or "slice"), a name indicating five-segmented antennae] and *Scutelleridae* [Latin *scutum* ("shield")]), squash bugs and the curious leaf-footed bugs (Family *Coreidae* [Greek *koris,* gen. *koreōs*—but Byzantine Greek gen. *koridos* ("bug," particularly "bedbug")]), grass bugs and box-elder bugs (Family *Corizidae* [Byzantine Greek *korizein* ("to be infested with bedbugs")]), seed bugs and chinch bugs (Family *Lygaeidae* [Greek *lygaios* ("gloomy" or "murky")]), assassin bugs or kissing bugs (Family *Reduviidae* [Latin *reduvia*, gen. *reduviae* ("hangnail," in Pliny, *NH*, XXX, 111)]), the child-delighting water striders, back swimmers, and water boatmen (respectively in the families *Gerridae* [Latin *gerres*, gen. *gerris* ("a little worthless fish," according to Pliny, *NH*, XXXII, 148) and Latin's *gerres* = Greek's *mainē* ("a sprat")—see Thompson, *Fishes,* 155], *Notonectidae* [Greek *nōton* or *nōtos* ("back") + *nēktēs* ("swimmer")], and *Corixidae* [a nineteenth-century Latinization of the Greek *koris* ("bug") into *corisa* and thence into *corixa*]). The giant water bug or toe-biters of the American South and West are in the family *Belastomatidae* (Greek *belos,* gen. *beleos* ["arrow" or "dart"] + *stoma,* gen. *stomatos* ["mouth"]—a name given by the English entomologist W. E. Leach [1790–1836] in 1815 to suggest the nasty-looking mouthparts), and the infamous bedbugs are about forty species grouped into four or five genera in the family *Cimicidae* (Latin *cimex,* gen. *cimicis* [the "bedbug"]).

Entomologists often divide the Hemiptera into two suborders: the *Heteroptera* (Greek *heteros* ["other" or "different"] + *pteron*), a name supplied by Latreille in 1810 to indicate distinctive variations between structures in the fore wings and hind wings and including shield bugs, squash bugs, assassin bugs, bedbugs, and the rest as immediately above; and the *Homoptera* (Greek *homos* ["one and the same" or "common"] + *pteron*), a large suborder of several thousand species that incorporates "bugs" as varied in size and habits as the large cicadas, the smaller leafhoppers and aphids (often called plant lice), and the numerous scale insects. Whether one knows cicadas by sight, everyone living in temperate North America has heard them in their loud choruses of shrill, rasping mating calls (the males) beginning on hot, sunny days of late spring and continuing through much of the summer. *Cicada* is the classical Latin word for one of the smaller European species that sang in summertime to the Romans, sometimes irritating sensitive poetic ears with the stridently loud and hoarse hot-weather racket (our word "raucous" descends directly from the Latin adjective *raucus* ["harsh," "strident," or "hoarse-sounding"], and Vergil, *Eclogues,* II, 12–13, complains *raucis . . . arbusta resonant cicadis* ["the trees ring with the strident cicadas"]). Occasionally Americans call these insects locusts (which they are not) or harvest flies (which they do not resemble), but the common "dog-day cicada" is one of the species in the genus *Tibicen* (Latin *tibicen,* gen. *tibicinis* ["one who plays a reed pipe, a *tibia*"]), a large black-and-green insect that grows (as an adult) to a length of fifty millimeters (about two inches long). Famous are the "periodical cicadas," especially the "seventeen-year locust" (*Magicicada septendecim* L. [Greek *magos* ("a wizard" or "magician") + Latin *cicada* + *septem* ("seven") + *decem* ("ten")]), which emerges as a nymph from the soil after thirteen to seventeen years of subterranean life feeding on the roots of plants. The nymph shortly becomes an adult, shedding its old "skin" almost intact, and the nymphal casts occur very commonly in June and July to fascinate children and to excite wonderment over how the small slit in the top of the thorax allows the fully grown cicada to escape.

Order *Neuroptera* (Greek *neuron* [here meaning "nerve"] + *pteron*) consists of about four thousand species, including the flutteringly beautiful, emerald-green lacewing (genus *Chrysopa* [Greek *chrysos* ("golden") + *ōps*, gen. *ōpos* ("eye")—so named in 1866 for the gold hue in the eyes of the adults by the German-American entomologist Hermann August Hagen (1817–93)]); lacewings feed on aphids, so their common presence reassures gardeners, especially those who raise flowers. Neuroptera as an order usually has several suborders: *Megaloptera* (Greek *megas*, gen. *megalou* ["big" or "large"] + *pteron*; in later Greek, the term *megalopterygos* ["with great wings"] appears but does not apply to creatures in nature) includes the large dobsonflies (genus *Corydalus* [Greek *korydalos*, a "crested lark" in Thompson, *Birds*, 164–68]), whose ten-centimeter (four-inch) length and wicked-looking three-centimeter (1.5-inch) mandibles (in the adult male) engender respect from beginning naturalists who see them near lakes and streams in the northern United States (dobsonflies are quite harmless, and the large larvae—called hellgrammites or conniption bugs—are avidly collected as bait by experienced fishermen, who know how bass and trout favor these formidable-appearing creatures as food): the snake flies or serpent flies are species in *Raphidiodea* (Greek *raphis*, gen. *raphidos* ["needle"]) represented by seventeen North American species, and the name provided by Linnaeus in 1758 called attention to the long, needlelike ovipositor of the female (snake flies raise their heads above the body level, similar to the manner of a snake making ready to strike; specimens I observed on the western slopes of Colorado were a little more than three centimeters long (about 1.25 inches), with polished "necks." *Planipennia* (Latin *planus* ["flat," "level," or "even"] + *penna* ["wing"]), in addition to the lacewings, includes the renowned ant lions or doodlebugs (Family *Myrmeleontidae* [Greek *myrmēx*, gen. *myrmēkos* ("ant") + *leōn*, gen. *leontos* ("lion")]), with species in the genus *Myrmeleon* (as weird larvae, equipped with long sicklelike jaws) fashioning those five-centimeter-wide cone-shaped pits in sand, which trap wandering ants by the dozens (once over the edge, the hapless ant simply slides down into the waiting jaws at the bottom of the pit). Adult ant lions resemble damsel flies (above under *Odonata*) but are far weaker fliers: whereas damselflies dart about, as do their cousins among the dragonflies, ant lions feebly flutter.

The most successful life-forms on earth are the beetles, grouped in the order *Coleoptera* (Greek *koleon* ["sheath"] + *pteron*). Among the 330,000 species (Imms, *General Textbook*, 10th ed., Vol. II, 816) of beetles presently catalogued by coleopterists are animals as large as a human hand (the Amazonian *Titanus giganteus* L. [Greek *Titan*, gen. *Titanos* (in Greek mythology, one of the offspring of Uranus and Gaea, who waged war against Zeus) + *giganteios* ("monstrous")], which can reach twenty centimeters in length [slightly less than eight inches]) and those so small as to be barely visible to the naked eye (the American feather-wing beetle in the genus *Nanosella* [Greek *nanos* ("dwarf") + Latin *sella* ("seat," "chair," or "stool")], is .25 millimeters long [roughly .01 inch]). The Brazilian *Titanus* is eight hundred times larger than its tiny American relative among the feather-wing beetles, yet the basic morphology and the structure mark them both as members of the Coleoptera. Beetles almost always have four wings, but the anterior pair are thickened to form two half-sheaths (hence the name of the order), which protect the posterior pair of wings, functioning as coverings usually meeting as a straight line down the back of the insect. These thickened or brittle wing-covers bear the name *elytra* (sing. *elytron* [Greek *elytron* normally meant "covering," but special meanings included a "case for a mirror," a "sheath for a spear," and a "case" or "jacket-cover" for one's bow or shield, as well as technical meanings among physicians and naturalists: *elytron* was the "sheath of the spinal cord" to the author of the Hippocratic *Joints,* XLV, 13, and Aristotle's *elytron* in *HA,* 532a23–24 is a "sheath" or "covering for the wings of a flying insect," almost exactly the adaptation of meaning for modern coleopterists]). The *elytra* of beetles are usually hard and brittle, sometimes leathery, and sometimes reduced in size from a full armor-coating for the second pair of membranous wings, neatly folded until flight is necessary.

When one of the larger beetles takes wing, the muted roar signals the relatively low frequency of wingbeat, but the largest American beetles in the genus *Dynastes* (Greek *dynastēs* ["ruler" or "lord and master"—so named for a "regal" appearance]) or unicorn beetles (six centimeters [about 2.5 inches] long) can fly rapidly enough to avoid slow-moving human collectors, especially those startled by a sudden and noisy takeoff. Familiar, to be sure, are the loud and raspy, low-pitched buzzings produced on summer screens and around outdoor lamps and streetlights by the overly common May beetles or June bugs in the genus *Phyllophaga* (Greek *phyllon* ["leaf"] + *phagein* ["to eat"]), some two hundred species in the United States east of the Mississippi, all about 2.5 centimeters (1 inch) long as adults and almost all colored coppery to dark brown. And growers of fine roses gnash their teeth when a hum comes from their rose beds in late July or early August anywhere in the eastern United States: that muted hum means swarming Japanese beetles in the genus *Popillia* (Latin *Popillius,* adj. of *Popilius,* the name of a Roman *gens* or clan or family). The nomenclator,

E. Newman, who provided *Popillia japonica* as the name for the most common Japanese beetle (accidentally introduced into New Jersey in 1916 on nursery stock from Japan), recalled from Roman history how the Popilian *gens* represented reactionary politics in the Late Roman Republic, with Caius Popilius Laenus murdering Cicero in 43 B.C. and with Publius Popilius Laenus, as consul in 132 B.C., persecuting the followers of the murdered Tiberius Gracchus. *Japonica* is a modern Latinization for "Japanese," so that the nomenclature for this widespread pest means "Japanese murder." Japanese beetles are in the subfamily *Rutelinae* (Latin *rutilus* ["glowingly orange or red" or "golden"]), the shining leaf chafers often yellow-brown, refulgent gold—and in the instance of the Japanese beetle, a beautiful metallic green bordering a burnished brown-gold pair of elytra. Among American native species in Rutelinae is the beautiful gold-and-black grape beetle (*Pelidnota punctata* L. [Greek *pelidnotēs*, gen. *pelidnētos* ("bloody extravasation" or something "ashen" or "livid") + neo-Latin *puncta* ("dot"), from Latin *pungere*, participle *punctum* ("to mark with small dots or spots)— Linnaeus must have received a mottled, gray-gold specimen]), as an adult reaching three centimeters (about 1.25 inches) long, easily recognized from the three black spots on each elytron; grape beetles are destructive pests on young grape leaves.

Among the beetles are some of the most striking animals in nature, and the antlerlike mandibles of the globally distributed stag beetles have excited wonder and interest since antiquity. Protected by law in much of Europe is *Lucanus cervus* L. (Latin *Lucanus* [usually "a native of Lucania" in southwestern Italy] + *cervus* ["stag" or "deer"]), which is a dark mahogany and reaches—the adult male—7.5 centimeters (2.75 inches) in length inclusive of the pincers (the female's mandibles are small by comparison, and she measures 4.5 centimeters [1.75 inches]). Male Asian stag beetles in the genus *Odontolabia* (Greek *odous*, gen. *odontos* ["tooth"] + *labis*, gen. *labidos* ["forceps" or "tongs"]), resplendent in their ambered-yellow-and-black elytra, grow to ten centimeters (four inches), the toothed-mandible of the generic name alone reaching 3.5 centimeters (about 1.25 inches). And the western slope Andean jawed stag beetle of Chile in the genus *Chiasognathus* (Greek *chiazein* ["to mark with the letter chi," that is, X] + *gnathos* ["jaw"]—thus the Latinate is "cross-jawed"), a refulgent insect with tawny elytra, has (in the male) a pair of inner-toothed, tonglike mandibles that are more than half the length of its eight centimeter (3.25 inches). American stag beetles are somewhat smaller: *Lucanus elephas* Fabricius is commonly six centimeters (about 2.5

inches) long in a muffled shiny dark brown (Latin *Lucanus,* as above, + Greek *elephos* ["stag" or "deer"]); *Pseudolucanus capreolus* L. normally is dark brown to blackish, and the males are four centimeters (1.5 inches) long (Greek *pseudēs* ["false" or "deceptive"] + Latin *Lucanus,* as above, + *capreolus* [a "weeding fork" as one reads in Columella, *Agriculture,* XI, 3.46]). Linnaeus's command of Latin enabled him to use *capreolus* as a "weeding fork" for this American species, even though the most common meaning of the word was "young of a European roe deer," and clearly his nomenclature could not be confused with *capra* ["goat"]. Even as small as our species are, they are frequently termed "pinching bugs" from the sharp "bite" administered to one's fingers when the insect assumes his head-elevated battle position.

Related to the Lucanidae (the family name for stag beetles, worldwide) are the equally famous members of the Family *Scarabaeidae* (Latin *scarabaeus* ["beetle" or "dung beetle"], cognative with Greek *karabos* ["horned beetle"]), with the Egyptian scarab (*Scarabaeus sacer* L. [*sacer* is Latin for "holy" or "sacred"]) a repeatedly essential sign in ancient Egyptian art and hieroglyphics (Greek *hieros* ["sacred" or "priestly"] + *glyphein* ["to carve"]). About fifty thousand species of scarab beetles occur around the world, including the June bugs, Japanese beetles, grape beetles, unicorn beetles, and several hundred other subfamilies. In the United States, dung-roller beetles (the American version of the Egyptian scarabs) often carry the common name of tumblebugs, and entomologists class them as subfamily *Coprinae* (Greek *koprinos* ["full of dung" or "filthy"]): large species are 2.5 centimeters (one inch) long, dull black with parallel striations running along the elytra. Tumblebugs provide a fascinating show as they work in pairs, chewing off a chunk of pasture manure and then slowly manipulating the dung into a ball, which they roll (with their hind legs) to a location some distance away; the adults quickly bury the manure ball, the female lays her eggs in it, and the emerging beetle larvae have a ready-made food supply.

Order *Siphonaptera* (Greek *siphōn* ["tube"] + *aptera* ["without wings"]) are fourteen hundred species of fleas, bloodsucking and wingless insects, whose jumping abilities border on the fantastic: "A flea jumping several inches up in the air would be comparable to a man jumping over a 30-story building" (Borror, Triplehorn, and Johnson, *Study of Insects,* 4). Along with sucking lice, cockroaches, and bedbugs, fleas in history are some of the most familiar—one could say intimate—animals to human beings, in spite of their small size (large fleas can grow to a length of five millimeters [.2 inch]), and have caused annoyance and transmitted death to humans and animals since prehistoric times. Fleas infest wild and domestic animals, and the cute scratchings of rabbits or squirrels with forepaws worrying their ears suggest the usual hundreds of fleas feeding on each creature. Hog farmers know too well how fleas can multiply where their porcine charges rest, and occasional counts of neglected hogpens indicate five hundred thousand fleas in each. Poultry have their own genus of fleas (*Echidnophaga* spp. [Greek *echidna* (usually "snake" or "viper" but also in classical Greek "treacherous friend") + *phagein* ("to eat"]) known simply enough as sticktight fleas or tropical hen fleas. The human flea is *Pulex irritans* L. (Latin *pulex,* gen. *pulicis* ["flea"] + *irritare* ["to provoke" or "to enrage"] with present participle *irritans* ["provoking" or "enraging"]), not necessarily specific to humans but also taking blood meals from hogs, poultry, dogs, rats, skunks, and a number of other animals.

Fleas are carriers of the dreaded bubonic plague or Black Death, transmitted usually from rat to human by the tropical rat flea, *Xenopsylla chepis* Rothschild (Greek *xenos* ["foreigner" or "stranger"] + *Cheops,* gen. *Cheopis* [the Greek name for Khufu, an Egyptian pharaoh of the Fourth Dynasty who built the Great Pyramid at Gizeh (about 2575 B.C.), as one reads in the famous account of Herodotus, *Histories,* II, 124–27]). Still endemic in rodent populations in various parts of the world—including the western United States—plague is caused by the bacillus *Pasteurella pestis* = *Yersinia pestis* (a Latinization of Louis Pasteur [1822–95], the famous French chemist and founder of modern microbiology, often called the author of the germ theory of disease + Latin *pestis,* gen. *pestis* ["plague" or "pestilence"]; and a Latinization of A. E. J. Yersin [1863–1943], the Swiss bacteriologist who discovered the plague bacillus in 1894 "at the beginning of the extensive pandemic of the disease which developed in Hong Kong in that year" [Faust and Russell, *Paristology,* 921]). Mortality before modern antibiotics was about sixty percent, and the terror provoked by bubonic plague in Justinian's Byzantium in A.D. 542 is vividly recounted by Procopius, *History of the Wars,* II, 22–24.

Although ancient medicine did not recognize the flea as a vector for the transmission of plague, Greco-Roman physicians clearly understood the diagnostic sign of the swollen lymph nodes in the groin (Greek *boubōn,* gen. *boubōnos* ["groin"] but pl. *boubōnes* ["glands" especially "swollen glands" as one reads in the Hippocratic *Aphorisms,* IV, 55, and—punningly—"swollen testicles" frequently in Attic comedy, commented on by Henderson, *Maculate Muse,* 125]), from which this killer pestilence has received its modern name. Enlarged lymph nodes (termed *buboes* in modern medicine) of the femoral and inguinal zones (the groin) appear among half the victims of the plague, followed by lesser incidences of swollen nodes in the axilla or armpit (about 22 percent), the neck (roughly 10 percent), and generalized nodal enlargement 14 percent), a modern clinical description paralleled by Procopius's account: "A *boubōn* swelling appeared, not only in that part of the body termed the groin, but also within the armpit, and sometimes alongside the ears as well as on the upper thighs" (*History of the Wars,* II, 22.17). And in the medical Greek of the Roman Empire occurs the term *boubōnokēlē* ("inguinal hernia"), one of the most common afflictions of middle-aged males in any century, corrected with a *boubōnophylax* ("truss for an inguinal hernia"), the treatment of choice before antiseptic abdominal surgery (accompanied with reliable anesthetics) in the twentieth century. Likewise, the plague bacillus has yielded in the twentieth century to antibiotics, and if quickly diagnosed and treated, bubonic plague victims have mortality rates of less than 5 percent.

About seventy-five thousand species make up the order *Diptera* (Greek *dis* ["twice"] + *pteron,* thus "two-winged"), the flies, gnats, midges, and mosquitoes. Sizes among the Diptera range greatly, from the gigantic Chinese crane fly, with its name *Tipula brobdignagia* (Latin *tippula* ["an aquatic insect," most likely the "water boatman"] + Latinized Brobdingnagian ["huge" or "enormous"], derived from the region in Jonathan Swift's *Gulliver's Travels,* where everything was of enormous size) given by the English entomologist J. O. Westwood (1805–93)—a fly that attains a wingspread of ten centimeters (four inches)—to the minute California insect often called a no-see-um in the genus *Leptoconops* (Greek *leptos* ["slender" or "small"] + *kōnōps,* gen. *kōnōpos* ["gnat" or "mosquito"]), which as a full-grown adult reaches a length of two millimeters (about .07 inch). Within the Diptera are efficient predators on other insects, and among the deliciously skilled robber flies is the Australian giant in the genus *Phellus* (Greek *phellos* ["cork"]), which is five centimeters (two inches) long with a wingspread of nine centimeters (3.5 inches). The larval forms of most species in Diptera are known as maggots, and anyone who has observed flies swarming around freshly dead animals will also recall how, within a few days, the carrion writhes with countless maggots as they feed in seeming waves on the rotting flesh. In nature, this garbage collection is essential, but the presence of organic waste upon which fly maggots feast also signals the presence of billions of bacteria, many of which engender disease in humans and animals. And yet paradoxically, the careful application of certain species of maggots to torn and festering wounds of soldiers on the Western Front in World War I allowed these terrible injuries to heal cleanly: maggots will eat only dead cells, carefully sealing off and avoiding those neighboring tissues that remain alive.

A *culex,* gen. *culicis,* to the Romans was a "gnat" or "midge," and the Latin survives as *Culicidae,* the family of Diptera that are the infamous mosquitoes. Only the females are bloodsuckers, but their enormous numbers in the tropics and in more temperate zones provide a common transmission of protozoan and viral diseases to humans. Malaria (see chap. 3, above) is given to humans by the mechanical transmission of *Plasmodium* spp. (chap. 3, above), parasitic protozoans that attack human red blood cells—*Plasmodium* passes part of its multistaged life cycle only in mosquitoes in genus *Anopheles* (Greek *anōphelēs* ["useless" or "harmful"]), and various species among the hundreds in *Anopheles* carry the classic "tertian fever" and "quartan fever" known since Greek antiquity. Species in the genus *Aedes* (Greek *aēdēs* ["disagreeable"]) transmit the virus of yellow fever to humans, and the same genus carries the virus of dengue fever as well as the phasmid nematode (above, chap. 3), which causes filariasis, commonly seen in the tropics in men with enormously swollen testicles.

Added to human and animal misery are afflictions carried by a number of genera in Diptera other than mosquitoes: Family *Tabanidae* (Latin *tabanus* ["gadfly" or "biting fly"]) includes the nasty deerflies (genus *Chrysops* [Greek *chrysos* ("golden") + *ōps,* gen. *ōpos* ("eye")]), implicated in the dissemination of *tularemia* (named after Tulare County, California, where the disease was first recognized) from wild animals to humans, and West African species in *Chrysops* carry the phasmid nematode *Loa loa* (*loa* is a native West African name for this "eye worm") from human to human (humans are the only host). Genus *Tabanus* (horseflies) has species that are vectors from animals to humans of *anthrax* (Greek *anthrax,* gen. *anthrakos* [usually "charcoal" but also "coal" as in Theophrastus, *On Stones,* 16, and also as in Aristotle, *Meteorlogica,* 387b18, a "precious stone colored dark red" (ruby, garnet, etc.)], allowing analogy in medical writing for "carbuncle" or "malignant pustule"), and *Tabanus* species in Central and South America, North Africa, the Middle East, and Asia fatally infect camels, horses, and dogs with protozoans in the genus *Trypanosoma* (Greek *trypanon* ["borer" or "auger"—a carpenter's tool, rotated by a thong, thus in Greco-Roman bone surgery, a "trepan" to bore holes in bone, particularly the skull] + *sōma,* gen. *sōmatos* ["body"]), engendering the disease known to veterinarians as *surra* (*sūra* is the Indic Marathi word for "wheezing"). Tsetse flies (*tsētsē* is Tswana for "fly") in the genus *Glossina* (Greek *glōssa* ["tongue"], suggesting the prominent feeding proboscis) transmit to humans the trypanosomes of the dreaded "sleeping sickness" of Central Africa, in which "in the absence of treatment, death is inevitable. . . . The population of [some] districts of Uganda, originally about 300,000, was reduced in six years to 100,000 by sleeping sickness early in this century" (Wilcocks and Hanson-Behr Manson, *Tropical Diseases,* 99). Fortunately, if diagnosed early African trypanosomiasis can be treated successfully with the antiviral drug suramin (from *sūra,* as above), and administration of pentamidine before one enters the "tsetse belt" of Central Africa confers limited immunity (about six months), but all antitrypanosomal drugs carry the risk of kidney damage. And one cannot leave the Diptera without mention of the family *Tephritidae* (Greek *tephrē* ["ash" or "ashes"], with adj. *tephroeidēs* ["like ashes" or "ash-colored"]), which embraces a number of genera among the "fruit flies," including agricultural worries like the apple maggot (genus *Rhagoletis* [Greek *rhax,* gen. *rhagos* ("grape" or "berry") and common adj. *rhagos* ("ruptured") + Latin *letum,* gen. *leti* ("death"), here in the modern form with ablative plural]), and the Mediterranean fruit fly (genus *Ceratitis* [Greek *keratitis,* gen. *keratidos* ("horned")]), so devastating to citrus crops in California.

Although not as numerous as the beetles, there are about 150,000 species among the very familiar butterflies and moths in the order *Lepidoptera* (Greek *lepis,* gen. *lepidos* ["small, skin-like fragment" in Hippocratic *Aphorisms,* IV, 81] + *pteron,* pl. *ptera*), some of the most beautiful creatures known. Lepidopterans undergo complete metamorphosis, and the larval stages (commonly called caterpillars) often occur in huge numbers, frequently becoming pests on both wild and cultivated plants ("phytophagous" is the fancy term) throughout the world. Many caterpillars are decidedly *not* beautiful, since they are clothed with spines, spikes, and occasionally brilliant colors to deter predators. Linnaeus's 1758 name for these insects reflected how one's fingers became covered with "dust" whenever butterflies and moths were handled, and under a magnifying glass the "dust" was revealed as thousands of tiny "scales," somewhat analogous to the scales of fish. Linnaeus thereby chose only one of the meanings available from classical Greek (*lepis* is collectively "fish scales" in Aristotle, *HA,* 486b21, and Herodotus, *Histories,* VII, 61, but "snake scales" in Nicander, *Theriaca,* 154), which include "onion skin," "flakes" of copper flying off in hammering (in Dioscorides, V, 78), and "flakes" of snow, as one reads in Theophrastus, *HP,* IV, 14.13. Externally, a quick observation of antennae indicates a moth or butterfly: moths generally carry fanlike or plumed antennae, whereas the antennae of most butterflies are slender.

Among the moths are a great number of destructive species, with the larvae damaging trees and crops often to the point of killing them. The larvae of the common European goat moth, *Cossus cossus* L. (Latin *cossus* or *cossis,* gen. *cossis,* nom. pl. *cosses* ["a worm or grub found in wood," in Pliny, *NH,* XI, 113]), attacks and bores large tunnels into many deciduous trees (alder, ash, birch, beech, elm, linden, maple, oak—among many), weakening these trees to other diseases. And the cosmopolitan carpenter worms in the genus *Prionoxystus* (Greek *priōn,* gen. *prionos* ["saw"] + *xystos* ["shaved," "whittled," "scraped," and similar meanings]) sometimes occur in such numbers that their galleries kill their hosts among North American fruit trees and other broad-leafed deciduous species. Some genera of moth larvae produce nettlelike irritation or urtication (Latin *urtica* usually meant "stinging nettle") of human skin, characterized by wheals or itchy rashes when these spine-laden caterpillars are touched; most familiar in the United States is the green-and-brown saddleback caterpillar in the genus *Sibine* (Greek *sibynē* ["hunting spear"]), slowly wiggling along the trunks and limbs of trees in the summer (saddlebacks are about 2.5 centimeters [one inch] long). The moths include the famous silkworm of China, named *Bombyx mori* by Linnaeus (Greek *bombyx* ["silkworm"] + Latin *morus,* gen. *mori* ["the black mulberry," which now bears the Linnaean label *Morus nigra*]), perhaps next to the honeybees the most important and beneficial insect in human history. Silk from the cocoons of *Bombyx* remains unmatched among elegant clothing anywhere. Related species, like the gorgeous and enormous American cecropia moth in the genus *Hyalophora* (Greek *hyalinos* ["shining"] + *phoros* ["carrying" or "bearing"]) have silk that is difficult to reel, so that the common moths cannot replace the Chinese *Bombyx,* whose silk is easily reeled. Once observed in the wild, the cecropia moth is unforgettable: mating adults have a wingspan of about fifteen centimeters (six inches), with wings of red-brown crossed outwardly by thin bands of white and centered in each of the four wings a white crescent brilliantly bordered in red. It is little wonder that beginning entomologists gasp in awe at cecropia moths, much as they might write poems to the gossamer beauty of another related species, the justly renowned, light emerald-green, long-tailed luna moth, *Actias luna* L. (Greek *aktaia,* gen. *aktaias* ["Persian royal robe"] + Latin *luna* ["moon"]), which can attain a wingspread of twenty centimeters (close to eight inches).

One of the loveliest sights in flower gardens is the rainbowed fluttering of our larger butterflies, seeking their nectar meals as they carry pollen from flower to flower in their essential role (along with bees and some flies) of cross-pollination. The familiar monarch or milkweed butterflies, orange-brown with bordered wings in black in turn spotted brilliant white, have amazing migration patterns; birds avoid them (the orange-and-black wings are distinctive "I'm inedible" signals) since monarch larvae feed on milkweeds as well as many species of nightshades, rendering both caterpillar and adult literally poisonous. Linnaeus named the monarch *Danaus plexippus* (Greek *Danaos* [a mythical king of Argos] + *plēxippos* ["striking" or "driving horses"—an epithet for certain heroes in Homer's *Iliad*]), perhaps an example of Linnaeus's "occasionally careless mythology" (Heller, *Linnaean Method,* 30 n. 60), and lepidopterists have proposed numerous synonyms to replace Linnaeus's odd coinage, but *Danaus* still appears as the genus in most butterfly guides. Familiar too are the magnificent zebra swallowtails in the genus *Eurydites* (Greek *euryedēs* ["spacious" or "broadseated"]) or *Papilio* (Latin for "butterfly"), which can have a wingspan of twelve centimeters (4.5 inches). Colors among North American butterflies range from brilliant emerald-greens through purples, oranges, reds, gradations of golds and yellows defying any artist's palette, blues of varying shades, and all possible tones of brown, gray, white, and black. So colorful are some tropical butterflies that some species face extinction from overzealous collectors of mounted specimens of these gorgeous animals: colors of the "scales" do not fade much, even after the death of the butterfly.

There are over 130,000 species in the order *Hymenoptera* (Greek *hymēn,* gen. *hymenos* ["thin skin" or "membrane"—especially that covering the brain and heart, as in Aristotle, *HA,* 494a29, or (among alternative meanings) "wing of an insect," as also used by Aristotle, *PA,* 682b18] + *pteron*), a name that was given by Linnaeus in 1758 and that neatly fuses these two meanings from classical Greek. These are the ants, bees, wasps, gallflies, sawflies, horntails, the graceful ichneumon flies, and similar insects. Wasps are familiar to anyone anywhere in the world, except the polar regions, and the pesky gold-and-black insects, displaying their prominent stingers, engender grouchiness and some fear from summer picnickers: wasp stings can cause a fatal anaphylactic reaction (Greek *ana* ["upward" and similar meanings] + *phylax,* gen. *phylakos* ["watcher" or "guard" or "sentinel"]) in hypersensitive individuals (bee stings likewise). The modernism *anaphylaxis* and its adjective *anaphylactic* borrow the Greek to suggest how the overreaction, leading to potential vascular collapse from bee or wasp stings, is the body's excessively protective mechanism reacting to hymenopteran venoms; the opposite modern coinage in toxicology is *prophylaxis,* that is, the development of immunity to venoms, toxins, and other allergy-producing agents. All wasps in the numerous genera carry this remarkably complex venom (which includes peptides, non-enzymatic proteins, enzymes, and amines—the last encompasses histamine), and the Family *Vespidae* (Latin *vespa* ["wasp"]) contains the very common paper wasp (genus *Polistes* [Greek *polistēs* ("founder of a city")]), whose queens are the only members of the colonies to overwinter and begin a new community in the spring (thus the Greek name for this genus). Subfamily *Vespinae* are the yellow jackets and hornets, and the genus *Dolichovespula* (Greek *dolichos* ["long"] + Latinized diminutive *vespula* ["little wasp"]) constructs large, cardboardlike nests (up to thirty centimeters in diameter [roughly twelve inches]): the spheroid is packed within by hundreds of hexagonal cells, made by the workers (workers and queens have stings; the caste of males does not) from the chewed wood or foliage that also forms the outer envelope of the nest. Family *Sphecidae* (Greek *sphēx,* gen. *sphēkos* ["wasp"]) are genera of solitary wasps, parasitic on other arthropods. Famous are the beautiful, thread-waisted mud daubers in genus *Sceliphron* (Greek *skeliphros* ["lean" or "dry" or "parched"]), glittering blue-black in the sun as they flit rapidly, seeking spiders to paralyze, to stock their underground nests built of mud (the hapless spiders serve as food for the wasp larvae emerging from eggs laid on the arachnids). Other related genera provision their nests with grasshoppers, beetles, cockroaches, flies, shield bugs, and leafhoppers, and thereby these wasps are essential in a natural control of many destructive pests. The largest American wasp is the common cicada killer in the genus *Sphecius* (from Greek *sphēx,* as above), which grow as large as small hummingbirds (up to six centimeters [2.5 inches]); as the common name indicates, *Sphecius* spp. stuff their nests with paralyzed cicadas.

Ants have been part of folklore and legend since the earliest times, and these occasionally voracious creatures often pique the imagination of science-fiction writers, who populate their miniature formican cities with organized cultures and warring leagues ruled by warrior queens of military genius in tactics and strategy. Ants are the family *Formicidae* (Latin *formica* ["ant"]) and are distributed all around the globe. Ant specialists call themselves *myrmecologists* (Greek *myrmēx*, gen. *myrmēkos* ["ant"])—not *formicologists*. (The plasticlike hard coating trade-named *Formica* means "in place of mica," and the proprietary name has nothing to do with ants [*mica* is an orthosilicate of aluminum and potassium, sometimes occurring in enormous plates from which "Muscovite windows" and isinglass still are fashioned]). Myrmecologists generally speak of their formicans in terms of subfamilies, convenient groupings of a number of related genera. Subfamily *Dorylinae* (Greek *dory*, gen. *doratos* ["shaft of a spear"]) are the horror movies' "army ants," eating everything organic—dead and living—in the paths of their frequent migrations. Tropical America has a single genus, *Eciton* (Medieval Latin *ecitum* ["danger"]), and the soldiers carry enormous mandibles, which are long, curved, and toothed; the queen is blind. Subfamily *Myrmicinae* (Greek *myrmēx*, as above) include the seed-feeding harvester ants in the genus *Pogonomyrmex* (Greek *pōgōn*, gen. *pōgōnos* ["beard"] + *myrmēx*), leaf-cutters among *Atta* spp. (Latin *atta* ["father," as said in respect by children, or an Etruscan word—in Sextus Pompeius Festus, *De verborum significatu* (ed. Lindsay, 11)—for "someone who walks on his tiptoes"]), and the fire ants in the genus *Solenopsis* (Greek *sōlēn*, gen. *sōlēnos* ["channel" or "pipe"] + *opsis*, gen. *opseōs* ["aspect," "view," or "appearance"]), introduced accidentally into the southern United States in 1918 from South America. Fire ant nests have large populations (often over one hundred thousand ants) and are hard-crusted and tall enough to damage agricultural machinery (the mounds can be a meter wide and a meter tall [three feet]). *Formicinae* (Latin *formica*, as above) is the subfamily containing the shiny black carpenter ants in genus *Camponotus* (Greek *kampē* ["bend" or "caterpillar"] + *nōtos* ["back"]), the workers of which can reach 2.5 centimeters long (one inch); unlike termites, carpenter ants do not feed on the wood they excavate from their tunnels and galleries. There are two American genera of slave-making ants: *Polyergus* (Greek *polyergos* ["hard-working"]) and *Formica* (the straight Latin for "ant"). To begin a new colony, a *Polyergus* queen raids the nest of another species, kills its queen, and the workers in the colony (frequently *Formica*) adopt their new queen; soon warring raids emerge from the *Polyergus* queen's captive colony, with workers who are soldiers, and they slaughter the workers in other nests, carrying back the pupae—some to be eaten, some to be raised as workers. Not surprisingly, "amazons" is the name often applied to *Polyergus*. In their turn, *Formica* spp. raid colonies of other *Formica* spp., seizing pupae, killing workers. The subfamily *Formicinae* also includes the genus *Lasius* (Greek *lasios* ["hairy," "woolly," or "shaggy"]), the always fascinating honeydew ants. *Lasius* carefully tend aphids, "milking" them, and during the winter, *Lasius* store aphid eggs within the nest, depositing the eggs in the spring on new leaves of plants as food for the hatching aphids.

The superfamily *Apoidea* (Latin *apis*, gen. *apis* ["bee"]) groups the numerous families and genera of bees, insects that not only gather nectar (honey is nectar concentrated by evaporation) but also collect pollen to provision their nests. Honeybees are the family *Apinae*, and the most famous species is *Apis mellifera* L. (Latin *apis* + *mel*, gen. *mellis* ["honey"] + *ferre* ["to carry"]), introduced into North America from Europe. Our common honeybee workers are usually about 1.25 centimeters long (.5 inch) and generally unaggressive, making them ideal as domesticated "beehived" insects, as contrasted with such species as the wild Indian honeybee, *Apis florae* Fabricius (Latin *flos*, gen. *floris* ["flower" or "blossom" with *Flora*, gen. *Florae*, the "goddess of flowers"]), whose workers are 1.90 centimeters (roughly .75 inch) long, with the queen a large 2.5 centimeters (one inch) long. Subfamily *Bombinae* (Greek *bombos* ["booming" or "humming"]) are the familiar bumblebees, ranging up to three centimeters (about 1.25 inches) long, commonly banded in yellow and black and incredibly industrious as they go about their tasks of gathering nectar and pollen from clovers and alfalfas and related plants (it is not possible to grow some varieties of red clovers in areas where there are no bumblebees). *Xylocopinae* (Greek *xylon* ["wood"] + *koptein* ["to cut"]) is the subfamily of carpenter bees, resembling bumblebees in superficial appearance but somewhat less "hairy." And the family *Megachilidae* (Greek *megas* ["big" or "large"] + *cheilos* ["lips"]) are the leaf-cutting bees, whose neatly cut circles and ovals of leaves line the cells of their nests (circular cuts form the partitions, ovals the sides), the circles and ovals often cut from rose leaves and other ornamentals, to the grumpy frustration of flower gardeners around the world. Most leaf-cutters are solitary insects.

Ants, bees, and wasps are known as "social insects" from their remarkable skills in home building for the thousands passing their lives in a "hive" or a "hill" (the latter for ants). Fine beeswax (Latin *cera*; Greek *kēros*) retained a valued place in medicine until the early twentieth century as an inert, semisolid vehicle for drugs applied to the skin (as thick ointments and plasters [wax is easily heated to make it runny, then quickly hardens and sticks in place]), and wax tablets, wax seals, wax models, wax for encaustic painting, and a number of other uses made *cera* an item of widespread commerce from very ancient times. Beehives in Egypt and Mesopotamia were common by 2500 B.C., so that bees have been "domesticated" by humankind from the earliest eras of civilization, supplying honey (Latin *mel,* gen. *mellis;* Greek *meli,* gen. *melitos;* "bee" in Greek was *melissa,* literally "honey-licker") for medicine and embalming. In addition to its legendary sweetness (thus an early metaphor in love poetry), Egyptians, Greeks, and Romans knew honey's properties in preserving organic matter. Pliny the Elder, *NH,* VII, 35, comments on the use of honey to preserve corpses (and there seems no sense of anything extraordinary); modern analysis has confirmed ancient knowledge: honey is extremely *hypertonic* (Greek *hyper* ["above"] + *tonos* ["stretching" or "tension"]), that is, it pulls water out of cells, and the pH of honey is about 3.91, making it quite acidic (pH is the modern symbol, first used in 1909, expressing hydrogen ion [H^+] concentration; pH 7 is neutral, with lower values suggesting increased acidity, higher values [to 14] indicating alkalinity). That pH also makes honey a good natural antiseptic, but as the Greeks and Romans applied honey salves and ointments, they were not only drying out festering wounds (albeit with the patient's complaints about the sting) but also—as we would say—applying a mild antibiotic brought into the honey by an enzyme, secreted by the bee's pharyngeal glands (details in Majno, *Healing Hand,* 117). And when Scribonius Largus, *Compositiones,* 82, mentions *propolis*—which he says his sources call *cera sacra*—as part of a wax salve for tumors, he is telling us that "bee glue" (*propolis* is the Greek word) was a common ingredient in Greco-Roman pharmacy. As Majno writes, bee glue is also "antibiotic.... Its main active principle is galangine, a flavonol, which now holds U.S. patent 2,550,269 as a food preservative" (*Healing Hand,* 117). In the case of the Hymenoptera, medical entomology in human history offers the positive aspects of healing drugs and the honeys storied from all eras (there are occasionally poisonous honeys, derived from drawing nectar from the flowers of poisonous plants), even as we learn more about the infrequently fatal effects of the venoms in the stings of wasps and bees.

Added to the ants, bees, and wasps in Hymenoptera are a goodly number of insects that are solitary in their habits, including the sawflies in the family *Tenthredinidae* (Greek *tenthrēdōn,* gen. *tenthrēdonos* ["wasp that nests in the earth," in Aristotle, *HA,* 629a31]).

Among species in the genus *Pristophora* (Greek *pristēs* ["saw" or "file"]) are the larch sawflies and spruce sawflies, whose galls (the reaction of trees to inserted eggs and larvae) cause widespread devastation in the forests of both North America and Europe.

SPIDERS AND THEIR COUSINS

Spiders are perhaps the most feared and loathed creatures, even as they provide a fascinating and generally harmless (to humans) aspect of nature's adaptations. Spiders and their kin are essential in the population control of insects, and without these eight-legged animals, the earth would shortly be overrun by masses of insects. Spider webs are among the most amazing engineering feats in all of the natural world, and their stringed beauty as coated by the morning dew and split into prismed colors by the rising sun (a sign of an unsuccessful night's hope for the stray flying insect: a rent web shows the lady found her food [most spiders one observes are females] and will return again another night to spin anew) is matched by the steel strength and technically superb coatings on the threads, entangling an insect evermore as it struggles. Witnessing the doomed grapplings of a housefly in the web of a rightfully honored house spider vividly illustrates why a few spiders are necessary in any home, anywhere in the world. Flies are attracted by human waste (rotting garbage or otherwise), and spiders are attracted by flies; together they function in a natural balance over time.

> Class *Arachnida* (Greek *arachnē* ["spider"]) includes spiders, scorpions, ticks and mites, harvestmen (the "daddy longlegs"), wind scorpions or solifuges, and whip scorpions. Arachnids have eight legs (contrasted to the six of insects), and unlike the huge numbers of species among insects, there are about thirty thousand species of spiders and about thirty-five thousand distributed among the other orders of Arachnida.
>
> All spiders are poisonous, but only two in North America are dangerous to humans: more famous of the two is the black widow, *Latrodectus mactans* L. (Latin *latro* ["robber"] + Greek *dēktēs* ["a biter"] + Latin *mactans* ["killing" or "deadly"]), which is the largest of the cobweb weavers or comb-footed spiders (Family *Theridiidae* [from the Greek *theridion* ("small animal")])—a gorgeous specimen I collected in Fresno, California, measured a full inch (2.5 centi-

meters) long, resplendent in her glossy-black, grapelike abdomen bellied with the famous red hourglass. Rarely biting man (widows are extraordinarily shy), *Latrodectus* causes about two deaths a year in the United States (usually children) with about four hundred cases a year reported in southern California alone. Spider venoms are complex mixtures of proteins, and the lethal fraction of widow poison is a peptide that interferes with neuromuscular transmission. Related species in *Latrodectus* (the brown widow and the red widow of Florida and the northern widow of the temperate United States) are less poisonous, although all such spiders should be carefully respected when observed and certainly suspected as residents in outbuildings. The genus *Theridion* (Greek "small animal," as above) generally have the bulbous abdomens characteristic of the larger widows, and our very common American house spider (genus *Achaearanea* [Latin *Achaei* ("the people of Achaea = Greeks") + *rana* ("frog")]) bears the widowlike abdomen even though she is a mere .3 inch long (8 millimeters) and carries bright brown, white, and pale orange patches and streaks swirling around her abdomen (hence the scientific name of the genus, reminiscent of painted ancient Greek pottery). Genus *Steatoda* (Greek *stear,* gen. *steatos* ["fat" or "tallow"]) also spins webs in our garages and houses, consuming welcome numbers of flies, mosquitoes, and ants, and the brown-and-gray mottles of her nine-millimeter (.4-inch) abdomen markedly resemble rancid animal fat or the tallow used to make home-manufactured candles.

Those horror-inducing, fulsomely hairy spiders that are sent crawling over the hero's body in adventure movies are usually the generally harmless and misnamed tarantulas of the American southwest. Arachnologists prefer to call these largest of spiders *mygalomorphs* (Greek *mygalē* ["field mouse"] + *morphē* ["form" or "shape"]) or "hairy" mygalomorphs (no arthropod has true hair, a possession only of mammals), placing these "tarantulas" in various genera according to anatomical structures. Common in Arizona and southern California is *Aphonopelma* (Greek *a-* ["without"] + *phonē* ["sound" or "voice"] + *pelma* [the "sole of a foot"], thus the "soundless sole of a foot," as descriptive of hunting habits), which reach hairy-legged lengths of seventy millimeters (2.7 inches). The giant bird spider of the Amazon basin is the largest spider in the world and ordinarily has a twenty-five-centimeter (10-inch) leg span attached to a nine-centimeter (3.5-inch) two-part body (all spiders have two basic body parts, the cephalothorax and abdomen, compared with insects' head, thorax, and abdomen). These enormous "tarantulas" occasionally catch small birds, lizards, and small snakes, but their bite is harmless to humans, producing only local effects.

The second American spider troublesome to man is the 2.5-centimeter (one-inch) brown recluse or fiddler spider (so known from a distinct violin pattern on the dorsal side of the cephalothorax) in the genus *Loxosceles* (Greek *loxos* ["crooked"] + *skelos* ["leg"]). *Loxosceles* venom contains at least a dozen proteins, and a bite produces an unusual necrotic lesion (Greek *nekrotēs* ["state of death" or "mortification"]), leading to sloughing and large tissue defects that can include muscle. Rare deaths as reported are from kidney failure.

Spiders display the gorgeous colors expected among terrestrial arthopods, and similar to the beetles and butterflies, spiders show a range that defies capture by the artist's palette. Added to the striking red and black (or brown and red) of *Latrodectus* are the brilliant yellow-and-black patterns of the zigzag web weavers of our *Argiope* spp. (Greek *Argiopē* [the name of a nymph], the white-striped athwart red-and-black bands of the common European ground-hunter genus *Pisaura* (Latin *Pisae,* gen. pl. *Pisarum* [a town in Etruria, traditionally a colony of Pisa in Elis (Greece, the district of Olympia)]), and hundreds of similar variations encompassing almost all colors known from the realm of insects and flowers. Even the reddish-brown yellows of the mygalomorphs are beautiful, even though "most people insist that they are revolted by the long legs and hairiness, but no one on record has ever objected to these same characteristics in a Russian wolfhound" (Buchsbaum et al., *Animals,* 360).

Far deadlier to man are the worldwide scorpions (Order *Scorpiones* [Greek *skorpiōn*]), which inflict death annually to hundreds of children and the elderly. Among the seven hundred species distributed on every continent except Antarctica are several that bring death in Mexico, North Africa, and Arizona and California; these are usually the small scorpions (United States and Mexico) in the genus *Centruroides* (Greek *kentrein* ["furnished with a sting"]), the bronzed-yellow sculptured scorpion with a normal length of six to seven centimeters (2.4 to 2.6 inches). Scorpion giants, like the coal-black, seven-inch (seventeen-centimeter) *Pandinus* spp. (from the Latin *pandare* ["to bend"]) of Egypt and the Near East have poisons no more toxic than that of a wasp, even though "the scorpion had an extremely sinister reputation among the ancients, and was regarded as the most dangerous of all venomous animals" (Beavis, *Insects,* 27).

Wind scorpions (Order *Solifugae* [Latin *solipuga*, Later Latin *solifuga* ("an animal which flees the daylight," in Isidore, *Origines*, XII, 3.4, and XIV, 6.40])—or "sun scorpions," since most live in deserts around the world—include about 130 species native to North America. Stingless and harmless to man, even though equipped with two pairs of enormous pincing *cheliceras* (Greek *chēlē* ["claw"] + Latin *cera* ["wax"]—hence the Greek name *tetragnatha* ("four-jawed ones," in Philumenus, 35.1–2)—these fascinating creatures can inflict a painful bite that sometimes becomes seriously infected. The common name *wind scorpions* mirrors their extremely rapid running "like the wind," and the 2.5-centimeter (one-inch) "running brown puffballs" are frequent in dry areas from Arizona to North Dakota. North African species are larger, and they prey upon scorpions (among many arthropods), neatly snipping off the stinger with its two pairs of cheliceras before consuming the hapless and defenseless scorpion.

Order *Uropygia* (Greek *ouron* or Latin *urina* ["urine"] + *pyx*, gen. *pygos* ["rump" or "buttocks"]) are about seventy species of scorpionlike animals (again without stingers) known as whip scorpions or, in the American South, as vinegarroons. The Louisiana vinegarroon, genus *Mastigoproctus* (Greek *mastix*, gen. *mastigos* ["whip"] + *prōktos* ["anus"]) grows to eight centimeters (three inches) long, and its tail or whip (usually arched over the animal as it moves about) can be ten centimeters (four inches) long. Spraying a mist of acetic acid (vinegar thus the common name) from a gland at the base of the tail both for defense and for seeking its prey (the acetic acid is part of the vinegarroon's solvent to dissolve the exoskeletons of its insect quarry), the metallic, brownish-black whip scorpions spend nocturnal lives seeking food by means of ground vibrations. Acetic acid is not the only chemical employed by whip scorpions as an exoskeleton dissolver: some tropical species use chlorine, formic acid, and similar substances.

Order *Acarina* (Greek *akari* ["a kind of mite, bred in wax," in Aristotle, *HA*, 557b8]) are about twenty thousand species of very small arthropods (thus the vernacular name *mites*) that include chiggers or harvest mites in *Trombiculidae* (from Greek *tromein* ["to tremble"] + Latin *culex*, gen. *culicis* ["gnat" or "midge"]), the scabies or mange mites in the suborder *Sarcoptiformes* (Byzantine Greek *sarko[p]tikein* ["to be born like lumps of flesh"] derived from Greek *sarx*, gen. *sarkos* ["flesh"] + Latin *forma* ["shape," "appearance," and similar meanings]), the hard ticks in the suborder *Ixodidae* (Greek *ixōdēs* [like "birdlime," thus "sticky" or "clammy"], derived from *ixos* ["oak mistletoe" or "birdlime prepared from mistletoe berries"]), the soft ticks in suborder *Argasidae* (from Greek *aergos* ["idle"]), spider mites, water mites, and similar specialized forms. Ixodidae (hard ticks) are transmitters of many serious human illnesses—including Lyme Disease, caused by a spirochete carried by a minute tick (arthritis in the knees is common), and Rocky Mountain spotted fever, carried by wood ticks in the genus *Dermacentor* (Greek *derma*, gen. *dermatos* ["skin" or "leather"]). Large specimens in Acarina are the wood ticks, familiar to anyone who has returned from a wilderness outing to discover several of these hard-shelled creatures comfortably nestled on one's legs or back or on the head among the hairs, quietly sucking blood meals. Unfed, a wood tick in genus *Dermacentor* is usually four millimeters (.2 inch) long, but bloated by a completed feeding, the well-fed *Dermacentor* has expanded to two centimeters (.8 inch). Ticks and their relatives are "the most dangerous of the arachnids . . . as they spread diseases that may be fatal" (Buchsbaum et al., *Animals*, 366).

Medical science continually learns new data about the arthropods and why their remarkable adaptations allow their survival even in the face of increasingly sophisticated human technologies. As scientists in parasitology and other fields of medical zoology probe the molecular wonders of insect chemistry or the biophysics of bloodsuckers from leeches to ticks, there will remain a constant requirement for labeling new discoveries. Greek and Latin will function as the ultimate quarry for these new names, and terminologies derived from the classical roots will retain their roles in precise specifications.

CHAPTER 5

BONES

IN naming the bones of the human body, anatomists since antiquity have easily provided analogies from commonly known objects in everyday life, from wedges to keys. Bones and their names also mirror a widely known stock of folk tales and mythological allusions, and when Renaissance anatomists sought labels for the bones observed in systematic dissections, they often drew on universally understood myths as taught from the heritages of classical antiquity. Yet bones represent one of the oldest studies of a medical nature because burial customs and earliest agricultural practices generally included a precise knowledge of how bones fit together and how bones survived the longest of a human being's mortal existence. One can argue that *osteology* (Greek *osteon* ["bone"] + *logos*) is the third-oldest aspect of the medical sciences, with the oldest being midwifery and the second oldest being pharmacy in its venerated form of herbalism.

From earliest times, necessity dictated that humankind gain skilled knowledge of birthing and its variations, as well as an equally skilled command of medicinal plants and substances that could enhance the rapid healing of maladies of mind and body. And since bone fractures were—and are—among the most ordinary of human accidents, detailed techniques of setting fractures were among the first medical arts to be practiced with reasonable assurance. Details of bonesetting in the Egyptian *Edwin Smith Surgical Papyrus* of about 1800 B.C. show a long history of previous development, probably going back to the ages when human beings emerged as a separate species. The scribe-surgeon certainly assumes much ordinary knowledge as he omits specifics of setting the fracture of a humerus (Egyptian *g'b* ["upper arm"]) even while he gives instructions for treatment: "Make two splints of linen; bind [the wound] with *ymrw* [an unknown medicinal substance]; treat it afterward with grease, honey, and lint until you see that a decisive stage has been reached (adapted from Breasted, *Edwin Smith*, I, 359).

Mistakes were also easily made, and unless the bonesetter knew the basic structures surrounding the humerus (muscles and which way they flexed or extended, in particular), healing of the fracture would occur incorrectly. Unlike the terse instructions from ancient Egypt, those of the bonesetters and surgeons of classical Greece ensured that readers and students alike understood that there was a "right way" to set fractures of the main bone of the upper arm. Long experience taught the importance of preparation for the correct healing of such a fracture, and the Hippocratic *Fractures,* VIII (of about 400 B.C.), begins a description of humerus fractures by noting how positioning the arm (extension or flexion) before application of bandages is essential; splints as such are to be applied after a week or nine days, and "a bone of the upper arm (*brachionos osteon*) knits usually after forty days" (*Fractures,* VIII, 38–39). Similar data are reported for treatments of numerous other bones and joints in these Greek tracts on fractures, works that are remarkable for detail and what modern physicians call "conservative therapies." By the fifth century B.C., Greek physicians and surgeons had precise knowledge of human bones and their attachments, as contrasted with a rather foggy command of various other internal anatomical structures of the human body. Bonesetting was an ancient skill, increasingly based on observations of human bones and their tendency to break and shatter in particular manners; long experience over hundreds of generations led to the documents we have in the form of the Hippocratic *Fractures* and *Joints,* still held in admiration by modern surgeons and doctors.

The Greek language did not have a single word *skeleton* that encompassed all the bones of the body but simply had *ta osta,* "the bones," which would be assumed "skeleton," as we would say. Our word *skeleton* comes from the Greek *skeletos* ("dried-up body" or "corpse"), and in the later Greek of the Hellenistic Era, the Roman Empire, *skeletos* usually meant "mummy." The first use of the word in English in its modern sense of "the bones" or "bony framework of the body" occurs in 1578 as *sceleton* in a commentary on Galen's bone lore, and *skeleton* (with its *k*) emerges in Thomas Browne's *Religio medici* of 1643. Brown wrote, "By continuall sight of Anatomies, Skeletons, or Cadaverous reliques" (*Religio medici,* I, 38). Alternative spellings included *scelleton, scaleton, skelton,* and *skeliton*—until *skeleton* became standard by the late eighteenth century.

There are 206 bones in the human adult, not counting the

smaller sesamoids (Greek *sēsamoeidēs* ["like a sesame seed"]), which occur irregularly in various tendons as they interact with given joint surfaces. The bones usually are grouped thus:

> Axial skeleton: vertebral column (26), skull (22), hyoid bone (1), the ribs and breastbone (25)
>
> Appendicular skeleton: upper extremities (64), lower extremities (62)
>
> Auditory ossicles (6)

Bone names frequently reflect analogies to common objects or shapes known to anatomists in late medieval Europe and in the Renaissance, and the Greco-Latin coinages often are clear enough, if one keeps in mind the borrowings in later Latin of Greek as thought appropriate.

SOME BONES OF THE SKULL

Occipital (Latin *occiput*, gen. *occipitis* ["back of the head"] = *ob-* + *caput* ["head"]). The term is rare in classical Latin (for example, in Persius, I, 62), but late medieval Latin revived the word for its exact meaning, and by the mid-sixteenth century, *occiput* had become standard in textbooks of anatomy for "the bone at the back of the head."

Parietal (from the Late Latin *parietalis* ["of walls"], derived from Latin *paries* ["wall"]). Renaissance anatomists saw this thick bone as a wall protecting the brain.

Frontal (from the Late Latin *frontalis* ["of the forehead"]).

Temporal (from vulgar Latin *tempula* ["the flattened region on either side of the forehead"]). Medieval farmers had also noted corresponding bones in the skulls of animals.

Sphenoid (Late Latin *sphenoides*, derived from the Greek *sphēnoēidēs* ["wedgelike"]). So this bone appears, wedged behind the socket of the eye.

Zygomatic (Late Latin *zygoma*, pulled from the Greek *zygon* ["yoke"]). By analogy, anatomists viewed this bone—the cheekbone—as a miniaturized yoke for a plow or a wheeled vehicle.

Nasal (the Latin *nasus* meant "nose," although Romans said *nasus* to mean "sharp wit" [as does Martial, *Epigrams*, I, 41.18]). Common also in Renaissance anatomy for "nose" is the Latin *naris* (sing.) and *nares* (pl.), so that anatomy texts print *nares* to indicate exactly "nostrils." In classical Latin, *nares* specified "openings" or "orifices" or "vents," almost always in the contexts of engineering or architecture (for example, Vitruvius, *On Architecture,* VII, 4.1).

- *Maxilla* (a Late Latin coinage from the classical Latin *maxillae* [pl., "jawbones"]). *Maxilla* is a diminutive form of classical Latin's *mala* (usually in the plural as *malae* ["cheeks" or "jaws"]), so that Renaissance anatomists could name the *maxilla* as the "lesser" of the two jawbones.
- *Mandible* (Late Latin *mandibula* ["lower" or "chewing jaw"], derived from classical Latin's *mandere* ["to chew"] + *-bula* [a suffix of means]).
- Various *foramina* [sing. *foramen*] are "holes" (Latin) allowing entrance and exit of nerves, arteries, and veins through the bones. The *foramen magnum* (Late Latin for "great hole"), for example, permits communication between the cranial cavity and the vertebral canal through this "great hole" in the occipital bone.

SOME VERTEBRAE

The basic term *vertebra* emerges in Late Latin as derived from classical Latin's *vertere* ("to turn"), and the *vertebrae* (pl.) came to mean "bones or segments of the spinal column" in anatomy texts by the early seventeenth century. *Spinus* is Latin for "thorn," and *columna* comes directly into English from Latin as a cognate. In the mind's eye, one is supposed to picture a "thorned column," a rather strained analogy unless one assumes the "thorns" are less sharp or pointed than those found in various stemmed plants (similar to rose thorns).

- The *first cervical* (from Latin *cervix,* gen. *cervicis* ["neck"]) *vertebra* "is named the *Atlas* because it supports the globe of the head" (Gray, *Anatomy,* 129). Roman anatomists had applied the name *Atlas* (Greek [gen. *Atlantos*]) to this bone by the second century A.D. (Pollux, *Onomasticon,* II, 132), and Renaissance anatomists simply retained the allusion to the classical myth of the Titan who held up the pillars of the universe.
- The *second cervical vertebra* is called the *epistropheus* (Greek for "turning on a pivot") or *axis* (Latin cognate with English) since it "forms the pivot upon which the first vertebra, carrying the head, rotates"

(Gray, *Anatomy*, 131). *Axis* became the standard name for this bone by the early nineteenth century, as recorded in the 1815 edition of the *Encyclopedia Britannica* (Vol. III, 289). In the medical Greek of the Roman Empire, *epistropheus* was the name of the first vertebra (that is, what is now termed the seventh vertebra) of the neck, in Pollux, *Onomasticon*, II, 131. By adopting *axis* in place of the confusing *epistropheus*, anatomists avoided the slippery label gained from classical and Renaissance texts: *axis* was always number two down from the head, whereas *epistropheus* might be number seven or number two.

The *seventh cervical vertebra* is the *vertebra prominens* (Latin *prominens*, gen. *prominentis* ["projecting"]) due to its distinctive and long *spinous process* (a Late Latin coinage for "thorny projection"). Each of the seven cervical vertebrae has a pair of *foramina* in its *transverse processes* (Late Latin for "projections lying crosswise"), and the presence of the foramina in the transverse process distinguishes the cervical vertebrae from the thoracic and lumbar vertebrae, which lack foramina in their transverse processes.

The *thoracic vertebrae* (twelve in number) display prominent transverse and spinous processes. Greek's *thōrax*, gen. *thōrakos* meant (in military parlance) that "covered by the *thōrax*," a soldier's chest and back as clothed in light or heavier armor. By the fourth century B.C., *thōrax* often was "chest" or our "thorax," as one reads in Aristotle, *HA*, 493a17; in the medical Greek of the second century Roman Empire, *thōrax* was a technical term for "chest bandage" (Soranus, *Bandages*, 33).

The five *lumbar vertebrae* are the largest segments of the movable parts of the vertebral column: *lumbar* derives from the Latin *lumbus* ("the parts of the body on either side of the spinal column between the diaphragm and the hipbone," in Pliny, *NH*, XI, 178). Traditionally, one can truncate this lengthy definition into the single word *loins*.

In the human adult, five vertebrae fuse to become the *os sacrum* (Latin "holy bone"), so called for unknown reasons. One can only speculate why Renaissance and earlier anatomists attached this name (in Greek it was the *hieron osteon* [likewise "holy bone"]). Perhaps someone recalled the lines of Vergil, *Georgics*, II, 476, and *Aeneid*, IV, 301, in which *sacrum* means something akin to "a sacred object" used in terms of a vessel or statue or symbol in ceremonials, and the unique appearance of this bone may have suggested some sort of link with ancient Roman religion. In Tacitus, *Annals*, II, 14, *sacrum* is a "sacrificial victim," and the odd shape of the bone perhaps was reminiscent of a crude version of antiquity's most common sacrificial "knife," a blade quite frequently fashioned from volcanic glass (obsidian) in natural curvatures similar to what one might see in this bone. A male sacrum is longer and more thin than that of a female, and the bone is one of the important markers in forensic medicine. "Sacred" or "holy" bone? Research on the question reveals how widespread was this label in antiquity (Greek, Latin, and Hebrew all have it), but the basic "why" has eluded scholars, as illustrated by Sugar, "How the Sacrum Got Its Name."

The *coccyx* (pronounced "cox-six," Late Latin derived from the Greek *kokkyx*, gen. *kokkygos* ["cuckoo"], from its likeness to the beak of a cuckoo) consists of four (sometimes five, sometimes three) rudimentary vertebrae, occasionally called *caudal* vertebrae (Latin *cauda* ["tail"]). Roman imperial physicians (for example, the second century A.D. Rufus of Ephesus and Galen of Pergamon) noted the cuckoo-beak shape of these four bones, but Pollux, in his *Onomasticon*, II, 183 (the same century as Rufus and Galen), tells us that the *sacrum* was termed in Greek *trētos kokkyx* ("a perforated cuckoo"). In this instance, the murky analogy of a cuckoo's beak to the four fused vertebrae above the coccyx was discarded for the much deeper tradition naming it the "holy" bone. "Cuckoo-beak" remained, however, the preferred tag for the four "tailbones."

BONES OF THE PELVIS

The five vertebrae of the sacrum and the normally four vertebrae of the coccyx form the rear or posterior portion of the pelvic girdle, or simply *pelvis* (Latin for "shallow bowl or basin," akin to Greek *pella*). Two other bones, the paired *os coxae* (Latin "bone of the hip")—sometimes called the *innominate* (Late Latin *innominatus* ["nameless" or "unnamed"]—form the lateral and front parts of the bony ring collectively termed the pelvis.

In classical Latin, *pelvis* almost always means "a shallow bowl made of a metal," as in Celsus's prescriptions for treatment of gout, which includes: "Sea water or strong brine is to be heated then poured into a shallow, metal basin" (Celsus, *De medicina*, IV, 31.4). In medical terminologies, the *pelvis* is a nineteenth-century coinage, first appearing in anatomy texts in the 1830s. By the time a twelfth edition of Dunglison's widely used *Medical Lexicon* was published in Philadelphia (1855), the author could write (651): "Pelvis . . . so called, because fancied to be shaped like an ancient basin." The analogy is strained, but the new name stuck and remains as an ordinary term.

Coxa in Latin has two basic meanings, depending on context: "hip" if one is speaking of a human being (as in Celsus, *De medicina*, VII, 27.1); or "haunch" if one is writing about animals. Latin's *coxa* was as vague as modern English's "hip," which includes the perceived projection of the hipbone as well as the upper part of the femur and the flesh covering the area. Classical Latin did, however, have a term that meant exactly "hipbone" (*coxendix*), and this term was quite common in the speech and writing of the late Roman Republic and early Roman Empire, as suggested by Pliny, *NH*, XX, 90, and Suetonius, *Augustus*, 80. *Coxa* meaning "hipbone" appears rather late in medical English, with William Smellie's famous *Midwifery* of 1752 (Vol. I, introd. sect. 34) being one of the first usages of *coxa* as "hip" or "hip joint": "The legs must be amputated at the coxa." Why the choice was not *coxendix* is lost, but *coxa* turns up in most anatomy books alongside "hipbone" and "innominate" (Gray, *Anatomy*, 258). *Innominate* as an alternative name also appears in the eighteenth century and becomes interchangeable with "hipbone" and "coxa" in the nineteenth. Why early-eighteenth-century anatomists should term the hipbones "nameless" is subject to pure speculation.

Each *coxa* is the product of a fusion of three bones, which are quite distinct in youngsters but which have become a single bone in the human adult. The three are called *ilium* (pl. *ilia* [Latin, "flank"]), *ischium* (pl. *ischia* [Latin borrowed from the Greek *ischion*, "hip joint" and in later Greek "lowest part of the hipbone"]), and *pubis* (*os pubis*: Latin *pubes*, gen. *pubis* ["pubic hair" or "groin"; here, "bone of the groin"]). The union of the three bones occurs in and around the *acetabulum* (Latin for "vinegar cup"), the large, cup-shaped articular cavity set near the center of the outer surface of the coxa; the *acetabulum* is the fitted cup receiving the *caput femoris* ("the head of the femur").

In classical Latin, *ilium* generally occurs in the plural *ilia* (as in Celsus, *De medicina*, IV, 1.12) and means "the side parts of the body extending from the hips down to the groin," a meaning narrowed slightly into "flanks" as used by Celsus here in the cited passage and by Pliny, *NH*, XI, 208. Another common meaning of *ilia* is "guts" or "innards," as one reads in Horace, *Epodes*, III, 4, a nuance borrowed by medicalese as the name for a section of the small intestine in its medieval Latin form of *ileum* (see chap. 9 below). *Ischium* is an eighteenth-century refashioning of the Greek plural *ischia* ("the hips"), borrowed rarely by classical Latin also in the plural (*ischia*, gen. *ischiorum*, so Aulus Gellius, *Attic Nights*, IV, 13.1). *Ischia*, however, were used by learned writers in the mid-seventeenth century to indicate "bones on which the body rests when sitting." By the middle of the nineteenth century, medical writers had forgotten that *pubis* was the genitive singular form of the feminine noun *pubes*, and this mistake has become standard as the name for this part of the coxa. Classical Latin's *pubes* had three basic meanings: "adult population" (the most common sense, illustrated by passages in Cicero, Catullus, Vergil, and Tacitus, among several); "the age of puberty" (the next most ordinary meaning, suggested by Celsus, *De medicina*, II, 1.19); and a third, uncommon connotation of "the pubic region" or "sexual parts" or "pubic hair," as met in the poetry of Ovid and Vergil, as well as the writings of Celsus, Pliny the Elder, and Apuleius. It is this last meaning that is preserved in modern English with *pubis* and the adjective "pubic," although the noun puberty carries through the second most common meaning (Latin, however, had its own *pubertas*, the direct ancestor of the English cognate-noun).

SOME OTHER BONES

The *sternum* (Late Latin, derived from Greek *sternon* ["breastbone"], but Homeric Greek's *sternon* means "breast" or "chest") has three parts: an upper *manubrium* (Latin "handle" or "haft"); a middle *gladiolus* (Latin "little sword") or *corpus sterni* (Late Latin "body of the breastbone"); and the lower *xiphisternum* or *xiphoid process* (Late Latin *xiphi-* derived from the Greek *xiphos* ["sword"]). Taken as a whole, the sternum bears some resemblance to an ancient Roman short sword, a *gladius*.

The *clavicle* (medieval Latin *clavicula* ["little key"], derived from Latin *clavis*, gen. *clavis* ["key"]) is one of the two bones known as the "collarbone"; each articulates with the sternum and a *scapula* (Latin "shoulder blade" or "shoulder") to form anterior aspects of the shoulder. The multifeatured scapula with its graceful ridges and knobs is a vivid example of how bones function as anchors, fulcrums, attachments, and insertions for muscles and ligaments. Prominent structures of the scapula include the ventral *coracoid process* (Late Latin *coracoides*, derived from the Greek *korakoeidēs* ["ravenlike" or "hooked like a raven's beak"—the Greek *korax*, gen. *korakos*, means "raven"]), which anchors part of the biceps muscle's origin, and the dorsal *acromion* (Greek *akrōmion* ["point of the shoulder"]), which is the outward end of the spine of the scapula, a major origination surface for the deltoid muscle.

The *humerus* (derived from Latin's *umerus* ["upper arm"]) is the long bone extending from the shoulder to the elbow. This is *not* a cognate of the English *humorous,* although one could certainly devise some appropriately groan-producing puns.

The *radius* (Latin for "staff" or "rod" or "spoke") is the bone of the forearm on the thumb side, whereas the *ulna* (Latin for "elbow," derived from the Greek *ōlenē* ["elbow" or "arm from the elbow downward"]) is the bone of the forearm opposite the thumb. The ulna's upper articular surfaces illustrate the frequent mechanical efficiency displayed by many bones as they articulate against one another (*articulate* here means "forming a joint," as derived from the Latin noun *articulus* [most commonly "joint"]). Prominent in the top of the ulna is the *semilunar notch* ("half-moon" from the Latin *semi-* ["half"] + *luna* ["moon"]), fitted for motion with the *trochlea* (Latin for "block and tackle") at the distal end of the humerus. The semilunar notch (also called the *incisura trochlearis* [Latin "notch for the trochlea"] or the *greater sigmoid cavity* [*sigmoid* means "shaped like the Greek letter sigma, written *C*"]) has an upper lip called the *olecranon* (Greek *ōlekranon* ["point of the elbow"]), the bony knob of the elbow known by the majority of American children as the "crazy bone"; and the lower tip of the semilunar notch is the *coronoid process* (Latin *corona* ["crown"] + *-oid* = "crownlike").

Although Aristotle, *HA,* 493b27, used *ōlekranon* to mean "point of the elbow," the term dropped out of medical Greek and Latin until being revived in the early eighteenth century. Its initial use in medical English appears in Ephriam Chambers's famous *Cyclopaedia* of 1728, followed shortly in Alexander Monro's *Anatomy of Human Bones,* 3d ed. (Edinburgh, 1741), 248. Galen, *Use of Parts,* II, 2.14, had written that Hippocrates had previously used *ankōn* (not *ōlekranon*) for "point" or "head of the elbow," and Galen's authority doomed the Aristotelian label to obscurity until its reapplication to human osteology in the eighteenth century.

The *carpus* (Late Latin as taken from Greek *karpos* ["wrist"]) or the *ossa carpi* (Latin "bones of the wrist") contains eight bones, arranged in two rows: the four abutting the radius and the ulna are the *navicular, lunate, triquetrum,* and *pisiform* (derived from Latin terms meaning "boat-shaped," "half-moon-shaped," "triangular," and "pea-shaped," respectively); and the four distal wrist bones are the *trapezium, trapezoid, capitate,* and *hamate* (in order as listed: Greek *trapezion,* diminutive of *trapeza* ["small table"], thus "very small table," but in geometry, "four-sided figure with no parallel lines," which is why this bone is often called the *greater multangular;* Greek *trapez-* + *-oid* ["like a trapezium," but in geometry, "four-sided figure with two parallel lines and two nonparallel lines"], which is why anatomists—to avoid this Greco-Latinate confusion—frequently term this small bone the *lesser multangular;* Latin *capitatus* ["with an enlarged head"]; and Latin *hamatus* ["hook-shaped"]).

Usually Greek *karpos* meant "fruit," but an alternative meaning in early Greek (Homer, as well as the Hippocratic *Fractures,* 3) was "wrist." Again the medical English of the eighteenth century pulled a term from the Greek and applied it to a particular structure, and Monro's *Anatomy of Human Bones,* 259, shows it in common use. Traditional anatomy texts term the bones of the wrist *ossa carpi* (for example Gray, *Anatomy,* 248). *Ossa* is the nominative plural form of the Latin neuter noun *os* (gen. *ossis*), and often at first sight *os* ("bone") is confused with *os* ("mouth" or "entrance"), also a neuter; only by knowing that the genitive of *os* ("mouth") is *oris* can one avoid mistranslating, even though the English *orate* preserves this essential difference, as contrasted to *ossify,* which is "to become bonelike" or, more commonly, "rigid." Frequently medical and biological terms reflect not only a nominative form of the original Latin or Greek but also a genitive (for example, *pubes, pubis,* as above), so that as one gains confidence in "translating" modern medicalese, there is a necessity to become familiar with both the nominative and the genitive forms in the declensions of Latin and Greek nouns. In the case of the *carpus* or *karpos* derivatives in modern medical and biological terminologies, *carpo-* almost always stands for "fruit" as it preserves the most ordinary meaning in classical Greek; *carpus* gives rise to *carpalis* ("of the wrist" in Late Latin), so that something labeled *carpal* will be related in some manner to a wrist, whereas a word like *carpology* would mean "study of fruits." Unhappily, botany's term *carpel* (from *karpos* ["fruit"] by way of the French *carpelle* ["a simple pistil assumed as a modified leaf"]) can engender uncertainty, but medicine's carpal terms are quite distinct from botany's carpels. That difference in the last vowel is essential.

The *metacarpus* (coined from the Greek *meta-* ["after" or "beyond"] + *carpus*) has five cylindrical bones, usually numbered in anatomy texts from the lateral side of the hand (the thumb side to the "pinky") as the *ossa metacarpalia I-V.* In the medical Greek of the early Roman Empire, *to metakarpion* meant one of the "bones forming the palm of the hand," as one reads in both Pollux, *Onomasticon,* II, 143, and Galen, *Use of Parts,* II, 4.

The *phalanges* of the hand, or *phalanges digitorum manus,* are the small bones of the fingers. Borrowed from the Greek *phalanx* (gen. *phalangos;* nom. pl. *phalanges* [*not* the expected "line of battle" or "heavy infantry in battle order," but "round piece of wood" or "log"—here assumed to be a diminutive in its adapted form—as used by Herodotus, *Histories,* III, 97]), *phalanges* appeared in medical English in the early eighteenth century. By the nineteenth century, *phalange* had become the singular of *phalanges,* and the original derivation (*phalanx* ["small log"]) was forgotten, engendering an understandable puzzlement from medical lexicographers. Dunglison's *Medical Lexicon* (1855), 661, reflects this quirky confusion: "*Phalanx, Phalange, Phalangoma* . . . A name given to the small bones which form the fingers and toes, because placed alongside each other like a phalanx." *Digitorum* is the genitive plural of the Latin *digitus* ("finger" or "toe"), and *manus* is the genitive singular of *manus* ("hand"). There are fourteen phalanges, three for each finger and two for the thumb. In older texts of osteology, the thumb is termed the *pollex* (gen. *pollicis*), the classical Latin word for "thumb" or "big toe."

BONES OF THE LEG AND FOOT

The *femur* (Latin for "thigh" [gen. sing. *feminis* or *femoris;* nom pl. *femora,* showing its neuter gender]) is the longest—and strongest—bone of the body and presents an almost perfect cylinder for most of its length. The ball-like *caput femoris* (Latin "head of the thigh," here adapted as "head of the femur") fits nearly into the hip socket called the *acetabulum* (above under "Bones of the Pelvis: Coxa") and functions as a classic ball-and-socket joint. Connecting the head of the femur to the main body of the bone (at an angle slightly more than 120°) is the *collum femoris* (Latinate for "neck of the femur"), an extremely compact section of bone that serves well in the efficient distribution of the weight stresses from the body's trunk into the bones of the leg and foot. At the juncture of the *collum femoris* and the upper part of the main body of the femur (sometimes appearing in Latin as *corpus femoris*) occurs a large and irregular, quadrilateral eminence called the *trochanter major* (Greek *trochantēr* ["one of two processes at the head of the thigh bone," in Galen, *Use of Parts,* II, 309, and XV, 8] + Latin *maior* [comparative of *magnus* ("great")], thus "greater trochanter"), which serves, among many functions, as the insertion of the gluteus medius tendon along with a partial attachment of the tendon from the great gluteus maximus muscle (see below, chap. 7: Muscles). The *tro-*

chanter minor (Latin's *minor* ["smaller" or "lesser"], thus "lesser trochanter") is a prominent protuberance at the juncture of the base of the femur's neck with its body.

The distal end of the femur also displays structures demonstrating the remarkable engineering and architectural functions of bones in the human body: roughly twinned knobs form the bottom end of the femur, knobs that bear the names *lateral* and *medial condyle* (Greek *kondylos* [usually "knuckle," as in Aristotle, *HA*, 493b28, but in later Greek, "knuckle of various joints," for example, that of the humerus and elbow, in Pollux, *Onomasticon*, II, 141]). *Lateralis* is Latin for "of the side" (the noun *latus*, gen. *lateris* ["side" or "flank"]), engendering the English *lateral*; and Latin's *medius* is "middle" or "of the middle," Englished as *medial*. A much more common meaning in classical Greek for *kondylos* was in the context of hitting someone (with the fists), as one reads in Aristophanes' comic play *Peace*, l. 123. Seventeenth-century English had the word *condyl* (the superfluous final *e* comes from the French form of the word), which meant exactly what the Greek word meant in the fifth century B.C.: "The stroke inflicted with the hand thus composed, hath from antiquity retained the name of Condyl" (*OED*, s.v. ref. to John Bulwer, *Chirologia, or the naturall language of the hand* [1644], 180). Just above the condyles on the femur are two *epicondyles* (Greek *epi-* ["upon"] + *kondylos*), also *lateral* and *medial*, which function as originations of the large gastrocnemius muscle and various ligaments of the knee joint; the larger condyles articulate with the tibia (below), beautifully distributing weight stresses, and the anterior surfaces of the condyles articulate with the patella (below).

The *patella* (Latin "small dish" or "small plate," rarely "kneecap") is regarded by some anatomists as one of the irregularly occurring sesamoid bones, since it develops in the tendon of the quadriceps femoris (chap. 7, below). The patella, or kneecap, shields the front of the knee joint and is—as many amateur and professional athletes know too well—subject to frequent injury, not merely from direct blows to the frontal surface of the patella but also from repeated wrenching of the legs in mechanically difficult postures at rapid or jerky speeds and motions. The knee joint is one of the most complex in the body, having eleven ligaments involved in various connections among femur, patella, tibia, and fibula; any of the ligaments yanked just too much in a wrong direction causes excruciating pain, and healing is slow. Latin's *patella* is the diminutive of *patina* ("shallow pan"), and *patella* as "kneecap" occurs rarely in classical Latin: Celsus in his *De medicina* is the first to record *patella* as "kneecap," although he writes *patellam vocant* ("they call it the patella" [VIII, 1.25]), suggesting he has gained his special term either from written texts or from medical informants. *Patella* entered medical English in the late seventeenth century.

The *tibia* (Latin for "shinbone") is the second-largest bone of the body, and unlike the cylindrical form of the femur, the shape of the tibia is *prismoid* (Greek *prisma* ["something sawed"], Latinized to *prisma* in the sixteenth century to mean—usually—"a transparent, solid body, frequently with triangular bases, employed for dispersion of light into its spectrum of colors"—thus English *prism* + *-oid* ["similar to" or "like"]). The top of the tibia is equipped with medial and lateral condyles (above, under *femur*), but the tibia's distal and medial end has a prominent medial *malleolus* (Latin "small hammer" = *malleus* ["hammer" or "mallet"] + *-olus* [a diminutive suffix]), which articulates with the talus bone of the ankle (below). The meaning of "shinbone" for *tibia* in classical Latin is fairly rare, with instances occurring in Celsus, *De medicina,* VIII, 1.26; Pliny, *NH,* XXII, 69; and the *Compositiones,* 162 (a book on drugs) by Scribonius Largus. Most ordinary as a meaning for *tibia* among the Romans was "reed pipe," a musical instrument. The term as "shinbone" came into medical English in the late seventeenth century.

The outer and thinner of the two bones of the lower leg is the *fibula* (classical Latin, using "pin," "clasp," "brooch," and several other rather ordinary meanings), which is the slenderest of the long bones. The *caput fibulae* ("head of the fibula" [Late Latin]) has several surfaces on its irregular quadrate form, one of which articulates with the lateral condyle of the tibia; the *caput fibulae* also displays a *styloid* process (Late Latin coinage from Latin *stilus* ["pointed writing instrument"], traditionally *stylus* from a false association by Renaissance savants with Greek *stylos* ["column"]), which does vaguely resemble a writing quill. The fibula's distal extremity includes a *lateral malleolus* (as above under *tibia*), which articulates in part with the talus bone of the ankle (below). Renaissance and Enlightenment anatomists were reminded of a tongue of a clasp when they saw the fibula—the tibia forming the other part of this bony "clasp." *Fibula* appears in Monro's *Anatomy of Human Bones,* 3d ed., 287, as a term commonly used in anatomy and osteology.

Modern osteology preserves only one part of the ancient meaning for *fibula,* which to Romans—if used to mean "clasp" or "brooch"—included both "tongue" and "clip" side (most Roman *fibulae* resembled modern belt buckles, with early versions that look like ornate paper clips). Yet in Roman medicine and widely practiced sexual customs, *fibulae* were most frequently "pins." Celsus tells us that "if a wound is gaping in the flesh with its edges not easily drawn together, sewing them together is unsuitable: then *fibulae* (the Greeks call them ancteres) are to be inserted, and they draw together the edges somewhat, and the resultant scar would be less broad" (*De medicina*, V, 26.23B); the "pin" would be passed through the wound margins, then fixed by a thread twisted around it in a figure eight. *Fibulae* also were commonly inserted into the prepuces ("foreskins") of actors and singers in the early Roman Empire, since it was believed that abstension from sexual intercourse preserved one's voice. Celsus, *De medicina*, VII, 25.3, terms this *infibulare adulescentulos* ("to put fibulae into the prepuces of young men"), commenting that such is done *interdum vocis, interdum valetudinis causa* ("occasionally for the sake of the voice, or sometimes for the sake of health"), implying that if young men's penises were "inoperable," there would be less inclination to frequent the ever present prostitutes. *Infibulation* is a learned term in modern English used to describe how various peoples customarily have performed surgical and other techniques on their youngsters (both male and female) to prevent sexual intercourse, and such customs evoked mirth from Roman poets, especially Martial, the composer of often lewd epigrams. The following is illustrative:

Fibula. Dic mihi simpliciter, comoedis et citharoedis,
   fibula, quid praestas? Carius ut futuant.
(*Fibula*. Tell me frankly, O fibula, what you provide to comic-actors
   and cithara-players? "That they fuck more expensively.")
                                        —Martial, *Epigrams*, XIV, 215

The expense was in paying to have the fibula removed. Modern osteology's *fibula* reflects the belt-buckle clasps of Roman antiquity, but the term has lost its splendidly Roman sense of sexual puns—unless one happens to be an anthropologist familiar with *infibulation*.

The *tarsus* (Late Latin from the greek *tarsos* ["flat of the foot," in Homer and Herodotus, and "ankle," in Galen, *Use of Parts*, III, 6]), or *ossa tarsi* ["bones of the ankle"]), has seven bones: *calcaneus, talus, cuboid, navicular,* and three *cuneiform* bones (numbered I–III).

The *calcaneus* (Late Latin derived from Latin's *calx*, gen. *calcis* ["back part of the foot" or "heel"]), or *os calcis* ("bone of the heel"), is the largest of the tarsal bones and has six surfaces on its rather irregular cuboidal form for insertion of a number of tendons and articulation with the talus and cuboid bones (below).

The *talus* (Latin for "ankle bone" or "ankle"), sometimes called the *astragalus* (from Greek *astragalos* [a "neck vertebra" in Homer, but "ankle bone" in Galen (Moore, ed. and trans.), *Introduction to the Bones,* 24]), is the second largest of the bones of the tarsus. Several surfaces of this unsymmetrical bone articulate with the tibia, fibula, calcaneus, and navicular. Older texts say the common name for the *talus* is the "hucklebone," and *talus* has become standard only in the twentieth century in medical English. This bone "sits atop the arch of the foot like a keystone" (Cartmill, Hylander, and Shafland, *Human Structure,* 302).

The *cuboid* (from Greek *cybos* ["cube"] + *-oid* ["like"]) bone, or *os cuboideum,* is on the lateral side of the foot, in front of the calcaneus. Resembling less a cube than a rounded pyramid, the cuboid articulates with the calcaneus, third cuneiform, and fourth and fifth metatarsal bones (below).

The *navicular* (above under *carpus* for "boat-shaped wristbone"), sometimes labeled the *scaphoid* bone (Greek *skaphē* ["boat"] + *-oid,* thus "boat-shaped" or "boatlike") or the *os naviculare pedis* ("the boat-shaped bone of the foot" [Latin *pes,* gen. *pedis* ("foot")]) to distinguish it from the same-named bone of the wrist, is on the medial side of the tarsus, in front of the three cuneiform bones.

The *cuneiform* bones (Latin *cuneus* ["wedge"] + *forma* ["shape" or "form"]), usually numbered I, II, and III from the medial to the dorsal, are roughly six-sided wedges of blunt shapes.

The *metatarsus* (*meta-* [Greek for "beyond" or "after"] + *tarsus*) has five bones, normally numbered from the medial as *ossa metatarsalia I–V.* The *os metatarsale I* is the metatarsal bone of the big toe, and so on in sequence.

The *phalanges* of the foot, or *phalanges digitorum pedis* (above under "*phalanges* of the hand" for *phalanges* and *digitorum,* and above under "*tarsus: navicular*" for *pedis*), are similar in number and arrangement to those of the hand, with two phalanges in the big toe and three apiece in the rest of the toes. Sometimes nineteenth-century anatomy books show the big toe as a *hallux* (coined Latin as corrupted from *allex,* gen. *allecis,* or *hallex,* gen. *hallicis*), a made-up term appearing first in the early nineteenth century. Given its confused and murky etymology, one assumes that *hallux* has dropped out of medical English, but not quite: "The elongated 'thumb' of the human foot—the big toe, or *hallux*—is tied tightly to the side of the second toe by a deep transverse ligament and is permanently adducted. Grasping is no longer possible, and the hallux's joints and muscles have been modified accordingly" (Cartmill, Hylander, and Shafland, *Human Structure*, 299).

Classical Latin's *alec* or *hallec* or *hallex* is the name for the sediment of an incredibly rancid (and highly prized) fish sauce called *garum*, as suggested by Cato the Elder's *Agriculture*, 58, and Pliny, *NH*, IX, 66. Food fanciers craved the stuff—perhaps as Martial, *Epigrams*, III, 77.5, writes *putri cepas allece natantis* ("onions swimming in rotten fish-sauce")—and it was well known as smelling like carrion. One ponders how fermented fish sauce, made from fish intestines, became medical Latin's "the big toe": late Roman and early medieval lexicographers began the lengthy history of erroneous association of *alec* with several similar-sounding terms, showing how even ancient etymologists were sometimes reduced to learned guesswork, much as are their modern counterparts.

Alternative meanings and associations for *allec* perhaps underpin this etymological quandary, but Isidore of Seville's *Etymologiarum*, XII, 6.39, says simply that *allec* is a kind of liquid sauce made from little fish, and Sextus Pompeius Festus, in his *De verborum significatu*, s.v. *hallus* (ed. Lindsay, 91), records that *hallus* = *pollis pedis* ("thumb" of the foot [but *pollis* is an alternative nominative form of *pollen*; Festus and his sources may have corrupted *pollex*, gen. *pollicis*, to the short-form *pollis*]). Festus, s.v. *allus* (ed. Lindsay, 7), however, wrote *allus* = *pollex* ("thumb" and "big toe") and added a muddled bit about how *hallesthai* in Greek reflects similar usage of what Festus calls *proximum digitum* ("next digit") in leaping or acting (probably twitching) against something (*hallesthai* is an infinitive form of the Greek verb *hallomai* and meant "to leap upon" in its most common usage). Du Cange's great lexicon of medieval Latin *Glossarium mediae* (s.v. *hallus*) shows that this word had become embedded in medieval commentaries as an equivalent of the Greek words *podos megas daktylos* ("a big digit of a foot"). And the introduction of *hallux* into medical English occurs late, almost as a kind of osteological afterthought: "The first [toe] is also called the Great Toe (hallux)" (*OED*, ref. Robert Knox, trans., *Cloquet's System of Human Anatomy* [1831], 161). Presumably, medical French had adopted *hallux* sometime before.

This digression on the peculiar etymological problems of how *hallux* became "the bone of the big toe" from Latin's *alec*, or "fermented fish sauce," illustrates an important aspect of medical and scientific derivations in English: it shows how *hallux* is, indeed, the exact term for "big toe" if one chooses a Latinate term, but it also shows that the underpinnings of Latin or Greek (or any other language) often are *not* the meanings adopted or adapted into modern medical English.

CHAPTER 6

NERVES

AN astonishing aspect of human anatomy is the nervous system, enabling us to exist in a marvelously varied world stuffed with colors and sounds, sensations and odors and tastes—all somehow translated into the interlocking, four-dimensional panorama that is human existence. Anatomically, one can easily demonstrate the nerves and the translation organ, the brain, but understanding exactly what the brain and nerves "do" remains beyond modern medicine and neurophysiology. Arguments about what and how the brain "works" and just what sensations "are" have raged since classical antiquity, and Clarke and Dewhurst's curiously murky summary of what was not known in the past and what still remains unknown (penned in the early 1970s) continues to be aptly pertinent: "The extensive literature on the localization of cortical function is still lacking in coherence and abounds with inconsistencies. It covers a wide range of disciplines and without mastery of all of them a balanced and critical appraisal is well nigh impossible." (Clarke and Dewhurst, *Brain Function*, 126).

Clarke and Dewhurst deliberately focus their quandary on problems in comprehending a minuscule facet of the brain's structure—tiny as viewed from the vantage of the gross anatomy of the brain—the cerebral cortex, literally the "bark of the brain" (Latin's *cortex* usually means "bark" or "rind"). Much is known about how this outer layering of the brain (sometimes simply termed *gray matter*) controls specific functions, and even more is known about the multiple interconnected pathways linking the cerebral cortex with other, more inward parts of the brain, parts that have primary roles in translating what is perceived by the senses into conscious recognition. There is far more here than what Restak likes to call "the enlightened machine" in his book *The Brain*. But how can one express what the brain does in terms other than mechanical?

Modern physics teaches that even the numberless neurons and their seemingly endless functions are quite limited in what they can do, however anatomists and physiologists might study them:

Knowledge derived from physics informs us that the world from which we obtain sensory information is very different from the world as we experience it. We know that the universe consists of electromagnetic fields, atomic particles, and the empty spaces that separate atomic nuclei from the charged particles that spin around them. The picture the brain creates is limited by the range of stimuli to which our senses are attuned, a range that renders us incapable of perceiving large segments of the electromagnetic spectrum. (Rock, *Perception*, 3).

Even within these severely restricted limits, one cannot state exactly what the nerves and brain "do" but can only provide an always circular definition, much as is given by Restak, *The Brain*, 7: "The brain is a collection of nerve cells. Nerve cells compose the brain." These definitions cannot tell us, either from the specifics of neuroanatomy or from the particulars of neurophysiology or neurophysics, what *is* the nature of sensation, or what *is* intelligence. Anatomy (or physics), for all of their precision, cannot answer "What is mind? or "What is soul?" or "What is seeing and perceiving?" All are basic questions, and all were posed early in the history of philosophy.

Human thinking (however defined, whatever one calls it) was deemed awesome by earliest humankind, and by the time of the beginnings of Greek philosophy in the thoughts of the Nature Philosophers in the sixth century B.C., there is clear indication of long pondering on why things are and why people perceive things as they do. Thales of Miletus (about 585 B.C.) taught that the world originates from water and that all things eventually return to their original state; by positing a primordial and eternal substance, Thales could thereby assume that his "eternal water" was divine and that objects and thoughts about objects were also divine, or as a later Greek proverb put it (attributed to Thales), "All things are full of gods." And early Greek—illustrated by the passage in Homer's *Iliad*, IV, 122—already had the word *neuron* (pl. *neura*) meaning "bowstring," among several definitions. A *neuron* literally was a "sinew" or "tendon" used to make bowstrings, strings for the lyre, sandal thongs, and similarly practical, tough, and twinelike cords. Homer's warriors knew well wnough what *neura* looked like, observing exposed tendons and sinews resulting from the battle wounds so graphically depicted by the poet. Yet *neura* included more than tendons, since many tendonlike structures were also called *neura* (alternatively *neurai*, with the feminine singular *neura*), those sinews obviously not linked to muscles.

Greek philosophy had a peculiar manner of asking essential questions about human life in its physical existence as part of the physical universe and then coupling these questions with those aimed at probing why a human being could and should be able to think about the cosmos and feel the emotions of music and poetry—perhaps evoked by sunsets, the birth of a child, the motions and colors of the sea, or literally thousands of daily experiences. Greek philosophy chose to examine these matters in a way that did not necessarily deny religion but that attempted to explain them through pure reasoning, through speculation leading to hypotheses and some kind of logical conclusion according to observable data. If one begins with Thales's speculations, one immediately notes that Greek thought assumed Nature (Greek *physis*, from which all *physico-* and *physica-* words emerge, with "physics" presumably *the* study of nature in its truest sense) was alive in all forms; thus, thought had a life of its own. But how to explain the origin of thought? Homeric Greek used *noos* (in later Attic Greek, *nous*) to mean "mind," "sense," "thought," and a wide swatch of corollary meanings, with an occasional inclusion of what we would term "feeling," as in our idiomatic "with all my heart." By the fifth century B.C., *nous* could also mean simply "reason" or "intellect," but thinkers debated how this power (Greek *dynamis*, hence derivative words like *dynamic, dynamo*, etc.) came to be and where in the body it properly would have its origins. Fifth-century Greek now also had a refined meaning for *epistēmē* (broadly, "skill" or "understanding"), which could become "knowledge" in the writings of Plato and Aristotle. If *epistēmē* was "knowledge" in the true sense, it would be by definition the opposite of *doxa* (usually, "opinion"), the normal manner of thinking criticized by Socrates (469–399 B.C.), his student Plato, and Plato's student Aristotle. Plato argued that the intellect had its seat in the brain, whereas Aristotle believed that the heart was the home of this power, due to how one "felt" emotions. The philosophic debate between Platonists and Aristotelians eventually led to systematic dissection, in an attempt to decide which theory was closer to the truth.

The whirlwind career of Alexander the Great (King of the Macedonians, 336 B.C. to his death at age thirty-three in 323 B.C.) included not only the rapid military conquest of Asia Minor, the Near East, Egypt, what is now Iraq, Iran, Afghanistan, and parts of central Asia and western India but also the shrewd establishment of cities at selected and strategic locations. Most of these new settlements were named, naturally enough, Alexandria, with the most important of the implanted Greek cities being the Alexandria in Egypt, which became the capital of the Greek-speaking rulers of Egypt, the Ptolemies (after Ptolemy I, a commander under Alexander), a dynasty lasting from about 305 B.C. to 30 B.C., with the death of the last of the Ptolemaic line, the famous Cleopatra VII. Ptolemaic Alexandria swiftly became a flourishing emporium and one of the most important intellectual centers in classical antiquity, due in large part to Ptolemy's open patronage of scholars, poets, and learned men of many varieties. At state expense, Ptolemy I (305–282 B.C.) and Ptolemy II (282–246 B.C.) sponsored the residence of famous scholars in the Alexandrian Museum ("Temple to the Muses"), flanked by the finest library then in existence. "Research" by the resident savants most often was study and commentary on the great literary classics of Greece, but occasionally some startlingly original work took place, as in the instances of anatomy and physiology.

The beginnings of modern approaches to anatomy and physiology emerged in the systematic dissection of human cadavers at Ptolemaic Alexandria by Herophilus (about 280 B.C.) and his younger contemporary Erasistratus. For the first time in history, anatomy was learned directly from human structures, not by analogous comparison with animals, as had been the case with Aristotle's dissections. Herophilus described the large divisions of the brain as *enkephalos* ("within the head," a term for "brain" first in Greek with Homer's *Iliad,* III, 300), differentiated from what he termed the *parenkephalis* ("beside the brain"); the two terms were earlier used for these structures by Aristotle in *HA*. Herophilus's *enkephalos* and *parenkephalis* later became the familiar Latin *cerebrum* and *cerebellum* (for derivations, see below), but he thought he had the "answer" to the long-simmering philosophical debate about the seat of the intellect: it was located in the "hollow cavity" (*anaglyphē kalamou*) of his *parenkephalis*. The later Latin translation of *anaglyphē kalamou* is *calamus scriptorius* ("hollow reed for writing"), quite vividly indicating Herophilus's immediate need to "coin" terms to describe something new he had observed in dissection. Ancient pens were, of course, hollowed reeds, so that Herophilus's analogy was to a common object in everyday use in contemporary Alexandria (modern anatomy texts still, on occasion, label the small cavity at the rear of the fourth ventricle as the *calamus Herophili* ["the pen of Herophilus"]). It was Herophilus who discovered that *neura* originated in the brain and that these tendonlike structures provided the body with sensations; moreover, Herophilus was the first to distinguish between what we call motor and sensory nerves. Yet almost as important as his discoveries from human dissection were Herophilus's attempts to provide precise names for the structures he observed, making him "a pioneer [in] . . . medical terminology. Before the Hellenistic period there is but scant evidence of the use of technical terminology in Greek medicine" (Longrigg, "Anatomy in Alexandria," 471). This struggle for precision in terminology in the medical and biological sciences thus has a lengthy history, going back at least to the dissections of Herophilus and Erasistratus at the Alexandrian Museum in the third century B.C.

The English word *nerve* is the Anglicized form of the Latin *nervus*, which had multiple meanings in classical Latin. Much as *neuron* (cognate in Greek with Latin's *nervus*) meant "sinew" or "tendon," among a number of things, so too *nervus* could mean simply "sinew" (for example, in Cicero, *Nature of the Gods,* II, 139, and Celsus, *De medicina,* II, 10.5). Another meaning for *nervus* was "plant fiber" (in Pliny, *NH,* XIX, 90 [borrowing this meaning from the *neuron* as "plant fiber" in Plato, *Politicus,* 280c]), and Horace, *Satires,* II, 7.82, uses *nervus* to mean "puppet string." Cicero, in his *Flaccus,* 13, however, has the plural *nervi* as "strength of mind," and Varro, *Agriculture,* III, 5.13, has *nervus* as the expected "animal tendon." Quite common too in ordinary speech was *nervus* as "penis," suggested by Juvenal, *Satires,* IX, 34. The analogy remains: cord, thong, bowstring, tendon, fiber, and the links with mental functions and the full range of human feelings.

THE BRAIN AND ITS PARTS

Names for various parts of the brain, first dissected and described by Herophilus in the third century B.C., generally suggest shape or function by analogy, although sometimes the terms come directly from Latin and retain basic earlier meanings:

> *Cerebrum* is classical Latin for "brain," in Cicero, *Tusculan disputations,* I, 19, in Vergil, *Aeneid,* IX, 753, and in a number of other writers. Other meanings for *cerebrum* among the Romans include "top of the head" (Pliny, *NH,* XXXII, 138), "seat of intelligence" (Lucretius, VI, 803), "anger" (Petronius, *Satyricon,* 75.6), and "terminal bud of a palm" (Pliny, *NH,* XIII, 36).

> *Cerebellum* is a Late Latin coinage from *cereb[rum]* + *-ellum* (a diminutive suffix), thus "little brain." Classical Latin's *cerebellum,* however, could mean simply "the brain" (Celsus, *De medicina,* II, 18.8; Pliny, *NH,* XXX, 112; and Scribonius Largus, *Compositiones,* 43) or "the seat of the intellect and senses" (Petronius, *Satyricon,* 76.1).

The cerebrum is encased inside an extraordinary triplicate layering of membranes, with added cushioning provided by two intermediate levels of fluids. The membranes are often termed *meninges,* a seventeenth-century medical Latin borrowing from the Greek *mēninx* (pl. *mēninges*). Aristotle, *HA,* 495a8, used *mēninx* to designate "the membrane enclosing the brain" in animals, and seventeenth-century anatomists realized how appropriate was the Latinized word, still employed today. Just beneath the bone of the skull is the first of these membranes, termed the *dura mater* (Renaissance Latin for "hard mother"). This curious name has nothing to do with origins in either Latin or Greek: late medieval Latin medical texts included a fair number of works translated from the Arabic, and *dura mater* is a literal translation of the Arabic *umm al-qalīdah* or *umm al-jāfīyah,* following the manner in Arabic of expressing relationships between things as "father," "mother," "son," and so on. *Dura mater* as a specific term, designating the tough, outer membrane of the brain and spinal cord, entered medical English as early as 1400. Immediately under the *dura mater* is a widely dispersed level of veins, which drain blood from the brain; collectively, these venous channels (which lack valves) are usually called the *dural sinus* ("cavity" or "hollow" of the *dura mater;* Latin's *sinus* [pl. also *sinus*] usually meant "the cavity or fold made by the looping of a garment," or simply "hollow," "depression," or "cavity").

The *arachnoid* is the second membrane encasing the cerebrum, and the name means "spider-web-like," coined from the Greek by anatomists in the mid-eighteenth century to suggest the delicate, wispy appearance of this membrane, which bridges the cerebrum's many fissures and crevices. Pulled from the Greek's *arachnoeidēs* ("cobweblike"), the term became standard, since it did describe this filmy, filament-filled but bloodless membrane. Underneath the *arachnoid* is the envelope of cerebrospinal fluid, described as "a clear watery fluid . . . [which] fills the ventricles of the brain and occupies the sub-arachnoid space" (Gray, *Anatomy,* 928). And the innermost, tightly wrapped, and highly vascular membrane encapsulating the cerebrum is the *pia mater,* a second example of a translation from Arabic into late medieval Latin. Here, *umm raqīqah* ("tender" or "thin mother") became *pia mater* ("pious mother"), a label that entered medical English by 1400 and that remains standard.

The cerebrum presents a cauliflower-like appearance, characterized by numerous *convolutions* (Latin *convolutus* ["something rolled up" or "coiled"]), or *gyri* (sing. *gyrus* [Latin for "circle" or "coil," derived from the Greek *gyros*]), which are elevations or ridges caused by the infolding of the cerebral cortex, suggesting why these coilings appear as *gyri cerebri* in older anatomy texts. The convolutions (or gyri) are separated by *sulci* (sing. *sulcus* [Latin for "furrow" or "groove" or "fissure"]), each named according to location or after the anatomist given credit for first describing it (for example, the prominent *sulcus lateralis* ["fissure of the side"] is sometimes still called the *fissure of Sylvius,* after Franciscus Sylvius [1614–72], whose dissections of the brain made him famous in his time). The cerebrum is divided into two halves by the *interhemispheric fissure* (Latin *inter* ["between"] + Greek *hēmi-* ["half"] + Latin *sphaera* ["globe," from Greek *sphaira* ("ball")] + Latin *fissura* ["cleaving" or "cleft"]), giving the brain its two *hemispheres* (the "right brain" and "left brain" of the popular literature). A very prominent fold of the dura mater which descends into and ensheaths the interhemispheric fissure reminded Renaissance anatomists of the curved sickle (Latin *falx*) wielded by individuals at harvesttime, so that *falx cerebri* became the label for this infolding of the dura mater.

Connecting the extension of the spinal column (the *medulla oblongata* [Latin's *medulla* ["marrow"] + *ob* + *longus* + *-ata,* to make "the elongated marrow"]) with the pathways and structures of the cerebrum is the appropriately named *pons* (Latin for "bridge"). Between the pons and the complicated inner recesses of the undersurfaces of the cerebral hemispheres are several structures in what some anatomists call the *midbrain*. Collectively, the medulla, the pons, and the midbrain function in carrying out *autonomic* missions (Greek *autonomos* ["with laws of one's own"]). For the midbrain, older texts of anatomy carry the labels *mesencephalon* (Greek *mēsos* ["middle"] + *enkephalos* ["within the head"]) or *diencephalon* (Greek *dia* ["between"] + *enkephalos*), and the current *midbrain* incorporates the formerly acceptable "middle brain" and "in-between brain." Among the many structures in the midbrain are:

> The *thalamus* (Greek *thalamos* ["woman's bedchamber" or simply "bedroom"]), which "translates" sense perceptions (except for smell) for the cerebrum.
>
> The *hypothalamus* (Greek *hypo* ["under"] + *thalamos*), a kind of control center for nutritional requirements, levels of bodily chemicals termed *endocrines* (see chap 12, below), and general coordination of the autonomic nervous system.

Some neurophysiologists consider the thalamus and hypothalamus as but two parts of what they term the *limbic* system (Latin *limbus* ["border" or "edge"]), a rather modern Latinate adaptation entering medical English in the mid-1950s. The *limbic* system is the ring of interconnected structures in the midline of the brain just below the cerebral hemispheres, more or less centered around the hypothalamus, and these structures have important (if poorly understood) roles in emotions and memory, as well as in *homeostatic* regulations (Greek *homoios* ["same" or "similar"] + *stasis* ["state of standing"], thus "maintenance of internal stability" in medical English). The lower arm of the paired limbics is termed the *hippocampus* (Greek for "sea horse"), a very strained analogy. A small knob of nerve *ganglia* (sing. *ganglion* [Greek for "swelling on a tendon"]) nestled next to the hippocampus is named the *amygdala* (Greek *amygdalon* ["almond"]), which does resemble an almond and which seems to have a role in expressions of fear and aggression.

THE CRANIAL NERVES

Beginning students of anatomy are always faced with the task of memorizing the names of the twelve cranial nerves in their proper order, an exercise traditional for medical students since the Renaissance. A common mnemonic (Greek *mnēmē* ["memory"]) nonsense line remains popular, and students of comparative anatomy, as well as first-year medical students, charged with mastering a cadaver's parts, retain this mnemonic almost indefinitely: *On Old Olympus' Towering Tops, a Finn and German Viewed Some Hops.*

All twelve in order begin with the *olfactory,* a name based on Latin's *olfactorium* ("a smelling bottle"), a meaning well defined in the Latin of the early Roman Empire as suggested by Scribonius Largus, *Compositiones,* 104. Anatomists have long assumed the analogy to a small, long-necked bottle in considering the shape of the "olfactory bulb," the enlarged end of each olfactory lobe from which the olfactory nerve originates. Modern physiologists do not completely understand how the sense of smell actually works, so that they often speak of olfactory sensations as "primitive."

Number two (the "Old" of the mnemonic) is the large *optic* nerve, so named from medieval Latin's *opticus,* in turn borrowed from the Greek *optikos* ("of" or "for sight"). This very prominent nerve, with its crossed pairing behind the eyes (the optic *chiasma* [named for the Greek letter *chi,* written *X*]), was from early times unmistakable regarding its function. Just *how* images were formed and sent out or received by the brain caused centuries of speculation and philosophical theorizing, but Greek and Roman physiologists and doctors were on the right track when they assumed something must "carry" an image (whichever way they chose to have it go—either from the exterior or from some mysterious imagery power within the brain).

The third cranial nerve ("Olympus") has the name *oculomotor,* a Late Latin coinage combining *oculo-* (*oculus* is Latin for "eye") and *motus* ("mover" [*motus* is a participle of *movere* ("to move")]). This complex cranial nerve innervates most of the muscles attached to the eyeball.

The fourth cranial nerve ("Towering") is the *trochlear,* in this instance derived from the Greek *trochileia* ("a block with pulleys" or simply "pully"). The trochlear is the smallest cranial nerve, and although it often does resemble a pully, variations among cadavers sometimes do not fit the presumed analogy. Even with wide differences in appearance, *trochlear* became the accepted label by the late eighteenth century. The nerve innervates the superior oblique muscle of the eyeball.

Contrasted with the tiny trochlear, the fifth cranial nerve ("Tops") is the largest of the twelve. The label *trigeminal* suggests its three branches (*trigeminus* is Late Latin, combining *tri-* ["triple"] with *geminus* ["twin" or "double"]), and one can translate this as "double-triple" or "twinned triple," indicating the pair of trigeminals, each with its three main divisions. The branches from the three major trunks of the trigeminal nerve innervate the face and provide sensory nerves to the mucous membranes and several internal structures of the head, as well as controlling the chewing muscles. The three major branches are named by their functions and location: the *ophthalmic* (Greek *ophthalmos* ["eye"]), the *maxillary,* and the *mandibular* (both above, chap. 5, under "Some Bones of the Skull"). Your friendly dentist aims his Novocain (procaine hydrochloride) usually at either the maxillary or the mandibular branch of the trigeminal, depending on whether your decayed teeth are in the upper or the lower jaw.

The sixth on the list ("a") is the *abducens,* a name derived from the Latin verb *abducere* ("to draw" or "to take away"). This is a small cranial nerve that innervates the lateral rectus muscle of the eyeball.

Number seven ("Finn") is the *facial* nerve, a label descending from Middle English as derived from Vulgar Latin's *facia,* ultimately stemming from classical Latin's *facies* ("face," "looks," "appearance"). The facial nerve is a complicated, multibranched, multigangliated, internally interconnected series of motor fibers having multiple functions including innervation of the salivary glands, the tear ducts, the soft palate, and the anterior two-thirds of the tongue.

The eighth cranial nerve ("and") is the *acoustic,* so termed from the Greek *akousis,* gen. *akoueōs* ("hearing"), with adjective *akoustikos* ("for hearing," "of hearing"), a nerve occasionally in the anatomy texts as the *vestibulocochlear,* a modern Latinate name that accurately reflects the acoustic nerve's two branches: the *vestibular* (Latin *vestibulum* ["forecourt" or "entrance"]; and the *cochlear* (Greek *kochlias* ["snail with a spiral shell"]). The two branches are those of hearing (the cochlear) and of balance or equilibrium (the vestibular). The "snail shell" label neatly captures the look of the bony cochlea of the inner ear.

The ninth cranial nerve ("German") is the *glossopharyngeal,* created by combining the Greek *glōssa* ("tongue") with Late Latin's *pharyngeus* (derived from the Greek *pharynx,* gen. *pharyngos* ["throat," in general]), so that the name says "tongue-throat." The term indicates how the nerve in its numerous branches innervates the posterior one-third of the tongue and various structures of the neck and throat, as well as neighboring conformations.

Latin's *vagus* ("wandering" or "the wanderer") is the tenth cranial nerve ("Viewed"). In dissection, this is exactly what one thinks of when the vagus nerve is traced along its enormously complicated and extended branches. Among several interconnected ganglia, the multiple branches of the vagus run into and innervate (among other parts) the muscles of the pharynx, the larynx, the heart, and the viscera of the chest and abdomen.

Number eleven of the cranial nerves is the *spinal accessory* ("Some"), or simply the *accessory* nerve, so termed from medieval Latin's *accessorius,* descending from classical Latin's *accessio* ("addition"). In dissection, the spinal accessory appears partially interwoven with the upper ganglia of the vagus, but the accessory nerve has separate paths to muscles of the pharynx, as well as to the trapezius and sternocleidomastoid muscles.

And the last of the twelve is called the *hypoglossal* ("Hops"), a name meaning "under the tongue" (Greek *hypo* ["under"] + *glōssa*). This is the basic motor nerve of the tongue.

Anatomical nomenclature for the cranial nerves is a good model to suggest how names for many parts of the body are coined and why these terms have had such lasting use in medical English. One kind of term will verbally depict what a nerve looks like (vagus, trigeminal, trochlear); once these nerves are seen in actual dissection, their names reinforce their appearances, and they become imprinted in the visual memory. A second type of name will loosely define a particular function (olfactory, optic, oculomotor, abducens, acoustic), so that when one connects the tasks of "smelling," "seeing," "eye-moving," "drawing away," and "hearing" with the names of these nerves, one receives a double memory reinforcement that implants both a context of motion ("smelling" and "seeing" are in a continuous process, as would be what an "eye-mover" would do) and a reinforcement of location and relation to other organs and structures (the nose, the eye, an eye muscle). A third kind of label immediately tells where the nerve is (facial, glossopharyngeal, spinal accessory, hypoglossal), also in a link with other structures (face, tongue and throat, the upper backbone, undersurfaces of the tongue), again reinforcing in the visual memory how and why these nerves function.

To be sure, all terms generally interlock these three objectives, but over the centuries, particular names have worn better than others, and modern medical English has incorporated just those terminologies that portray or define what antomists and physicians presume as "primary" functions. The optic nerve, for example, speaks instantly of seeing—its primary function, as opposed to its location behind the eyes or its appearance as contrasted with other nerves. Yet the vagus, even with its essential role in autonomic regulation and functioning of various upper viscera, remains most vivid in the minds of medical professionals as they reflect on its strange, seemingly confused wanderings in and out of ganglia and in and out of several important organs and structures in the neck and upper chest. One could have named this nerve from one of its basic roles, but since the vagus has so many innervations, a single and functional label would omit many of its other fundamental roles. "The wanderer" encompasses the full appearance and also indicates that this nerve goes here, goes there, and impinges on a number of locations and physiological tasks. In the case of the vagus, leaving the name indicative of its appearance is simple and descriptive.

Smaller nerves, or nerves limited in their expanse or length, can thereby receive names best descriptive of their location, so that the hypoglossal says precisely where one will find it. Yet with the facial nerve, the range of branches might cause one to wonder why this large complex of subthreads should be collectively known as "the facial." Medical English replies that since the "face" is familiar, "facial" is appropriate for its multitudinous functions and multiple innervations. Medical nomenclature seeks simplicity, even as it borrows descriptives and depictions most often from Greek and Latin; that simplicity must connect in some way with what the doctor and anatomist experience daily in practice or in dissection, and the names must transmit a vivid sense of function, place, relationship, or appearance. Medical terms must designate as clearly as possible single things—and only single things.

NERVES OF THE BODY

Traditional anatomists generally class the cranial nerves as part of the *peripheral* nervous system (Greek *peri* ["about," "around," "surrounding," or "enclosing"] + *pherein* ["to bear"]), but most novitiates in anatomy learn the brain and the cranial nerves as a unit (Greek also has *periphereis* ["circumference"], engendering the Late Latin *peripheria,* coming into English as *periphery*). The central nervous system usually includes the brain and the spinal cord, both ensheathed in the meningeal layers described above for the brain. The spinal cord (sometimes still called by the Renaissance Latin *medulla spinalis*) is an extremely elongated extension of the medulla oblongata, and as a "central nerve" for the body, it has the primary task of connecting all peripheral nervous functions with brain-directed responses. Except for its lower tapering to a point (the *conus medullaris* [Greek *kōnos* (pine cone") = Latin *conus*] + *medulla* ["marrow"]) at the second lumbar vertebra, the spinal cord has an average diameter of about one centimeter (.4 inch), and its length is about forty-five centimeters (about eighteen inches [Gray, *Anatomy,* 836, says it weighs about thirty grams or slightly less than one ounce]). Below the conus medullaris, the spinal cord continues down for about twenty centimeters (eight inches) to the first segment of the coccyx as a delicate thread called the *filum terminale* (Latin *filum* ["thread" or "string"] + *terminalis* ["marking a conclusion" or "marking a boundary"]). The vertebral canal (each of the twenty-six vertebrae [see chap. 5 above] has a central hole, or *foramen*) encloses the spinal cord in a cylindrical structure that is both an armor protecting the fragile nervous tissue and also a remarkably flexible pipe equipped with openings, ligaments, and cushions (the often troublesome intervertebral discs) allowing a clear connection between peripheral nerves and the brain while also enabling the body to have its basic support from the backbone (a skilled teacher of anatomy once likened the vertebrae collectively to a "ridgepole" for the body).

Exiting from intervertebral *foramina* (pl. of *foramen*) are thirty-one pairs of spinal nerves, each connected to the spinal cord by three *radices* (Latin *radix* ["root"]), the names of each reflecting specific relationships and neural activities:

Radix anterior: Latin's *anterior* meant "earlier" or "previous," as a comparative form of *ante* ("before" or "in front"), with *anterior* descending into medical English to mean "toward the front plane of the body:" Sometimes the radix anterior is called the *ventral* root (Latin's *ventralis* was a "money belt," as recorded in Justinian's *Digest,* XLVIII, 20.6 [of the sixth century], quoting Ulpian [a jurisconsult of the third century], derived from the basic noun *venter* [usually "belly" or "abdomen"]. In medical English *ventral* means the "front" [anterior] of the human body, and in some texts of neuroanatomy, the radix anterior has the label *motor* root (see *movere* under *oculomotor* nerve, above).

Radix posterior: Latin's *posterior* was "coming after in time" or "later" or "further back," as a comparative form of *posterus* ["later" or "next"], and *posterior* came into English in the sixteenth century to mean "behind," with medical English's special nuance "toward the back plane of the body." Sometimes the radix posterior is termed the *dorsal* root (*dorsum* is "back" in classical Latin, with the derivative medieval Latin adjective *dorsalis* emerging in English as *dorsal* [meaning "back"] by the 1540s), and medical English *dorsal* means "situated toward the posterior plane of the body." A few texts call the radix posterior the *sensory* root (Latin *sensus,* gen. *sensus* ["sensation," "feeling," "understanding"], and *sensus* is also the passive perfect participle of *sentire* ["to feel"]).

Sympathetic root: Greek's *sympathēs* meant "affected by like feelings," and the Late Latin derivative *sympatheticus* came into English in the 1640s as *sympathetic.* Until recently, a "sympathetic nerve" in medical English was more or less the same as an "autonomic nerve" (see under *medulla oblongata,* above), but currently neurophysiologists distinguish between sympathetic and *para*sympathetic nerves (Greek *para* ["beside," "by," or "beyond"]), thus outdating this equivalence (sympathetic nerves stimulate the beating of the heart, the dilation of the pupils of the eyes, and similar actions, whereas parasympathetic nerves act in opposition). Occasionally in older texts of anatomy, one finds the sympathetic root called the *gray ramus communicans* (Latin *ramus* ["branch"] and *communicans* [the present participle of *communicare* ("to share with," "to link," or "to impart")]). The fluidity of nomenclatures for the origins of the spinal nerves suggests the struggle for precision among neurophysiologists and neuroanatomists, but each of the "old" and "new" names for the "roots" continually mirrors a borrowing from Latin or Greek.

Contrary to the notion that nerves are simple and thonglike, running from a beginning point in the spinal cord to an end point somewhere in the periphery of the body, an examination in dissection generally reveals a complex intercrossing of nerves, sometimes to the point where anatomists call such crossings and recrossings *plexus* (sing. also *plexus*), a seventeenth-century coinage meaning "network," pulled from the Latin suffix *-plex* (more or less "fold"), derived in turn from the verb *plectere* ("to twine" or "to plait"), with its participle *plexum*. The major plexus are the following:

The *cervical* (Latin *cervix,* gen. *cervicis* ["neck"]) involves spinal nerves that merge into cervical nerves numbered I through V.

The *brachial* (Latin *brachialis* ["belonging to the arm"]) interconnects cervical nerves IV through VIII and thoracic nerves I and II.

The *lumbar* (Latin *lumbus* ["the loins"]) intertwines thoracic nerve XII and lumbar nerves I through V.

The *sacral* (see *os sacrum* in chap. 5, above) weaves together lumbar nerves IV and V, sacral nerves I through V, and the coccygeal nerve.

The *pudendal* (Latin *pudere* ["to fill with shame"], with *pars pudenda* ["the genitals"]) entwines sacral nerves and their branches numbered II through IV.

Within the extended autonomic nervous systems (both sympathetic and parasympathetic), are also the *cardiac* plexus at the base of the heart, close to the arch of the aorta, and the extremely entangled *celiac* plexus (Greek *koiliakos* ["of the bowels"], akin to *koilos* ["hollow"], which becomes Latinated as *coeliacus*), in turn leading to about eleven smaller plexus that include nerve networks in the diaphragm (*plexus phrenicus*), the liver (*plexus hepaticus*), the spleen (*plexus lienalis*), the kidneys (*plexus renalis*), and the testes or ovaries (*plexus spermaticus*). The celiac plexus is widely known as the *solar* plexus, so called by mid-eighteenth-century anatomists because of the "raylike" appearance of its fibers.

The branches and subbranches of nerves as they proceed beyond the roots in the spinal nerves, or the various plexus, generally do have a thonglike appearance—at least the larger ones do. In dissection, a great challenge is tracing the course of smaller and smaller nerves, from trunks to branches; almost all peripheral nerves receive their names according to location—for example, *dorsal scapular,* *suprascapular,* and *subscapular* for three nerves serving the musculature of the shoulder blade. To illustrate how anatomists designate nerves, one can choose a single extension of branches from a plexus; following the courses of two nerves that emerge from the brachial plexus exemplifies the process.

The *axillary* (Latin *axilla* ["armpit"]) is the last branch of the posterior cord of the brachial plexus before the posterior cord becomes the *radial* nerve (for its destination, see *radius* in chap. 5, above); the brachial plexus has three main cords, networking cervical nerves IV through VIII and thoracic nerves I and II. The axillary nerve—the posterior cord's final branch—itself divides into posterior and anterior branches, supplying the *teres minor* and the *deltoid* (see chap. 7, below, "Muscles").

The second and much more involved illustration is the *median* nerve (*medius* [masc.] or *medium* [neuter] is Latin's "middle"), which is the fusion of the brachial plexus's two other major cords, the *medial* (Renaissance Latin's *medialis* ["middle"], drawn from *medium*) and the *lateral* (classical Latin *latus,* gen. *lateris* ["side" or "flank"], with adj. *lateralis* ["of the side"]). The median nerve has no branches above the elbow, but below the elbow the nerve has eight main branches, including the *volar interosseous* (Latin *vola* ["hollow in the palm of the hand or sole of the foot"] + *inter* ["between"] + *osseus* ["bony"]), which innervates the radial half of the *flexor digitorum profundus,* the *flexor pollicis longus,* and the *pronator quadratus. Volar* is a nineteenth-century coinage (*OED* states that the first printed instance in English appeared in an 1814 translation of an Italian manual on hernias), and Dunglison's *Medical Lexicon,* 8th ed. (1855), 910, has the clipped entry: "*vola,* palm—v. manus, palm—v. pedis, sole." The clarity of this "new" term convinced anatomists, so that by the 1870s the term had become standard. *Volar interosseous* says very succinctly "on the palm side, between the bones," that is (more vaguely), on the underside of the lower arm between the radius and the ulna. Once *volar* became widely accepted, anatomists could apty describe *all* aspects of this part of the arm as *volar,* including surface structures.

Similar comparisons apply to the nerves of the legs and the trunk of the body; most are named by location or relationship to other anatomical structures. The Greco-Latinate terminologies, although occasionally not derived from strictly classical roots, certainly enable parts and structures to be labeled precisely. Sometimes, when anatomy and physiology texts describe parts in "plain English," that plain English precedes a "translation" into the usually more succinct Greco-Latinate terms found in most textbooks of anatomy.

CHAPTER 7

MUSCLES

MODERN English has an amazing knack of borrowing terms from other tongues, or pulling names and phrases from subterranean levels, and then either adapting the sharply defined meaning of the foreign word or blurring any deep historical or cultural nuances into a gray fuzz of everyday expressions. We all know what *muscle* means when the word occurs in everyday speech or nontechnical writing; we spend no time reflecting why the term for "little mouse" in classical Latin (*musculus*) should have become the bland word encompassing a little less than half of a human body's mass or the word immediately associated with "strength" or "exertion." Yet the etymology of *muscle* suggests how words always mirror living languages and how words in those languages and their historical successors (and ancestors) generally reflect supple change, sometimes from the general to the specific, sometimes from the precise to the woolly, sometimes both. *Muscle* in English is an example of the last: it is simultaneously a most common, yawn-producing word and a term specific in anatomy for particular structures.

A *mouse* in Latin was *mus*, gen. *muris*, and there are numerous examples of *mus* or a similar rodent in the writings of the late Roman Republic and the early Roman Empire, ranging from Cato the Elder's handbook *On Agriculture* of about 160 B.C. to Pliny's *Natural History* of A.D. 77 (to name but two). Not only did the authors of works on farming and the wonders of nature consider mice and their cousins and the repeated problems endured by Roman farmers from grain losses, but also nontechnical writers frequently made allusion to *mures* (the plural) as part of ordinary life, taken for granted in proverbs and poetry. Without a second thought, Cicero penned in his *Nature of the Gods*, II, 157: *neque enim homines murum aut formicarum causa frumentum condunt* ("men do not store wheat for the sake of mice or ants"). The masterful hexameters of Vergil, *Georgics*, I, 181–82, included: *seape exiguus mus / sub terris posuitque domos atque horrea fecit* ("often the small mouse / underground builds his home and his granaries"). This is the Roman mouse, fuzzy and bland, so ordinary that further comment does not follow.

Vergil's *exiguus mus* fits neatly into his carefully crafted lines, but the requirements of poetry in all languages differ from the needs of everyday speech. Most tongues have a natural tendency to use one word in place of two or more with the same meaning, and the addition of a diminutive suffix to a basic noun achieves this with *musculus* ("little mouse," *mus* + *-culus*) in Latin. Diminutives are very useful in many contexts (our word comes from the Latin verb *deminuere* ["to lessen" or "to make smaller"]). A little or young duck becomes *duckling,* a small or insignificant book is singleworded as *booklet,* and a model of the human body ("little man") receives the simplified *manniken*. Much as the examples from modern English diminutives demonstrate, other languages have also given suffix forms (here German, Latin, and Danish respectively), but Latin's innate suppleness is illustrated through its *-ulus* and *-culus* (for example, *homunculus,* literally "diminutive human being," supposedly made in a flask by alchemists, as one reads in late medieval Latin) and *-ellus* (for example, *novellus* [*novus* ("new") + *-ellus*], "young" or "tender"). Latin's *-ulus* thereby allowed *musculus* = *mus exiguus,* so that Cicero, *Republic,* III, 25, could write "little mice [here *musculi*] emerging up from plowed fields," and Pliny, *NH,* II, 227, could set down a tale about some "little mice born in the water" of a famous Greek spring (*nascuntur aquatiles musculi*). But most important for the history of the word in medical terminologies is the *musculus* mentioned in the context of a "tendon" (*nervus*), an "artery" (here, *arteria*), and a "bone" (*os*) by Celsus, *De medicina,* V, 26.3B, and a drug (*medicamentum*) for *musculi* in Scribonius Largus, *Compositiones,* 101. "Little mice" in the body?

Musculus evoked in readers and speakers alike a mental picture of a small creature with a longish nose, a fat spindlelike midsection, and a long tapering tail (*mus* could also mean "rat" or even larger rodents like the marmot). By analogy, the mouse shape was quite indicative of what Roman anatomists and doctors might see: muscles frequently display "bellies" which "thin" on either end of their attachments to various bones in the form of ligaments and tendons. Greek and Roman religious officials, supervising ceremonial sacrifices of animals, would also observe these "mouse-like" structures, as would Greek and Roman gymnastic experts (and there were as many then as there are now), who would note that these *musculi* connected bones to bones and suggested how given motions of the body came about, from running and jumping to lifting heavy weights and grasping a writing instrument.

MUSCLES AND ANATOMY

Among the many self-proclaimed accomplishments of Galen of Pergamon (A.D. 129–after 210), perhaps the most famous philosopher-physician of classical antiquity, was his skill in the theory and practice of gymnastics. Not only had Galen improved the diet and instituted appropriate exercises for gladiators in his charge at Pergamon in the 150s, but he also became an acidic critic of the professional athletes of his day (especially boxers and wrestlers, who were—so he writes—uniformly stupid). Galen was, moreover, a skilled comparative anatomist and performed many dissections on numerous animals, usually pigs and monkeys (his "monkeys" were Barbary apes, a very close cousin to our Rhesus monkeys, and Barbary apes in those days were still fairly common in North Africa and the Mediterranean regions of southern Europe). In his dissections, Galen had discovered a number of interesting things about what muscles "do," as illustrated by his account of the flexor surface of the forearm:

> ... the first muscle seen is on the surface of the middle of the forearm ... You will see ligaments lying across the articulations, both on the inside and on the outside of the limb. Under them lie the heads of the tendons, on the inner side those that flex the fingers, on the outer side those that extend them. On either side of the ligaments on the inner side is a muscle flexing the wrist. The one is on a line with the little finger, the other with the index finger. On the outside, there is the single muscle in the forearm which extends the wrist as well as two in the radius [ulna] both moving the wrist. The latter also move the thumb ... The heads [tendons] of all the muscles on the outside which I have described have ligaments around them transversely. (Galen, *Anatomical Procedures,* I, 5 (Greek text in Galen, ed. Kühn, Vol. II, 244–45), adapted from Singer, *Galen on Anatomical Procedures,* 13).

Galen's "first muscle seen ... on the surface of the middle of the forearm" is the *palmaris longus* (Latin *palma* + *-aris* ["measuring the width of a palm (hand)"] + *longus,* cognate with English), which has the following description in a widely employed textbook of human anatomy:

The Palmaris longus is a slender, fusiform muscle, lying on the medial side of the [Flexor carpi radialis]. It arises from the medial epicondyle of the humerus by the common tendon, from the intermuscular septa between it and the adjacent muscles, and from the antebrachial fascia. It ends in a slender, flattened tendon, which passes over the upper part of the transverse carpal ligament, and is inserted into the central part of the transverse carpal ligament and into the palmar aponeurosis, frequently sending a tendinous slip to the short muscles of the thumb. Action—Flexes the hand. Nerve—a branch of the median nerve, containing fibers from the sixth and seventh cervical nerves. (Gray, *Anatomy*, 501.)

One may not notice on a first reading that Galen's description is that of a Barbary ape and that the implicit assumption is as startling as it is fundamental in the history of anatomy: by simple analogy, Galen presumes the muscles of his monkey are close enough to those of a human being that they present structures and functions close enough to *be* human muscles. Galen's use of comparative anatomy to analyze human anatomy has its modern counterpart, demonstrated by the following "updated" description:

We still have the palmar aponeurosis just under the skin of our palms. But the finger-flexing muscles and the five fingertip tendons no longer attach to it. The only remnant of the old reptilian setup is a vestigial and sometimes absent little muscle—*Palmaris longus*—that runs down from the humerus's medial epicondyle to insert on the palmar aponeurosis. In early mammals, the five digital tendons attached to the fingertips became detached from the underside of the palmar aponeurosis and gained direct attachments to the finger-flexing muscles in the forearm. The proximal edge of the old palmar aponeurosis was thickened to form the flexor retinaculum, underneath which our liberated digital flexor tendons slide in and out of the palm. In our monkeylike ancestors, the forearm musculature attached to those tendons became more finely subdivided, thus making it possible to flex one digit without flexing all of them. (Cartmill, Hylander, and Shafland, *Human Structure*, 260.)

Galen, Gray, and Cartmill and his colleagues all address several questions regarding form and function among muscles: What do they present as basic appearances? What do they "do"? What do they "do" in relationship with other nonmuscular structures? Why are they formed as they are? How does form fit function? Galen's approach was that of Aristotle: comparative anatomy with analogy as a watchword on both form and function. Gray's views are those common in the mid-nineteenth century (the first edition of his *Anatomy, Descriptive and Surgical,* appeared in London in 1858), with various "systems" laid out (bones, joints, arteries, veins, etc.) for practical application by surgeons, then in much want of good anatomical knowledge. This approach is explicit in Gray's preface; the first sentence reads, "This work is intended to furnish the Student and Practitioner with an accurate view of the Anatomy of the Human Body, and more especially the application of this science to Practical Surgery" (as quoted by Goss, *Henry Gray F. R. S.,* 22). Cartmill, Hylander, and Shafland represent what might be called the revival of the "comparative approach," the modern analogue of the anatomy performed by Aristotle and Galen, with the added details of purely human origin. One notes in the brief quotation on the palmaris longus from *Human Structure* that the anatomists now insert appropriate details of embryology and paleontology on reptiles, vaguely mentioned early mammals, and simian ancestry for humans to indicate how structures "came to be," thereby explaining both what they look like and why they do what they do.

Nevertheless, all three anatomy texts say basically the same things, with an essential focus on specific parts, structures, and functions. The two modern anatomies make this vivid, even as *Human Structure* attempts to use fewer of the traditional Greco-Latinate terms than are found in Gray's *Anatomy.* And although Cartmill and his fellow authors reintroduce some data from comparative anatomy, the basic focus remains almost identical:

. . . the muscle under consideration is called the *palmaris longus.* It "originates" (that is, it "begins") on the humerus's medial epicondyle (see chap. 5, "Bones," under *femur*) and runs down the inner superficial ("surface") aspect of the forearm with a fusiform belly (Latin *fusus* ["spindle"]) and ends by a long tendon (from Latin *tendere* ["to stretch"]) inserted (that is, "ends") into the transverse (Latin *transversus* ["lying across"]) carpal (Late Latin *carpus,* derived from Greek *karpos* ["wrist"]) ligament (medieval Latin *ligamentum* ["band" or "tie"]) and into the palmar (Latin *palma,* as above) *aponeurosis* (Greek *apo* ["from" or "away"]

+ *neuron* ["sinew" or "tendon"]). *Aponeurosis* (used by both modern anatomy texts as quoted) is a curious and initially confusing term, unless one knows the multiple meanings of *neuron* in Greek—including "tendon" or "sinew." In anatomical terminology, the word means a fibrous sheet or expanded tendon, which provides attachment to muscle fibers and serves as either the point(s) of origin or insertion of a flat muscle (the long tendon of the palmaris longus is flattened), and an aponeurosis sometimes functions as does a *fascial* layer (Latin *fascia* ["band" or "bandage"]) sheathing muscles, additionally attaching to another muscle or bone or ligament.

Terminology clearly shows muscles "do" the following: connect bones without making such links rigid; tie bones together through ligaments and tendons to enable particular movements to take place (the palmaris longus is a *flexor* [from Latin's *flectere* ("to bend")] of the wrist); ensure through attachments, usually by ligaments, that the freely movable joints (where two bones "join" [here Middle English, derived from the Latin *iungere* ("to join")] articulate ("join together" from Latin's *articulare* ["to be jointed"]) and move only so far that the multiple structures (bone + cartilage [Latin *cartilago* ("gristle")] + ligaments + tendons + muscles and fascia) retain a basic, quasi-rigid form for the body as a whole. In traditional gross anatomy, *joints* and *articulations* are treated as synonyms; in the freely movable joints, the surfaces of the bone ends are completely separate from one another, with the bones that are forming the articulation often expanded to facilitate their connections, and the articulating surfaces are covered by cartilage and encased by capsules of fibrous tissue. The *synovial* membrane (Late Latin *syn* [from Greek ("with")] + *ovum* ["egg"], thus "eggwhite-like")—the inner lining of the capsule—secretes synovial fluid, which acts as a lubricant for the joints. Ligaments generally strengthen the joints, and the ligaments extend between the bones that form the joints.

Anatomists call the human skeleton an *endoskeleton,* as contrasted with the *exoskeletons* of insects and many arthropods. Modern anatomists generally tend to "explain" their observed structures through developmental anatomy, using the traditional techniques of comparative anatomy to suggest why structures seen in the human body are related to similar (and dissimilar) structures in other mammals, as well as in birds, reptiles, and occasionally amphibians. "Function" is thereby assumed to be part of a developmental pattern, traced through an evolutionary track and documented by both embryology and fossil finds. And when the authors of *Human Structure* "explain" the palmaris longus as a "remnant" of a reptile's musculature, they are linking the "function" of this small muscle to the manner of use by such reptiles as alligators and crocodiles. The "form" of the present muscle in humans is thus subservient to its former "function."

Myology (Greek *mys* ["mouse" or "muscle" and sometimes "whale," "filefish," "jerboa," and "mussel"] + *logos*) is the special study of muscles. There are about 360 muscles listed separately in anatomical references, added to 70 groups of muscles that act together (often given the specific label *musculi*), and there are about 30 designations for the muscles that move through the intestinal tract, circulate the blood, and contribute to the operation of internal organs. The study of muscles involves far more than mere form: one considers how muscles "work" in terms of *histology* (Greek *histos* ["warp fixed to the beam of a loom," that is, the "web of a loom"] + *logos*; in modern medicine, *histology* emerged as a word in the 1850s to describe the "study of microscopic structures of organic tissues"), how muscles respond to the commands of the central nervous system through an elaborate electrochemical process involving muscle spindles (myological equivalents of sense organs enabling muscles to measure strain, thereby allowing the establishment of proper tension) and the release of *acetylcholine* (an early-twentieth-century coinage combining Latin *acetum* ["vinegar"] + Greek *hylē* ["matter," "substance"] + Greek *cholē* ["bile"] + Latin suffix *-inus* ["of the nature of" or "made of"]) from motor nerve endings to transmit impulses across *synapses* (sing. *synapse,* from Greek *synapsis* ["point or line of junction"]), and several other physical and chemical actions. Another approach to the study of muscles is through *kinesiology* (Greek *kinēsis* ["movement"] + *logos*): understanding the interrelationships among physiological activities and muscular anatomy that delinate how the body moves. Simply memorizing muscle names cannot ensure a comprehension of why muscles do what they do, but their names reveal aspects of form and function, as well as what anatomists in the past—and present—presume to be clear descriptives.

THREE MUSCLES AND THEIR NAMES: GASTROCNEMIUS, SARTORIUS, STAPEDIUS

The carefully worded summary in Gray's *Anatomy*, 405, deserves quotation to suggest how anatomists think of muscles, as well as to illustrate how muscles have received their names:

> The muscles are the organs of voluntary motion, and by their contraction, move the various parts of the body. The energy of their contraction is made mechanically effective by means of the tendons, aponeuroses, and fasciae which secure the ends of the muscles and control the direction of their pull. They form the dark, reddish masses that are popularly known as flesh, and account for approximately 40 per cent of the body weight. They vary greatly in size. The Gastrocnemius forms the bulk of the calf of the leg; the Sartorius is nearly 2 feet in length, and the Stapedius, a tiny muscle of the middle ear, weighs 0.1 gm and is 2 to 3 mm. in length. In addition to these muscles, which are properly called voluntary, skeletal or striated muscles, there are other muscular tissues which are not under voluntary control, such as the cardiac muscle of the heart and the smooth muscle of the intestine.

This spare synopsis embraces essential elements of what muscles do and what structures allow the muscles to function and mentions the largest and heaviest muscle (the gastrocnemius), the longest (the sartorius), and the smallest (the stapedius) to indicate variations in size as well as action. Gray's examples are also exactly apt to illustrate the nomenclature of muscles, since each of his three names is rooted in Greek or Latin:

> *Gastrocnemius* is a Late Latin derivation from the Greek *gastroknēmē* or *gastroknēmia* ("calf of the leg," as one reads in Aristotle, *HA,* 494a7, and Galen, *Anatomical Procedures,* II, 7 [ed. Kühn, Vol. II, 316]). In Greek, the word meant literally "stomach" or "belly of the leg between the knee and the foot." Greek and Roman anatomists, and their Renaissance successors, again used analogy to name this very important and prominent muscle, which arises (originates) in two heads connected to the condyles of the femur by strong, flat tendons and has its insertion on the *calcaneus* (see chap. 5, above) by means of the famous "Achilles tendon" (*tendo calcaneus*), so called from the tale of Achilles' death from an arrow to his heel, as recorded in Greek legend by Quintus Smyrnaeus (*fl.* in the fourth

century A.D.) in his epic poem the *Posthomerica*, III, 62, as well as in other texts (the *Posthomerica* is sometimes known by its English title, *The Fall of Troy*). Oddly enough, current writers in American English will occasionally use *hamstring* to describe the cutting of the Achilles tendon, to suggest the crippling effect on someone's ability to walk from this nasty punishment meted out to escaped slaves in badly researched historical novels. The historic reality is far worse: slaves in Roman times, and in the *antebellum* (Latin "before the war") American South, indeed were *hamstrung*, but the tendons cut were those at the back of the knee (*hamm* is Old English for "bend of the knee"), essential tendons that act to flex and rotate the leg. If a novelist was to use *hamstring* correctly, the term would indicate severing three major tendons at the rear of the knee: the lateral hamstring tendon of the *biceps femoris* (Latin *bis* ["twice"] + *caput*, gen. *capitis* ["head"] + *femur*, gen. *femoris* ["thigh"], thus "two-headed thigh-muscle"), which inserts onto the head of the fibula (see chap. 5, above); the lengthy tendon of the *semitendinosus* (Latin *semi* ["half"] + Greek *tenōn* ["sinew" or "tendon"], which in medieval Latin became linked with Latin's *tendere* ["to stretch"], thus a muscle that is "half-tendon"), which is inserted onto the upper part of the medial surface of the body of the tibia (see chap. 5, above); and the triple tendons of the *semimembranosus* (*semi*, as above, + Latin *membrana* ["skin" or "parchment"], thus a muscle that is "half-a-parchment," so named from its origin, which expands into an aponeurosis [as above under *palmaris longus*]), which are inserted into the medial epicondyle of the tibia, the lateral condyle of the femur, and into the fascia (also as above) covering the *popliteus* muscle (Latin *poples*, gen. *poplitis* ["knee joint" or "back of the knee"]). Hamstringing a slave meant crippling for life, a punishment reserved for only the most recalcitrant of the recaptured runaways. A crippled slave would be useless to a master.

Sartorius has a dual derivation: Latin's *sartor* ("one who hoes") and the verb *sarire* ("to weed" or "to wield a sickle") suggested one aspect of this muscle, likened to the shape of a small harvesting sickle, since it curves obliquely from the front of the hip to the inner side of the tibia; and Latin's *sarcire* ("to patch" or "to mend" [participle as *sartum*]) gave rise to English's *sartor* ("tailor"), first documented by the *OED* as appearing in 1656. *OED* notes that the sartorius (the muscle) is so named (first appearing in print in 1704) because it was "concerned in producing the crosslegged position in which a tailor sits at his work." In formal, modern English, one can still say that someone is dressed in "sartorial splendor," although well-dressed gentlemen might not know if it is an insult or a compliment.

Stapedius is derived from the presumably Latin *stapes* ("stirrup"), but since the Romans did not use stirrups, the usual dictionary definitions are partially incorrect. One meets *stapes* as "stirrup" first in fourteenth-century Latin (Du Cange, *Glossarium mediae*, VII, 583, col. 1), and *OED* opines that *stapes* is an alteration of the medieval Latin *stapha* (Italian *staffa* ["stirrup"]) combined with Latin's *stare* ("to stand") and *pes* ("foot"), the new word indicating how one mounted a horse in late medieval times. Latin's *scandere* (one meaning was "to jump on a horse") reveals a lack of a "step" from which the rider swung his body over the horse's back from our assumed one-footed (usually the left) standing position. Military technology in the West lacked stirrups until about the ninth century (for this fascinating tale, see White, "The Origin and Diffusion of the Stirrup," in *Medieval Technology* 14–28), so that the famous mailed cavalry of the medieval knights was a fairly late innovation in medieval warfare. Once *stapes* = Italian *staffa* was commonly "stirrup," the word was used to describe anything that looked like a stirrup. Renaissance anatomists regularly scrutinized the works of Galen for omissions and errors, and since he had not described the tiny bones of the inner ear (the *auditory ossicles*) in his *Introduction to the Bones*, sixteenth-century anatomists quarreled over claims of discovery of these ossicles. The texts from the time show that Giovanni Filippo Ingrassia (*c.* 1510–80) was the first to see and describe the stapes (1546), in spite of the assertion by Bartolommeo Eustachi (*c.* 1505–74), in his *De auditis organis* (1563), that he was the first to discover this tiny bone.

The *stapedius* is the tiny muscle inserted into the posterior surface of the neck of the *stapes*, the smallest bone in the body and the innermost of the three tiny bones of the *tympanic* cavity (Greek *tympanon* ["drum"]). The stapes does markedly resemble a miniature stirrup, whereas the *malleus* (the outermost bone of the three) only faintly resembles a ball peen hammer (Latin *malleus* ["hammer" or "mallet"]), and the middle ossicle, named the *incus* (Latin for "anvil"), even more remotely looks like an anvil. One supposes that once *hammer* had been applied as a name for the outer ossicle, the notion of *anvil* would occur by analogy from commonly observed blacksmithing. The *stapes*, however, is unmistakable in its shape, and the term entered medical English by 1670.

As intriguing as the etymologies of Gray's three muscles are, most muscles have received Greco-Latinate names according to basic forms, functions, and location within the body. With some practice and a growing familiarity with Greek and Latin terms for "head," "back," "side," "flat," "large," and "small," for various shapes including rectangles and triangles, and for the names of the bones, one soon begins to understand the terms, in many instances, without recourse to an unabridged dictionary to determine derivations. A good example of how the usual mechanics work in word formation for muscle names is the *sternocleidomastoid:* one knows immediately that the *sternum,* or breastbone, is involved; one also recognizes the *mastoid* process (Greek *mastos* ["breast"], thus here "breastlike") at the base of the skull; but one may not recognize that *-cleido-* comes from the Greek *kleis* ("key"), equivalent to the Latin *clavis* (also "key"), which immediately indicates that the muscle is connected to the *clavicle,* or collarbone. Three bone names label this lateral cervical muscle that passes obliquely across the side of the neck, originating on the sternum and clavicle by two heads and inserting onto the lateral surface of the mastoid process.

A SAMPLING OF MUSCLES: NAMES AND WHAT THEY SAY

Trapezius (Greek *trapezion* ["small table"]) is a name describing the pair of muscles that cover the upper and back part of the neck and shoulders; taken together, these flat muscles do roughly resemble the geometrical shape known as a *trapezium* (from the same Greek word), that is, a four-sided figure with no parallel lines. Most anatomy texts, however, detail the trapezius as a single muscle, denoting it (as does Gray, *Anatomy,* 485) as a flat, triangular muscle. *Triangular* does not = trapezius, but two joined triangles certainly do.

Semispinalis capitis Latin *semi* ["half"] + *spina* ["thorn" or "back"] + *caput,* gen. *capitis* ["head"], here "half the back of the head") is a deep muscle of the upper back that originates by tendons from the tips of the transverse processes of the upper seven thoracic and the seventh cervical vertebrae, as well as from the articular processes of the sixth through the fourth cervical vertebrae; the tendons unite to form a fairly wide muscle to insert on the occipital bone of the skull. It is not quite "half the back" but is about half the length of the series of deep transverso-spinal muscles, so that the name describes both location and relationship to other muscles of similar structure and location.

Splenius capitis (Latin *splenium* ["patch" or "plaster"] + *caput,* as above) does look like an old-fashioned plaster (a drug applied to the skin in the form of a poultice capable of sticking to the skin at body temperature); it originates from a cervical vertebra and four of the thoracic vertebrae and ascends to insert neatly onto the occipital and temporal bones of the skull.

Deltoid (Greek *delta* [the fourth letter of the Greek alphabet, written like a small triangle as a capital letter]; here, "like a delta") is the thick, triangular muscle covering the shoulder joint in the rear, the front, and laterally. The shape is the name.

Teres minor and *major* (Latin *teres* ["rounded and cylindrical"] + *minor* ["smaller"] and *maior* ["larger"]) are two neighboring muscles running from the scapula to the humerus. One could call these the "lesser and greater cylinders" from their appearance.

Levator scapulae (Latin *levare* ["to raise"]) says exactly what this muscle does: raises the shoulder blade.

Rhomboideus minor and *major* (Greek *rhomboeidēs schēma* ["four-sided figure with only the opposite sides and angles equal"], as contrasted with Greek *rhombos* ["lozenge," that is, a "four-sided figure with all the sides, but only the opposite angles, equal," in Euclid, *Elements,* I, def. 22]) reflects nineteenth-century anatomists' attempts to provide a precise name for these two parallel muscles originating from the thoracic and cervical vertebrae and inserting onto the spine of the shoulder blade. Note that the name is "like a rhombus," *not* a rhombus, and *rhomboid* accurately tells what these muscles are in form.

Latissimus dorsi (Latin *latus* ["broad" or "wide"], comparative *lator,* superlative *latissimus* ["broadest"] + *dorsum* ["back"]) is indeed, as the name says, "the broadest one on the back."

Serratus anterior (Latin *serra* ["saw"], with adjective *serratus* ["notched"], + *ante* ["before"], comparative *anterior* ["previous"], here "more forward") is also sometimes labeled *serratus magnus* (Latin for "the great saw-toothed one"), but the important aspect of its appearance is its exaggeratedly notched look as it thinly spans the upper and lateral chest between the upper eight or nine ribs and the scapula; the "tips" of the sawtooths originate from the outer surfaces and superior borders of the ribs.

Subclavius (Latin *sub* ["under" or "beneath"] + *clavis* ["key"]) denotes the location of this muscle "under the collarbone," originating from the first rib and inserting on the underside of the clavicle.

Pectoralis major and *minor* (Latin *pectus,* gen. *pectoris* ["breast," "heart," "feeling"] + *maior* and *minor*) are two muscles (*minor* is beneath *major*), with the pectoralis major a superficial muscle, shaped like a fan and familiar to everyone as *the* muscle that covers the upper chest; exercise buffs frequently brag to each other about their "fine pectorals."

Intercostales externi and *interni* (Latin *inter* ["between"] + *costa* ["rib"], with *externus* and *internus* cognates in English) tell by their names that these forty-four muscles (eleven external intercostals and eleven internal intercostals on either side) extend between the ribs.

Gluteus maximus and minimus (Greek *gloutos* ["buttock" and "rump"] + Latin *maximus* ["biggest"] and *minimum* ["smallest"]) are two of the ten muscles that function in the complicated area from the top of the hip and the rear portions of the upper leg. The gluteus maximus is the "biggest rump," familiar to all from its superficial position, whereas the gluteus minimus (the "smallest rump," rather a misnomer here) lies under the *gluteus medius* (the "middle rump"), which together span the gap between the crest of the ilium and the greater trochanter (see chap. 5, above). Other muscles in this group of ten include the *piriformis* (sometimes spelled *pyriformis* [Latin *pirum* ("pear") + *forma* ("shape" or "appearance"), thus "the pear-shaped one"]), the *obturator internus* and *externus* (Latin *obturare* ["to stop up" or "to close"], suggesting how these muscles appear to fill up the cavities of the bony pelvis, even though they act to rotate the thigh laterally), the *gemellus superior* and *inferior* (Latin *gemellus* ["little twin"], diminutive of *geminus* ["twin"] with *superior* ["higher," comparative of *superus* ("upper" or "situated above")] and *inferior* ["lower," comparative of *inferus* ("situated below")], two small bundles of muscle that aid the obturator internus in laterally rotating the thigh), and the *quadratus femoris* (Latin *quadratum* ["square"] + *femur,* gen. *femoris* ["thigh"], a muscle, more rectangular than square, that extends between the trochanter and the lower crest of the hip, again acting to rotate the thigh laterally).

Superficial muscles of the face and scalp often suggest by their names "where they are" or "what they do." The following are illustrative:

Occipitofrontalis (Latin *occipitium* ["back of the head"] + *frons,* gen. *frontis* ["forehead" or "brow"]) describes this large muscular sheeting that allows us to raise our eyebrows, wrinkle the forehead, and widen the eyes if we wish to express horror or surprise.

Auricularis anterior, superior, and *posterior* (Latin *auricula* ["ear"], with adjective *auricularis* ["of the ears"]) are three muscles—sometimes vestigal—in front, above, and behind the ear; those who can wiggle their ears have fully operative auricularis muscles.

Levator palpebrae superioris (Latin *levare* ["to raise"] + *palpebra* ["eyelid"] + *superior*) says this muscle "raises the upper eyelid."

Orbicularis oculi (Latin *orbiculus* ["ring" or "circle" or "small disc"] + *oculus* ["eye"]) describes this muscle, encircling the eye, which enables one to close the eyelids.

Corrugator (Latin *corrugare* ["to make wrinkled"]) draws the eyebrow down and toward the middle of the forehead, making those familiar vertical wrinkles when one frowns. Sometimes the corrugator is called the "muscle of suffering," since the same wrinkles appear when one is sad or distressed.

Compressor naris (Latin *comprimere* ["to squeeze together"], participle *compressum,* + *naris,* gen. *naris* ["nostril"], pl. *nares* ["nose" = "two nostrils"]) allows one to narrow the openings to the nasal passages (Latin *nasus* also means "nose").

Buccinator (Latin *bucca* ["cheek"] and *buccinator* [usually spelled *bucinator* ("trumpeter")] enables air distending the cheeks to be forced out between the lips, essential to play the tuba, baritone, cornet, and similar instruments—the "brasses."

Masseter (Greek *masētēr* ["chewer"], pl. *myes massētēres* ["muscles of mastication"] in Galen, *Anatomical Procedures,* IV, 2 [ed. Kühn, Vol. II, 421–22]) is one of the most powerful muscles in the body. The force applied by the incisors can reach twenty-five kilograms and by the molars up to ninety kilograms—thanks to the masseter, which originates on the zygomatic arch and inserts onto the *ramus* (Latin for "branch") of the mandible. It is little wonder that human bites are often very nasty wounds.

Platysma (Greek for "plate," something "wide and flat") is the broad and thin muscle that layers like a sheet from the upper part of the shoulder to the corner of the mouth, covering parts of the sternocleidomastoid, pectoralis major, and deltoid as it ascends upward and obliquely medial along the side of the neck. "Wide and flat" it is as it draws open the corners of the mouth when one expresses horror.

Risorius (Latin *risus* ["laugh"]) originates in fascia over the masseter and inserts into skin at the corner of the mouth. We smile and laugh as the risorius raises the corners, an action also producing the related expression of scoffing (Latin's *risor,* gen. *risoris* ["scoffer"]).

Muscles of the hands and feet usually state through their names exactly what they are supposed to do, and with bone nomenclatures in mind, one can immediately "translate" such terms as *flexor digitorum profundus, flexor pollicis longus, flexor digitorum superficialis,* and *extensor carpi ulnaris,* among many similarly descriptive names. By contrast, the muscles controlling the three-dimensional motions of the eyeball all have names denoting their forms and positions relative to each other and relative to the globe of the eye itself, namely *rectus superior, rectus inferior, rectus medialis, rectus lateralis, obliquus superior,* and *obliquus inferior. Rectus* is Latin for "straight," so that the eyeball has four "straight" muscles positioned above, below, in the middle, and on the outer side; *obliquus* is "slanting" in Latin, with the two "slanting" muscles of the eyeball positioned at the upper and medial side of the eye socket and in the anterior margin of the socket.

Terminologies in myology, especially for names of muscles themselves, almost always are drawn from Latin, with some terms borrowed from Greek. Unlike many of the pseudo-Latinized (from Arabic and other tongues) nomenclatures that turn up in other systems of the human body, muscle names have retained the stamp given them early in the history of European anatomy, a history that ranges from classical antiquity through the eighteenth and nineteenth centuries, and the Latin names remain standard throughout the world. Muscles must be described usefully from the attitude of function ("what does it do?") or from the vantage of form ("what does it look like?"), usually by analogy, or from the stance of position ("where is it?"), normally in relation to other structures, especially bones and other muscles. Latin and Greek provide specifics in nouns, adjectives, and verbs (and their derivatives)—particular terms that indicate precise form, function, or place. Because the names applied to muscles, especially since the Renaissance, have generally been well chosen from Greco-Latinate words, these terms have weathered anatomical debates for five hundred years and are still accepted in modern anatomy and medicine.

CHAPTER 8

BREATHING AND HOW IT WORKS

FROM the beginnings of conscious recognition of mortality, human beings have wondered and speculated about why breathing is so essential to life. Was there something in the air that was so necessary for existence that one could store it for only a few minutes? Did the air contain good and bad spirits, which turned the life process itself on and off? And how did the air taken in become part of the body's living functions? Just what *was* air, anyway? Did the lungs have anything to do with the transfer of the life-forces into the body? And was there some link between a human soul and the breath that engenders life? Note how these basic questions span the spectrum of human inquiry from pure religion to pure philosophy, with anatomy, physiology, physics, demon lore, and similar approaches sandwiched among the layers. Note too that these questions rest at the foundations of human questioning and that such questions are universal among all cultures and all historical eras (and presumably prehistoric eras as well).

Among the ancient Greeks, there was much ingenious theorizing about how breathing worked. Typical of the most clever thinking about air and breath, in the centuries before Aristotle performed dissections on animals to "see the parts," are the words of Empedocles (c. 450 B.C.), who shows how pre-Socratic philosophers often expressed complicated problems with metaphor and poetry:

Thus do all things breathe in and out; for there are tubes of flesh, left by the blood, stretched over the outermost part of the body, and over the mouths of these the exterior surface of the skin is pierced through with close-set furrows, in such a fashion that blood lies hidden within, but a clear path for air is cut through by these channels. When the delicate blood runs away from these, air seething with fierce flood rushes in; when it flows back, it breathes out in return. (Aristotle, *On Respiration*, 473b9 [quoting Empedocles of Acragas], translated by Furley and Wilkie in "Introduction," *Galen on Respiration*, 3.)

We instantly perceive how the Greek genius for pure reasoning functioned here as it struggled to explain how and why life existed, with blood and breath integrated as fundamental necessities. Empedocles had *not* seen such channels, but the pores of the skin (occasionally visible on certain parts of the body) may have suggested to the philosopher how breathing *could* function, especially since blood also had "tubes" and since air gained entrance to the body through "tubes" as well. That Empedocles intuited some aspects of modern pulmonary physiology cannot be denied, but Greek biological thought before Aristotle generally did *not* necessarily base itself on actual observation of form or function in living bodies. What was important to Empedocles was explaining *an* idea for breathing, using a simple and single observation: breathing and blood were necessary for life. The presence of "tubes," even though invisible, would certainly explain the process. Empedocles stands in the sturdy tradition of many pre-Socratic philosophers who reached brilliant heights using pure intellect, essential in contemplating the ancient beginnings of physics, mathematics, and science as a whole.

Aristotle's determined curiosity about form and function in the world of nature led to a series of dissections and vivisections that he and his students performed in the 350s B.C. through the 330s. Human dissection was not included, illustrated by Aristotle's assertion of a single lung in man, contrasted with the bifurcated lungs found in birds and other animals: "The lung [*ho pneumōn*] indeed tends to be doubled in all the animals in which it occurs: but among the animals which bring forth their young alive, the separation is not similarly obvious, least of all in man" (Aristotle, *HA*, 495a35–37). This statement is curious when one notes that the most common term in the Greek of Aristotle's day for "lungs" was the plural *pleumones* (sing. *pleumōn*, gen. *pleumonos*), suggesting that the dual structure of lungs in general was embedded in ordinary speech and literature. His choice of the word to designate the lung, *pneumōn,* gen. *pneumonos*, may reflect Aristotle's interests in what moderns think of as physiology. *Pneumōn* (here, "lung") is closely akin to *pneuma*, gen. *pneumatos*, pl. *pneumata*, a term frequently employed in fifth- and fourth-century Greek to mean "wind," "breathed air," "breath," "breathing," and "respiration" (especially among the medical writers) and even "farts," as instanced by Aristotle or one of his students in *Problems,* 948b25.

Not surprisingly, the Victorianism "to break wind" descends directly from this special meaning in Greek, equivalent to the Latin *flatus* (usually a "blowing of wind," "breath," "act of breathing," sometimes "aroma" or "scent," and "wind from the intestines" = "farting"), whence modern medicine's *flatulence*. Aristotle's choice of *pneumōn* is quite deliberate, particularly since he carefully speculates on the nature of air and how such air becomes "vaporized" (the verb is *pneumatopoiein*), leading to questions of the sustenance of life itself. By the time of Erasistratus (fl. 260 B.C.) and the famous dissections of the human cadaver at Ptolemaic Alexandria, Aristotle's term had taken on increased significance. Erasistratus asserts (as quoted by Galen, *Use of Parts*, VI, 12) that the left ventricle of the heart conveys *pneuma*—here something close to "breath of life"—as distinguished from blood. Aristotle's *pneuma* had evolved into a kind of "pneumatology" to explain life itself to some Hellenistic and later Roman medical theorists.

Learned debate in classical antiquity continued not only about the manner in which animals and humans breathed and how respiration was essential for life but also about how the voice was produced and how breathing and speech were interrelated. Galen believed that dissection settled the matter, even though his dissections were on animals. First he emphasized anatomy to delineate the mechanics of breathing:

> . . . I pointed out all the muscles by which breathing and speech are generated . . . The muscles move certain organs which give rise to respiration and speech, but the muscles themselves in turn require for their motion the nerves from the brain; and if you block any of these nerves with a ligature, or cut it, you will immediately render motionless the muscle that the nerve entered . . . unforced inhalation is brought about by one set of organs, muscles and nerves, and forced inhalation by another set. I call unforced inhalation of animals in good health and engaged in no violent movement, and I call forced that which occurs in certain affections and violent exercises . . . in my work *On the Motion of the Thorax and Lungs*, I demonstrate that when the lungs are moved by the thorax and distended as it expands, they draw the outside air in, and this is inhalation; but when they are contracted by its contractions, they force the air they contain into the windpipe and mouth and thus expel it, and that is exhalation. (Galen, *On the Doctrines of Hippocrates and Plato*, II, 4.30–37, slightly modified from the translation by De Lacy, *Galen on the Doctrines of Hippocrates*, Vol. I, 123, 125.)

But Galen, in his *Doctrines* summary, has not directly addressed the basic questions of how and why breathing takes place, unless one assumes such an account was in his *Motion of the Thorax* (a tract that has not survived). Yet the indefatigable Galen has left us with an explanation of the process and purposes of breathing in a work that has reached us, and until the eighteenth and nineteenth centuries, after the nature of combustion and the nature of gasses were well understood, the following served to explain the physiology of breathing:

. . . we breathe for the regulation of heat. This, then, is the principle use of breathing, and the second is to nourish the psychic pneuma. The first is brought about by both parts of breathing, both in-breathing and out; to the one belong cooling and fanning, and to the other, evacuation of the smoky vapor; the second is brought about by in-breathing only. That some portion of the air is drawn into the heart at its swelling, filling the space produced, the size of the swelling proves sufficiently. And that there is breathing into the brain has been shown in another work of ours, in which we discuss the *Doctrines of Hippocrates and Plato*. (Galen, *On the Use of Breathing*, V, 8, translated by Furley and Wilkie in *Galen on Respiration,* 133.)

After William Harvey's demonstration of the closed circulation of the blood in 1628, physicians rejected the notion that "some air" entered the heart, and there were increasing doubts regarding Galen's concepts of how the brain "breathes." But although new explanations of the gross aspects of vascular physiology satisfied some problems better than the Aristotelian-Galenic theories, more and better interpretations of how air is used by the body to sustain life awaited the labors of seventeenth- and eighteenth-century chemists and physicists as they slowly came to understand the nature of gasses. Along the way, research into gasses gradually undermined the classical Greek concept of the four elements, culminating in 1783 with Antoine Lavoisier's demonstration that water was not an element. Once water was shown to be a combination of oxygen and hydrogen, physicists and chemists glimpsed a process of combustion in the body and in how the body "used" oxygen.

Aristotle, Erasistratus, Galen, and many other figures in Greco-Roman medicine and anatomy were well aware of the organs and parts of the body related to breathing, even while speculation continued on why and how they worked as they did. In today's concepts of respiration physiology, many of the anatomical structures retain nomenclatures from Greek and Latin, traced in several instances back to the works of Aristotle, the Alexandrian anatomists, Galen, and others from antiquity. The following list begins with the upper respiratory tract:

> The *nose* is a cognate of Latin's *nasus*, as well as the Sanskrit *nāsā*, German *Nase*, and Danish *neus* (for *naris* ["nostril"], see chap. 7, above, under "A Sampling of Muscles").
>
> *Nasopharynx* combines Latin *nasus* with Greek *pharynx* ("throat").
>
> *Larynx* (pronounced "lair-inks") is Greek for "gullet," which consists of the following (from top to bottom):
>> The *glottis* and *epiglottis*: *glottis*, gen. *glottidos*, is Greek for "mouth of the windpipe," in Galen, *Use of Parts*, VII, 13; the added prefix *epi-* is Greek "over" or "on." The glottis is the opening at the upper part of the larynx, between the vocal cords. The epiglottis is a thin, valvelike cartilaginous flap that covers the glottis when one swallows, thus preventing food and liquid from entering the larynx.
>> The *hyoid* bone takes its name from the Greek *hyoeidēs* ["shaped like the letter upsilon"], which becomes in its Late Latin form *hyoides* ["*U*-shaped" or "like a *U*"]. The capital Greek letter *upsilon* was written as *Y*, so that the name slightly misrepresents its Greek origins, or as Gray, *Anatomy*, 185, puts it, the hyoid bone "is shaped like a horseshoe."
>> *Thyroid* is the English form of the Late Latin *thyroides*, derived from the Greek *thyreoeidēs* ("shaped like a shield"), a name applied by Galen to the thyroid cartilage in *Use of Parts,* VII, 11.
>> The label for the *cricoid* cartilage stems from the Late Latin *cricoides*, derived from the Greek *krikoeidēs* ("shaped like a ring").

The nose, nasopharynx, and larynx are all lined by what medical jargon calls the *vascular mucous membrane,* covered by *ciliated columnar epithelium.* These triplicate nomenclatures give some exact particulars nestled within the Latin or Greek origins of the words:

> *Vascular* emerges from the Latin *vas,* gen. *vasis,* pl. *vasa* ("vessel," "dish," or "duct") + the diminutive suffix *-culum* ("small" or "little"), thus *vasculum* ("little dish" or "little vessel"), from which

Late Latin derived *vascularis,* that is, "provided with vessels or ducts to convey fluids" (blood, lymph, sap [in plants], and the like).

Mucous comes from Latin's *mucus* ("snot" or "phlegm") + suffix *-osus* ("full of" or "characterized by"), thus *mucosus* ("slimy" or "mucous").

Membrane is Latin for "skin" or "parchment."

Ciliated is pulled from the Latin *cilia,* sing. *cilium* ("eyelashes" or "eyelids"), derived from the verb *celare* ("to conceal"), thus *ciliated* means "having an eyelash- or hairlike surface."

Medical English's *columnar* means what it did with Latin's *columna:* "column" or "pillar," here in the microscopic sense.

Epithelium derives from the Greek *epi* ("over" or "on") + *thēlē* ("nipple" or "teat"), from which Late Latin created epithelium to mean "a surface or cavity-lining tissue that protects or secretes or a similar function in the living body."

The lower respiratory tract consists of the *trachea, bronchi,* and *lungs:*

Trachea is a medieval Latin "short form," derived from the Greek *tracheia artēria* ("rough artery" = "windpipe"). Until Galen demonstrated, through a simple ligature experiment, that blood was indeed in the arteries as well as in the veins, Greek and Roman physicians widely believed that "arteries" contained only air or some sort of etherial substance like *pneuma;* thus the "rough artery" (empty in dissection, as were the major arteries originating from the heart) was simply one of the largest and distinct of the whole class of "arteries" in the body. Galen's double-ligature experiment is a model of simplicity: "for we tie exposed arteries in two places, and then cut out the middle and show that it is full of blood" (Galen, *Blood in the Arteries,* VI, 5, trans. Furley and Wilkie in *Galen on Respiration,* 169).

Bronchi (sing. *bronchus*) is Latinized Greek from *bronchos,* which meant "windpipe." Many Greek and Roman medical writers used *bronchos* as a synonym for *tracheia artēria* (above), although occasionally medical Greek used *bronchos* to mean "throat," as in the Hippocratic *Aphorisms,* VI, 37 (of about 350 B.C.) and the *Acute Diseases,* I, 6, by Aretaeus of Cappadocia (about A.D. 100).

Lung comes to us from Middle English *lunge,* a cognate of German's *Lunge.* Etymologists suggest that *lunge* is cognative with Middle and

Old English *lēoht* and *līht*, becoming modern English's *light* ("not heavy" or "of little weight"). The lungs are so named because they were observed to be "light in weight" by farmers and butchers in comparison with other internal organs of animals.

Separating the thoracic cavity from the abdominal cavity is a sheet of hypaxial muscle called the *diaphragm* (pronounced "die-ah-fram" from Greek *diaphragma*, gen. *diaphragmatos* ["partition" or "barrier" in ordinary writing, but also the "muscle dividing the thorax from the abdomen" in some authors, exemplified from the fourth century B.C. by Plato in his *Timaeus*, 70a, and from the second century A.D. by Galen, *Use of Parts*, IV, 14]).

Each lung is covered by *visceral pleura*, whereas *parietal pleura* lines the "wall" of the chest, the *mediastinum,* and the diaphragm; the parietal pleura becomes continuous with the visceral pleura at the *pulmonary hilum:*

Viscera (sing. *viscus*) is Latin for "internal organs." To the Romans, *viscus* usually meant "flesh," but in medical English, *viscus* quite often is a single organ.

Pleura (sing. *pleuron*) is Greek for "ribs"; borrowed into Late Latin, it becomes *pleura* (sing.) and *pleurae* (pl.) to designate "a thin serous membrane covering the lungs and folded back as lining of the corresponding side of the thorax."

Mediastinum became the Latinate name in the mid-sixteenth century for the partition between the two thoracic cavities as formed by the two inner pleural walls, a partition containing all the thoracic viscera except the lungs. Latin's *mediastinus* (more commonly spelled *mediastrinus*) meant "a servant employed on general duties," which is what is intended by Renaissance anatomists who borrowed the term to suggest in metaphor what this partition did: performed the "general duties" for thoracic viscera except the lungs. The Renaissance metaphor is, of course, meaningless to modern doctors or pulmonary physiologists, but the label remains.

Pulmonary emerges from Latin's *pulmo,* gen. *pulmonis* ("lung"), becoming Renaissance Latin's *pulmonaris* ("having to do with lung functions").

Hilum is classical Latin for "a minimal quantity" or the "least bit," borrowed by mid-seventeenth-century anatomists to mean "a little thing." The hilum of the lung is where the structures that form the root of the lung enter and leave, and the hilum of any anatomical part is that place at which nerves, vessels, and such enter or exit. Botanical Latin uses *hilum* to designate the mark or scar on a seed caused by its separation from its funicle, that is, its stalk.

Our common word *respiration* enfolds multiple nuances in its own etymology, a history vividly indicating the ongoing and continuous shifting of how "breathing" was understood. *Respiration* comes from the Middle English *respiracioun,* in turn derived directly from the Latin *respiratio,* gen. *respirationis,* which had at least three basic meanings in classical Latin: "the act of recovering one's breath after it has been impeded," as in Seneca the Younger's *Letters,* LVI, 1; "pausing to take one's breath in speaking," in Cicero, *Orator,* 53, and Quintilian, *Institutio oratoria,* VIII, 9.11; and "emission of vapor, or exhalation," as one reads in Cicero, *Nature of the Gods,* II, 27. By the time of Apuleius (about A.D. 120–80), the word *respiratus* (gen. *respiratus*) as extracted from the verb *respirare* ("to recover one's breath") had come to mean simply "the process of breathing" (Apuleius, *Metamorphoses* [*Golden Ass*], IV, 15).

As usual, classical Latin employed a limited number of words to convey a wide range of meanings, suggested by context and intended nuance by a particular writer. Latin early used prefixes and suffixes to refine meanings and nuances of common terms, so that by employing *re-* ("reversal" or "backward movement") + *spirare* ("to breathe"), a speaker or writer of Latin could express a "backward breath." From *spirare* and its participle *spiratum* also arose the masculine noun *spiritus* (gen. also *spiritus*), which could mean—especially in the early Roman Empire—simply "breath," that is, "the air breathed into and expelled from the lungs," as illustrated by passages in Celsus, *De medicina,* I, preface 15, and Scribonius Largus, *Compositiones,* 184. *Spiritus* was one of those elastic words that met varying needs according to the requirements of different authors. For Ovid (43 B.C.–A.D. 17), *spiritus* was exactly the "non-corporeal part of the human being" = "soul" = "spirit," as indicated in his *Tristia,* III, 3.62, a meaning reflected in Apuleius's *Golden Ass,* VI, 17. That wispy or delicate or gossamer or vaporous combination one understood as *spiritus* could thereby become the misty, diaphanous, and rarified sense called smelling, so that Lucretius (95–55 B.C.) could use the word to specify "odor" in the beautifully written poem in defense of Epicurean theory: *De rerum natura,* III, 222. To Pliny in *NH,* II, 10, *spiritus* is simply "air."

In later legal Latin, *spiritus* became a technical term to indicate the "nature" or "dominating quality" of something or someone, as set down by the jurists Julius Paulus (about A.D. 210) and Sextus Pomponius (roughly A.D. 117–80), both quoted in the great compilation of Roman law, the *Digest,* assembled under the direction of the emperor Justinian in A.D. 533 (specific passages are *Digest,* VI, 1.23.5 [Paulus], and XLI, 3.30 [Pomponius]). What Roman law encapsulated was the precise yet very pliable concept incorporated in *spiritus,* a concept of that something that "defined" a thing or person while remaining flexible according to demands in particular cases, rulings, and instances of both legal precedences and current law. The law recognized how *spirare* was essential for life, and one's legal *spiritus* was one's basic nature, whether it meant moral or physical qualities. In ordinary Latin, *spirare* was likewise an expression of the process of life itself, and *respiratio* was an essential aspect of that quasi-mystical existence. *Spiritus* in popular parlance could easily slide into notions of the soul, which is what *spiritus* almost always means in medieval Latin.

The restatements of pulmonary function provided by twentieth-century respiratory physiology and anatomy are especially instructive in comparison with the theories of Empedocles, Aristotle, and Galen, reflections of the long history of definition and redefinition of what breathing "is" and what it involves. There are, to be sure, vast differences between ancient and modern, but the striking retention of a Greco-Latinate vocabulary indicates again, in another way, just how deep are the heritages of both the words and their changing historic contexts. Note the easy employment of Greek and Latin terminologies adapted into the following standard summary, contained in a widely used text of medicine:

The rich blood supply [of the mucous membrane] ensures that the inspired air enters the lungs at body temperature and fully saturated with water vapour. The cilia, aided by the layer of sticky mucus covering them, have the important function of trapping foreign particles and bacteria, and propelling them towards the pharynx. The whole respiratory epithelium down to the terminal bronchioles is equipped with cilia, which probably play an important part in the prevention of respiratory infection . . . The larynx, in addition to being the organ of voice production, has the function of preventing particles larger than can be dealt with by the cilia from reaching the lower respiratory tract. This it does by means of the cough reflex. (Davidson, *Practice of Medicine,* 304, 306.)

Modern physics tells us why the "parts" promote breathing:

In health the two pleural layers are separated only by a thin film of lymph, but between them there is a negative (subatmospheric) tension. This results from the natural tendency of the lung to recoil towards the hilum, a property given to it by the rich supply of elastic fibers in the bronchi and blood vessels. (Ibid., 308.)

And our explanation of "why" breathing takes place:

Respiration means the transport of oxygen from the atmosphere to the cells and, in turn, the transport of carbon dioxide from the cells back to the atmosphere. (Guyton, *Medical Physiology,* 456.)

CHAPTER 9

EATING, DIGESTION, ELIMINATION

> ... so long as you speak of the north and south ends of the human machine you may go pretty nearly as far as you like ... when you enter the intermediate region you must watch your every step ... a long word [using polysyllabic Latin or Greek names] is considered nice and a short word nasty.
> —RUPERT HUGHES, The Latin Quarter in Language (1937)

ALTHOUGH much has changed in social manners and mores (pl. of Latin *mos,* gen. *moris* ["custom"]) since Hughes's day, and especially since the leftover prudery of the Victorian age typical in the 1930s, Americans often are uneasy when blunt words occur in print or in speech describing eating and what happens thereafter. Food is one of two basic needs among human beings (the other is sex, for which see chap. 10, below), and because eating *is* basic, there is a universal tendency to clothe foods and their consumption, as well as the ultimate forms of consumed nutrients, in wrappers of custom, religion, taboo, and euphemisms. If an American archaeologist is offered the great delicacy of beetle grubs (usually larvae) to be crunched raw for an afternoon snack among the Bedouins of the Middle East, there may be a normal cultural gagging, perhaps insulting to one's hosts. One can argue, of course, about the rich protein sources of ants, grasshoppers, June bug larvae, and the like, but North Americans generally cannot "stomach the thought," to use a common psychological metaphor. Yet those same Americans may happily consume raw fish and seaweed, as Japanese culinary customs become more prevalent. Some citizens gag on raw oysters, others gobble them in vast numbers, while some of us who live in the upper Midwest may wonder why Louisiana catfish or Russian Sturgeon eggs catch the increasing fancy of food snobs from coast to coast.

Until the enormous cultural mix-up characteristic of the world after 1945—a grand amalgam (some might call it homogenization) that blended many bits of formerly insular habits—each culture or nationality defined what was "good" food, and each had its notions about "good manners at the table." Sometimes, however, no matter how such customs are practiced, culture-based prejudices reveal through their etymologies the shifting biases of these assumptions, suggesting how these biases always change over time, slowly in the distant past and faster in the dizzying fluctuations in the West since World War II. Sometimes those variations will swing from the poles of the overly repressive to the generally free, as illustrated by the ordinary vocabulary of sixteenth- and seventeenth-century English as contrasted with nineteenth- and early-twentieth-century words thought "acceptable" (this latter is the infamous "Victorian era"). Our Victorian foremothers and -fathers certainly knew how to suppress and be repressed, and their instincts about food words and elimination words were accurate, since they were most worried about matters of sex. By looking at the etymologies of some basic foods, one can occasionally see muted sexual content:

Milk is a common four-letter word, coming to us from Old and Middle English, a cognate of German *Milch* and kin to other Indo-European "milk words" including Latin's *mulgere* ("to milk"). In classical Latin, *lactans* means "giving milk" whereas *lactatio* means "allurement," with the root verb *lactare* generally suggesting "to entice" or "to lead on." Roman males found "lactating" women very sexually attractive.

Bread emerges from Middle English *breed* and Old English *brēad* ("fragment," "morsel," "bread"), and our word is a cognate of the German *Brot*. There is interplay among *bread, bred, breed,* and similar words in English, with Old English *brēdan* ("to nourish") simply reinforcing the historical sense of double meanings. *Bread* is made from wheat (the usual North American name) or corn (the British English for "wheat"), with *wheat* coming from Middle English *whete* (akin to German *Weizen*) and *corn* from the Middle English for "grain." In Latin, *panis* ("bread" or "food") does not have any sexual overtones.

Meat is derived from the Middle English *mete,* which also provides *meet* in now archaic English meaning "suitable," "fitting," or "proper." Latin's *caro,* gen. *caronis* or *carnis* ("flesh" or "covering of the body" or "meat"), could be used to insult someone, if one attached *putida* ("carrion") to *carnis.* Yet English preserves an underlying sexual nuance in "carnal pleasures" or "carnal knowledge," with the sexual or sensual meaning of *carnal* first recorded in English about 1400 (*OED*, s.v. def. 3).

In writing or speaking about the other end of the digestion process, that is, the products of elimination, one can find many ways of not saying what one is actually saying in polite speech. Such matters can be called *feces* or *dung* or *manure* or—for the particularly squeaky—*defecation* or *feculence*. The most common super-euphemism of all is to *have a movement*. To display an education in classical languages, one can say, with a straight face, *excrement, excreta, egesta, ejecta,* and even *ejectamenta*. In the presence of old-fashioned schoolmarms, there is always the retreat into *waste* or *waste matter*. If the excreta chance to be in liquid form, there is the polite *urination* or *micturition* and even *making water* in what the English still call a *water closet* (abbreviated as WC). These are a few of the currently proper words to use in polite conversation and presumably in proper writing; the contrast is striking between the verbs used in the euphemistic *have a movement* and the far blunter *take a shit*: common speech allows one full control.

The word histories of some of these pseudo-euphemisms in modern English indicate shifting nuances, often linked to social classes (self-professed or otherwise):

Feces is derived from the Latin *faex* or *fex*, gen. *faecis* or *fecis*, pl. *faeces*, usually meaning "dregs" (in wine) or, if applied to persons, "scum," as in Juvenal, *Satires*, III, 61, and Apuleius, *Golden Ass*, VIII, 24. The shift in meanings from "dregs," "sediments in wine," or "wine-lees" occurred in medieval Latin and thus came into Middle English, which provides *feces* (pronounced "feesees") with its current definition. All modern English words, medicalese or not, with a *-fec-* root generally reflect some contextual sense of "solid waste" or bowel function.

Dung is a puzzle to etymologists, with "root uncertain," as stated by Skeat, *A Concise Etymological Dictionary*, 156. The term emerges from Anglo-Saxon from Swedish *dynga* or Danish *dynge* and is a cognate of German's *Dung*. The word has been associated for a millennium with farming practices, and one can still say *dung* as a verb, meaning to spread manure (see immediately below) on a field or a garden. In his *Origins*, 170, Partridge connects the word with Old High German *tunga* or *tunc*, with the sense of an "underground chamber covered with dung," suggesting the "mucky" reality of medieval dungeons.

Manure is another polite word, with an etymology leading back into the late Roman Empire, in which Vulgar Latin (*vulgus* ["the rabble"]) used *manu opere* ("to work by hand"), which evolved into the Old French *manuevre*, with a variant *manouver* ("to till the soil"), borrowed into English as *manure* ("to fertilize"). Since one had to be of the untutored rabble to "work with the hands," such a person worked the soil and spread the fields with animal (and human) excrement by hand. The nobilities of late Rome and the Western medieval kingdoms never performed such duties; such was "beneath them," so that *manure* has a history of class distinction. Farmers worldwide still "manure" their fields, and the word remains polite as long as there is the rural context.

Urine and the act of *urination* comes to us from Middle English (through Old French), which borrowed *urina* directly from the Latin; the word is a cognate of the Greek *ouron*. Late Latin brought forth *urinarius*, which becomes medical English's *urinary*, and the Late Latin verb *urinare* gave birth to several terms, including *urination* (the proper noun) and *urinate* (the proper verb). From classical Latin through modern English, *urine* (*urina*) has retained a neutral sense, a bland word exciting little embarrassment even among most Victorians. *Micturition* is a late extraction from the Latin *micturire*, a rare verb—so we read in Juvenal, *Satires*, VI, 309 and XVI, 46— that meant "to want to urinate." The first recorded use of the educed *miction* is in 1663, and medical writers since the mid-seventeenth century have almost always misused *micturition*, which is not merely the act of urination but the "morbid frequency of voiding the urine" (*OED*, s.v.), in other words a pathological condition. Yet the term remains a polite, if incorrect, way of saying "pissing."

The once proper words *shit* and *piss* remain part of the so-called lesser levels in English-speaking countries. Partridge, *Origins*, 617, suggests that *shit* and *shite* (a variant) are akin to Old High German *scīzan* and Old Norse *skīta*, in turn linked to Old High German *sciozzan* ("uninhibited excretion"), hence German *schiessen*. All these words are connected to what becomes *shoot* in English. By contrast to the assumed crudity of *shit* by the late eighteenth century, one can cite the perfectly proper use by Caxton in his 1484 *Fables of Aesop*, X, 15, "I dyde shyte thre grete toordes," or a 1527 manual on distilled water that instructs, "an ounce from them that spetteth blode, pysseth blode, or shyteth blode" (*OED*, s.v.). Modern French's *merde*, by contrast to the obscure origins of English's *shit,* comes directly from classical Latin's *merda* (pl. *merdae,* the usual form used by the Romans). Martial (c. A.D. 40–c. 104) shows how the word was employed neatly and with humor in his *Epigrams,* I, 83:

> *Os et labra libi linguit, Manneia, catellus:*
> *non miror, merdas si libet esse cani.*
> (Your puppy, Manneia, licks your face and lips:
> I'm not surprised, if a dog likes shit.)

And if one wishes to sound learned and yet pleasantly obscene in modern English, one can easily coin terms from Latin's *stercus* (as in the perfectly proper *stercoraceous,* a fancy word drily defined as "constituting of, or pertaining to, feces") or Greek's *kopros,* which has given us paleontology's *coprolite* (defined as a "fossilized turd" by a well-known professor of geology), as well as psychiatry's *coprolagnia* (sexual stimulation from the thought or sight of feces) and *coprolalia* (defined by psychoanalysts as "excessive use of scatological language"). *Scatology* ("the study of excrement") is another learned term derived from Greek's *skōr,* gen. *skatos* ("dung," "ordure," or "excrement"), providing medicine's *scatoscopy* ("diagnostic examination of fecal matter") and *scatoma* ("a colonic or rectal tumorlike mass of feces"). Lest it be misunderstood that earlier cultures were always freer with their words and less class-conscious about scatological matters, one should contemplate the uproarious puns on such terms in the plays of Aristophanes (c. 457–c. 385 B.C.), for which see Henderson, *Maculate Muse* especially chap. 6.

OED repeatedly notes that *piss*-words are "not now in polite use." Yet the rich history of our tongue sports such delights as *pissprophet* (a physician in the seventeenth century who rendered diagnosis from the examination of someone's urine), *pissabed* (a sixteenth-century name for the dandelion, thanks to its diuretic properties), and *pisspot* (a common word in the fifteenth and sixteenth centuries), later becoming the euphemistic *chamberpot.* Partridge, *Origins,* 498, tells us that *piss* owes its origins to the Vulgar Latin *pissiare* and is thus a cognate of Italian's *pisciare,* and he offers his speculation that the verb ultimately derives from ancient Hittite's *pisan* ("a vessel for water") and that the word itself suggests the sound of urination. John Wyclif's 1388 translation of the Bible (here II Kings 18.27) shows how proper this term once was in English: "Thei ete her toordis, and drynke her pisse with you." And Geoffrey Chaucer's famous *Canterbury Tales* of 1386, in mentioning what Socrate's shrewlike wife thought of her husband's philosophy, writes simply enough that she "caste pisse upon his heed [head]" (*The Wyf of Bathe*, 729). Chaucer's English is mirrored in what dictionaries now define as "vulgar" or "slang" in modern English, as in *to take a piss* (urinate), *to be pissed off* (be angry), and merely *pissed* (intoxicated). The etymology of such words shows a consistent division between what is thought to be "proper" (most often "upper-class") speech and writing through the centuries, and the "vulgar" expressions of everyone else. One wonders what would have been the "vulgar" word for *piss* in Wyclif and Chaucer's day.

TO EAT, TO DIGEST, TO ELIMINATE: THE PARTS

If shifting cultural values cause the invention of euphemisms for the products of digestion and their ultimate destination, the names given from Greek and Latin for the parts of the digestive system have few shades of meaning; in fact, the nomenclatures are those that must be specific (as usual). Again the role of analogy is prominent as one proceeds through the digestive tract, beginning with the first action, the chewing of food by the teeth, which in normal adult dentition includes thirty-two permanent teeth (sixteen per jaw):

> *Incisors* (eight): a Late Latin derivative from Latin's *incisus* ("cutter").
>
> *Canines* (four): from Latin *canis* ("dog") and the adjective *caninus* ("doglike"), thus the "dog teeth." Often the canines are called *cuspids,* extracted from the Latin *cuspis* ("point"), which tells that these teeth have single projection points, or *cusps.* Latin's *cuspir* ("to spit") gave the English *cuspidor* (spittoon).
>
> Premolars or *bicuspids* (eight): teeth with two cusps.
>
> *Molars* (twelve): derived from the Latin *mola* ("millstone") and *molaris* ("grinder").

All *dental* words ("dentistry," "denture," etc.) are derived from the Latin word for tooth (*dens,* gen. *dentis*), which occasionally in classical Latin meant "ivory." Sometimes a Latin word has survived almost intact among dentists, as in the term *dentifrice,* which is Latin's *dentifricium* ("tooth powder"), a substance the Romans used to clean their teeth by rubbing them (Latin's *fricare* ["to rub"]).

Among other structures, the *mouth* (Middle English *mūth*, cognate of German's *Mund*) contains the following:

- The *tongue* (Middle English *tunge,* but akin to Latin's *lingua* ["tongue," "speech," or "language"]) is connected to the floor of the mouth by the *frenulum linguae* (Latin *frenum* ["bridle"] + *-ulum*, thus "little bridle"), so that the name of this part translates as "the little bridle of the tongue," limiting its movement. The surface, or *dorsum* (Latin for "back"), of the tongue (*dorsum linguae*) has a centered and shallow groove dividing the left from the right sides, a groove called the *sulcus medianus linguae* (Latin *sulcus* ["furrow"]), and the dorsum is covered with numerous *papillae* (Latin *papilla* ["nipple"]), some of which bear on their surfaces the taste buds, especially the eight to twelve *vallate papillae* (Latin *vallum* ["rampart" or "ridge"]) on the anterior surface of the dorsum.

- The *salivary glands* (Latin's *saliva* is "saliva" or "spittle," and *glans*, gen. *glandis,* usually meant "nut" and sometimes "acorn") occur in three pairs and carry the names *parotid, submandibular,* and *sublingual* glands. *Parotid* is Late Latin derived from the Greek *para* + *ōtikos* (thus "near the ear"), which tells the location of this gland; *sub-* is the common Latin prefix for "under," so that the other two salivary glands are located "under the mandible" and "under the tongue." An *enzyme* (Byzantine Greek *enzymos* ["leavened"]) in the saliva called *ptyalin* (Greek *ptyalon* ["spittle" or "saliva"]) has the property of converting starch into *dextrin* (Latin *dexter* ["right" or "right-handed"] + *-inus* ["of or pertaining to"]), thus in biochemistry "a mix of gummy carbohydrates, exhibiting dextrorotatary properties, obtained by the partial hydrolysis of starch." This modern biochemical definition bristles with Greco-Latinate terms:

    Carbohydrate emerges from Latin's *carbo,* gen. *carbonis* ("charcoal" or "embers"), + Greek's *hydōr,* gen. *hydatos* ("water"), + Latin suffix *-atus* (basically "function"). In his complete rejection of the ancient theory of elements, Antoine Lavoisier (1743–94) posited that one of his "new" elements was *carbone* (the French for "coal" or "charcoal"), a term borrowed almost immediately into chemical English (1789), with English *carbon* appearing first in print by 1813. Carbon in the new chemical system was often basic in oxidation of organic matter, so that when in the 1860s chemists discovered that sugars, gums, starches, and cellulose contained only carbon, hydrogen, and oxygen (the hydrogen and oxygen in proportions to form water), a fresh word was needed to describe this class of substances, and *carbohydrate* entered English by 1869. Carbohydrates are essential sources of energy in the human body. *Sugar* comes into English from Arabic *sukkar* or *sukhar,* through medieval Latin's *succarum* or *zucara* and medieval French *sucre. Gum* derives ultimately from the Greek *kommi* ("gum" or "acacia resin"). *Cellulose* is mid-eighteenth-century Latinate created from Latin's *cellula* ("small room," sometimes "a prostitute's cubicle") + the suffix *-osus* ("rich in" or "full of"), so that this common term in botany and advertisements for healthy foods translates as "full of small rooms" or "rich in prostitutes' cubicles," distantly analogous to the modern definition of cellulose: "an inert carbohydrate making up most of the cell walls of plants, occuring ordinarily in wood, cotton, paper, and similar materials." All this to define *carbohydrate* . . .

Dextrorotatory shows how physics and chemistry often fuse to describe properties of substances: here the term means "rotating or deviating the plane of polarized light, while one looks against the oncoming light." *Dextro-* is from the same Latin *dexter* as above, and *-rotatory* stems from the Latin verb *rotare* ("to spin" or "to move in a circle") and the noun *rota* ("wheel") + the suffix *-torius* (the Latin *tor* generally denoted "agents"). As a modern adjective, *dextrorotatory* means literally "[something] causing [something] to move in a circular path to the right-hand," the basic property embedded in the name *dextrin.*

Hydrolysis, by comparison with the complicated underpinnings of the word *carbohydrate,* is quite simple: *hydro-* is derived from the Greek water word as found above under *carbohydrate;* and *lysis* is Greek for "loosing," "releasing," or "emptying." In ancient Greco-Roman medical writing, *lysis* generally is "remission" (of a fever or disease), the opposite of *krisis.* In the 1870s, chemists concocted *hydrolysis* as a pseudo-Greek term, pulled from two ancient Greek words, to describe a particular chemical decomposition, in which water reacts with a compound to make it into other compounds or substances.

Ptyalin also has the property of converting starch into *maltose,* which along with *dextrin* begins the process of digestion. *Maltose* came into English in the 1860s formed from the common English *malt* (usually "germinated barley grains, used in brewing and distilling," derived from Old English *mealt* and Old Norse *malt* [giving German *Malz*], showing kinship with English *melt*—which is what *malting* grain seemed to do) + the Latin suffix *-osus* ("rich in" or "full of"), so that this white, crystalline, water-soluble sugar has the name "rich in malt." *Starch* emerges from Old and Middle English words that meant "to stiffen," which is why some executives insist on "starched shirts" for social occasions and why one can enjoy the wordplay on "stiff-necked stuffed shirts." Nutrient starches (the white, tasteless solid carbohydrate) are important in rice, corn, wheat, beans, potatoes, and many vegetables.

Continuing downward through the digestive tract, one proceeds through the *isthmus faucium* (Greek *isthmos* ["neck of land"] + Latin *fauces* [a feminine plural meaning "upper part of the throat"]), the opening by which the mouth communicates with the pharynx, past the epiglottis and into the gullet or *esophagus* (Greek *oisophagos* ["gullet"]). The esophagus opens into the stomach through the *cardiac orifice* (Greek *kardia* ["heart"] + late Latin *orificium* ["mouthlike opening"]); *stomach* comes directly from the Latin *stomachus* ("gullet" or "stomach"), but most *stomach* terms in medical English emerge from Greek *gastēr*, gen. *gastros* ("paunch," "belly," and sometimes "womb"), for example *gastritis* ("inflammation of the mucous membrane of the stomach"), *gastrology* ("study of the structure, functions, and diseases of the stomach"), *gastrolith* (literally "stomach-stone" [Greek *lithos*, "stone"], redundantly defined as "a calculous [Latin *calculus* ("pebble" or "stone")] concretion in the stomach"), and dozens of other *gastro-* words in medicalese.

Viewed from the front of the body, the stomach has as the upper part of its structure a hollowed, quasi-hemisphere (the "top" of the stomach), called by anatomists the *fundus,* which in Latin means "bottom." This adaptation by eighteenth-century anatomists owes its use to the manner in which anatomical Latin employed *fundus* is description of other organs (the eye, the bladder, the uterus, and others), so that the stomach's *fundus* was indeed its "base" and that part most distant from its major opening, the *pylorus* (see below), leading into the small intestine—*if* one approached dissection coming from the direction of the head. It is likely also that an anonymous but deeply educated Renaissance anatomist knew that classical Latin had the rare term *fundula* or *fundulum,* which meant "cul-de-sac," "blind alley," and sometimes "blind gut" (indeed rare words, since they are listed in the *De lingua Latina,* V, 145, 111, by Marcus Terentius Varro [116–27 B.C.], one of the most learned individuals of the late Roman Republic), so that *fundus* might be pulled to mean "blind gut" here. Latin's *fundus* ("bottom" or "base") also had its relative in *fundamentum* ("foundation"), which evolved into Middle English's *fondement* ("buttocks," "anus," and other closely aligned meanings), a sense preserved in the rarely used modern word *fundament*. Victorian doctors were fond of this term: unless one knew the word, would anyone know what the learned physician in 1871 actually intended when he said, "The end may be attained by the pressure of a warm cloth against the fundament" (*OED*, s.v. def. 3)?

Below the *fundus* of the stomach occurs the "body" (the *corpus* [Latin for "body"], pl. *corpora*) of the stomach, followed by the *pyloric vestibule* and *pyloric antrum*, which leads into the *pylorus*, connecting the stomach with the first part of the small intestine. *Pylorus* is Latinated Greek (*pylōros* ["gatekeeper"]), and the two previous divisions of the stomach translate as "forecourt" or "entrance to the gate" (Latin *vestibulum*) and "cave" or "cavity of the gate" (Late Latin *antrum* from Greek *antron*). The pylorus is equipped with a *pyloric valve,* a muscular ring that controls entrance of the contents of the stomach into the upper part of the small intestine. The pyloric valve is often called the pyloric *sphincter* (a Late Latin creation from the Greek *sphingein* ["to hold tight"]). The main digestive enzyme of the stomach is known as *pepsin* (Greek *pepsis* ["softening," "ripening," or "changing by means of heat" or "fermentation" or "cooking," and among Greco-Roman medical writers "digestion"—all this for the trade name *Pepsi*), which, in the presence of hydrochloric acid as secreted by the parietal cells of the stomach, functions to split proteins into proteoses and peptones. The resultant substance is called *chyme* (Late Latin *chymus* from Greek *chymos* ["animal juice" or "humor" in Galen, *Crisis Days,* I, 12 (ed. Kühn, Vol. IX, 595)]), which looks murky and milky and is a semifluid or paste. The chyme moves into the small intestine by a process termed *peristalsis* (Late Latin combining Greek *peri* ["around"] + *stalsis* ["contraction"]), physiologically progressive waves of contraction and relaxation.

The pyloric sphincter is the beginning of the small intestine (Latin's *intestina* [neuter pl. of *intestinum*] meaning "entrails" or "guts"), which—from the pylorus to the colic valve (the beginning of the large intestine)—averages about seven meters in length (about twenty-two feet) in the adult human. The small intestine has three basic parts: the *duodenum,* the *jejunum,* and the *ileum*. Our term *duodenum* is a fourteenth-century Latin "short form" for medieval Latin's *intestinum duodenum digitorum,* in turn a translation from the Greek *dōdekadaktylos* ("twelve fingers long"), a name given to this portion of the small intestine by Herophilus in about 280 B.C. in his dissections at Ptolemaic Alexandria, as quoted by Galen:

From the portal veins of the liver a large vein grows out and extends obliquely both to the lower parts and other parts of a living being, especially along the middle of the growth called "twelve fingers long" by Herophilus. And he gives this name to the beginning of the intestine, before it twists into convolutions. (Galen, *Anatomy of Arteries and Veins,* 1, Greek text ed. and trans. Heinrich von Staden, *Herophilus: The Art of Medicine in Early Alexandria* (Cambridge: Cambridge University Press, 1989), 209.)

After this [sc. first part of the intestine], which is twelve fingers long as Herophilus said correctly, the intestine bends downward into convolutions in many folds with a host of many blood vessels. This part they call the "fasting" intestine [sc. *jejunum*] because it is always found to be deprived of food. (Galen, *Anatomical Procedures,* VI, 9, ed. and trans. von Staden, *Herophilus,* 209.)

Galen's "fasting intestine" (Greek *nēstis*) is Latin's *ieiunum* ("empty," "hungry," or "fasting"), which has become the Latinated medicalese *jejunum*. Modern English preserves a piece of this meaning in the adjective *jejune* ("dull," "childish," and "uninformed," among several meanings). *Ileum* is a later Latin derivation from the Latin *ile* (neuter pl. *ilia*), meaning "guts" or "side of the body from the top of the hips to the groin" (the latter in Celsus, *De medicina,* IV, 1.12).

The small intestine connects with the large intestine through the *colic valve* (or *ileocecal valve*) at the point where the *cecum* and *colon* are joined. The beginning of the large intestine is a large, blind pouch placed below the colic valve; the pouch is termed the *cecum* (pronounced "seekum," a "short form" for the Latin *intestinum caecum* ["blind gut"]), and attached to the end of the cecum is the *vermiform appendix* (Latin *vermis* ["worm"] + appendix ["supplement," "appendage," or "hanger-on"]), the site of the very common *appendicitis* ("inflammation of the worm-shaped hanger-on"). Above the cecum, the large intestine or *colon* (Greek *kōlon* ["limb"]) runs upward as the "ascending" colon, then twists at the *hepatic* flexure (Greek *hēpar,* gen. *hēpatos* ["liver"], with adj. *hepatikos*) into the "transverse" colon, and then twists again downward at the *splenic* flexure (Greek *splēn,* gen. *splēnos* ["spleen"], with adjective *splēnikos* ["of the spleen"]) into the "descending" colon, to curve into the *sigmoid* colon (the Greek letter *sigma* [our *S*] was written in medieval Greek as *C,* thus "sigmoid" means "like the letter sigma"). Twisting again to the rectosigmoid junction, the digestive tract ends in the *rectum* (Latin *rectus* ["straight"]), and solid waste is eliminated at the *anus* (Latin for "ring"), equipped with a powerful, voluntary sphincter. It is here that *hemorrhoids* occur (Greek *haimorrhoia* ["bloody discharge"], with *haimorrhoïs,* gen. *haimorrhoïdos,* pl. *haimorrhoïdes* ["veins liable to discharge blood," especially hemorrhoids and piles]).

The digestive system also includes the *liver* (from Middle English *lifer,* a cognate of German *leber,* akin to Greek *liparos* ["fat"]) and the *pancreas* (Greek *pankreas,* gen. *pankreatos* ["sweetbread" or simply "pancreas"]). Through the pancreatic duct, which empties into the duodenum, the pancreas secretes enzymes that digest all three major kinds of foods (proteins, carbohydrates, and fats). For proteins, the major enzyme is *trypsin* (Greek *tripsis,* gen. *tripseōs* ["rubbing" or "friction," and in Greco-Roman medicine "massage"]); for carbohydrates, the enzyme from the pancreas carries the name *amylase* (Greek *amylon* ["starch" among several meanings; *amylos* literally meant "not ground at the mill," thus the "finest flour"] + the modern chemical suffix *-ase,* namely the "suffix in the names of enzymes"); and for fats, the pancreatic enzyme is named *lipase* (Greek *lipos* ["fat"] + *-ase*). The liver secretes *bile* (Latin *bilis* ["bile," "gall," "anger," "displeasure"]), which is stored in the *gallbladder* (Middle English *galla* ["something bitter"] + *blaeddre* ["blister," "pimple," or "something blown up"]). The bile is important for digestion, not for any enzymes present but for its bile salts, which contribute to the *emulsification* of fat globules (Latin *emulsus* [from *mulgere* ("to milk")], thus "milked out") so that they can be digested by the lipases. The gallbladder has a common duct joined with one from the liver, which enters the superior portion of the duodenum.

Liquid waste is collected from the bloodstream by the two kidneys (*kidney* is of uncertain origin, perhaps from the Middle English for "egg-shaped"). Most *kidney* words in medical English come from the Latin *renes* (masculine pl. [sing. *ren*]), which are "kidneys." Thus a *renal calculus* is a "kidney stone." Urine is collected in the numerous *glomeruli* (Late Latin derivation from Latin *glomus,* gen. *glomeris,* + diminutive suffix *-ulus* [thus sing. *glomerulus*], meaning "little ball of yarn or thread") and sent into the renal *pelvis* (Latin for "basin," akin to Greek *pellis* ["bowl"]). From the renal pelvis, the urine flows into one of the two *ureters* (a Late Latin creation from classical Greek *ourētēr,* with the basic Greek verb *ourein* ["to piss" or "to urinate"]), which lead into the urinary bladder. Stored for a short time, the urine is excreted through the *urethra* (from the same Greek roots as above), controlled by a voluntary sphincter.

CHAPTER 10

SEX

IN 1915, H. L. Mencken published a short and acerbic essay on terms used for the human body; the essay, "The Interior Hierarchy," appeared in a journal called *Smart Set*. Mencken stands as one of the fine wits in American literature, and he had a deft ability to lampoon pompous behavior, enjoying with special relish jabbing holes in the notions of "proper" and "improper" words. In summarizing his World War I–era thrusts at the then reigning bluebloods of the language, Mencken wrote:

> . . . I undertook to arrange the parts of the body in eight classes, beginning with the highly respectable and ending with the unmentionable. Into the highest class I put the heart, brain, hair, eyes, and vermiform appendix; into Class II, the collar-bone, stomach (American), liver (English), bronchial tubes, arms (excluding elbows), tonsils, ears, etc.; into Class III, the elbows, ankles, teeth (if natural), shoulders, lungs, neck, etc., and so on. My Class VI included thighs, paunch, esophagus, spleen, pancreas, gallbladder, and caecum, and there I had to stop, for the inmates of Classes VII and VIII could not be listed in print in those high days of comstockery. (Mencken, *The American Language*, 659–60.)

In 1945, Mencken could assume everyone would know and easily remember what was meant by *comstockery,* which now, in the last decade of the twentieth century, is a rarely used term. Anthony Comstock (1844–1915) was an American writer and self-proclaimed arbiter whose prudery and overzealous condemnation of "improper" art and writing gained the widespread derision of many American readers and fellow authors even while he was cheered on by other readers who shuddered at the encroachments of filthy words and even dirtier pictures of naked women and men painted by the brushes of corrupted European artists. By 1905, *comstockery* had entered the language as a word to mean exactly what Comstock was doing: overzealously censoring, on moral grounds, works of literature and the fine arts, especially mistaking simple and openly honest works for lewd ones. Mencken could laugh in 1945, but in 1915 his point was that he could not laugh, let alone expect to have his words appear in print describing parts between the belly-button and somewhere on the upper thighs. Euphemisms abounded in 1915—as they do today—but as Mencken remarks, one could mean anything one wanted in using such phrases as *illicit relations* or words like *soliciting*. Essential were double meanings, and nonnative speakers of both American English and British English continually find amusement and occasional frustration encountering such words and phrases as *screw* (American English, "to copulate"; British English, "amount of salary or wages" [among several meanings], with *screwed* usually meaning "drunk"), *bum* (American English, a "tramp" or "worthless person"; British English, "buttocks"), *knocked up* (American English, "be made pregnant"; British English, "to awaken someone in the morning" [again among several meanings], with a commonly heard Oxbridge sense of "to score runs rapidly at cricket," followed by *knockup* [noun], a "casual game at tennis"), *pecker* and *cock* (American English, both "penis"; British English [as in *keep your pecker up*], "maintain one's courage" and [as in *old cock*], "nonsense"; simply enough, a *cock* is a "rooster"), and dozens of others. A shrewd writer like Mencken could exploit these differences as he "explained" just what the English might mean but not what the Americanism might mean. Euphemisms about sex and sexual functions always lead to careful subterfuge, and our ancient forebears also indulged in this practice:

There is only one possible reference to the sexual organs in [Vergil's] *Aeneid,* at 3.427 . . . where *pubes* refers to the pubic area of Scylla. The original sense may have been "pubic hair" . . . It would thence have acquired the secondary sense "area covered by the pubic hair, external genitalia" . . . Lucretius' subject led him to deal with sexual matters in book 4 [of *De rerum natura*]. His terminology is of some interest, because it can be assumed that he chose euphemisms. *Loca* (*loci*) and *pars* are his most common words for the male and female genitalia . . . *Loca* (neuter or masculine) was an old Latin euphemism for the female parts, in the sense either of *cunnus* (first at Cato, Agr. 157. 11) or *uterus* (note the remarks of Pliny, *Nat.* 11. 209), or of the two words indiscriminately . . . The euphemistic tone of *loca* is shown not only by its presence in Lucretius, but also in a variety of polite genres, such as the philosophica of Cicero (*Nat.* 2. 128), elegy (Ovid, *Ars* 2.719, 3.799), and often in medical writings . . . the most general of anatomical terms, *corpus* is [sometimes] by implication used of the female parts (uterus/vagina) . . .

Corpus could be used indifferently of the penis . . . testicles . . . and *cunnus*. (Adams, "Anatomical Terminology in Latin Epic," 51.)

Adams notes that clever euphemisms are not confined to Lucretius and Cicero but are embedded in the language itself, suggested by the crusty Cato the Elder. More interestingly, in light of frequent modern medical squeamishness, is Adams's conclusion that such euphemisms are common in the Latin medical writers (although "medical writers" are represented only by Cornelius Celsus and Pliny the Elder). It is, however, most important to notice how even the presumably racy authors (Ovid and Petronius) *also* employ euphemisms, a point similar to the emphasis indicated by Mencken for the early twentieth century.

There is a universal tendency by human beings to mask the realities of sex and reproduction—next to the drive for nourishment, the strongest biological drive for humanity—in complex cultural and social customs that seek to "regulate" both an introduction to sex and the process of procreation itself. Many clichés, euphemisms, and inwardly understood phrases appear encrusted among all cultures on the topics of sex and reproduction. Thus in studies of sexual "initiation rites," there are genetic lines (either male or female) held more important than the "act" on its own terms. Sexual drive intends to produce children, but all cultures have devised dodges and attempts to avoid either pregnancies or paternity. In law, these dodges encompass legal parlance speaking of "legitimacy" and "illegitimacy" (as if the child did not exist), as well as the profession of prostitution (regulated, ignored, persecuted, or valued). The Romans insisted early in their legal history that wills should be carefully drawn (specifics are in the *Twelve Tables,* traditionally dated to about 450 B.C.) so that bloodlines and property could ideally stabilize the passage of generations, and the questions of who got what rested on "legitimacy," the legal definition of sex and the production of children. Euphemisms are natural in Roman law (and in any legal system), but the law sought stability within the unpredictable chaos of human passions.

Modern American English displays a dazzling variety of euphemisms concerning sex, and one can almost say politely "have *intercourse,*" or "*copulate,*" or "*engage in coition*" or "*coitus,*" or even more mildly "form a sexual union," "make love," "*fornicate*" (somewhat impolite), or "have carnal knowledge of someone." Should we not wish to express the function quite so directly, we can "have mates," "have commerce," "have congress," "enjoy intimacy," and "have relations." Dipping into ordinary speech with its raft of metaphors, someone can "sleep" with someone (of either sex) or "go to bed with someone." Considered obscene—but not widely—are euphemisms including "to screw," "to mount," "to board," and "to hump" (the last three from the male perspective).

If a *pregnancy* should result from any of the actions listed above, there are dozens of ways English can muffle this too, clothing it in layers of nice-nellyisms. One can say "be in a family way" and be readily understood, and one can "anticipate a blessed event" and likewise be understood. The woman is, of course, "with child," or "expecting," or if a learned manner is sought to describe the "coming event," she is *gravid*—and if birth is imminent, she is *parturient*. In common English, one can state that the woman is "big" or "heavy" or even "laden." Only in "with child" is the fact acknowledged that pregnancy produces a baby.

Men continue to "sire" children, and late-night stand-up TV comedians (whose job it is to wiggle and worm their way around verbal taboos without giving offense to the mythical moral majority) suggest something of the processes they call *insemination* and *pollination*, but few use *spermatize, fertilize, fructify,* or *fecundify*. The loudly proclaimed openness about matters sexual (with "sex education" beginning late in grade school) has produced its own kind of awkwardness among preteen children: TV comics can bring howls of laughter with condom jokes, but young children who might know exactly how to use this *prophylactic* (a word rarely used in the last decades of the twentieth century) do not feel comfortable in speaking about what goes into the condom. Moreover, there are only rare jokes about *masturbation*, although sexologists and psychologists say everyone (male and female) indulges. And with the repeated focus in newspapers and magazines on sexually transmitted diseases, there is continual reference to *syphilis, gonorrhea, genital herpes,* and AIDS (the acronym for *Acquired Immunodeficiency Syndrome*). If a writer chooses to consider the moral, legal, and medical questions enveloping *contraception* and *abortion*, quite frequently the popular press will devote much space to these medical questions, which are political ones as well. Sex-for-hire on both sides of the gender fence has its own vocabulary, as does *pornography,* and *prostitution* flourishes today as it has throughout history.

These "function" words mirror sex in its multiple varieties, and sexual English indicates the normal and usual concern about who-does-what-with-whom, as well as the particular and culture-bound precepts of what is "proper." In the late twentieth century, it is sometimes difficult to determine what is "proper," since we live in an era when many of the older assumptions concerning "aristocratic" and "educated" values have vanished. Doubtlessly, the future holds an emergence of a new "upper class," with a set of standards to be maintained in public and often flouted in private.

The etymologies of words in sexual English, as well as those that describe the anatomical parts essential in preserving our species, reflect most often the complicated and nuanced function (as defined culturally), followed by the form (by contrast, easily explained through analogy and the borrowing of Greek and Latin words):

Copulation comes from Latin's *copula* ("a bond or fastening," with a subliminal sense of "intimate connection" [among people]). In classical Latin, *copulatio* meant simply "the act of combining," with the adjective *copulatus* (here masculine) sometimes a "close" or "intimate" friendship. A Roman wishing to speak of sexual intercourse would often use *concubitio* or *concubitus,* with the masculine *concubinus* meaning "a homosexual lover" or "catamite" as in Catullus, 61.123, and Martial, *Epigrams,* VIII, 44.77, with the feminine *concubina* becoming English's *concubine. Copulatio* was bland, as is *copulation.*

Coition is the learned English form of Latin's *coitus,* alternatively *coetus.* Both have similarly bland meanings, with a single exception. When a Roman used *coitus,* he or she normally meant "coming together," "meeting," or "encounter," or if one was interested in astrology or astronomy, one could use *coitus* to signify "the conjunctions of heavenly bodies" (the nominative plural of *coitus* is also *coitus*), especially of the sun and the moon at new moon, as in Pliny, *NH,* II, 44, and XVI, 190. Tree experts spoke of *coitus* as "grafts" (that is "joinings"), again as Pliny says in *NH,* XVII, 103, and physicians said that *coitus* were "reunions" or "unitings" of injured tissues, as noted by Celsus, *De medicina,* II, 10.18. The "proper" Latin also included euphemisms of (or on) *coitus* on its own: botanists well understood that some plants were "fertilized" (*coitus* in Pliny, *NH*, XVII, 11), and such "fertilization" could become "sex" or "sexual union" in Ovid, *Metamorphoses*, VII, 709.

Intercourse in modern English is a semieuphemism, generally meaning *coitus*. *Intercourse* descends from the Latin *intercursus*, meaning "the action of running between" or "interposition," and *intercursus* in medieval Latin became "communication" or "trading." In English, *intercourse* is a lately introduced metaphor for "sex," with the first printed examples appearing in 1798 and 1804 (*OED*, s.v. def. 2d).

Fornication is famous (or infamous): Matthew, V, 32, reads (in the translation known as the *Jerusalem Bible*), "Everyone who divorces his wife, except for the case of fornication, makes her an adulteress." The key phrase in the *koinē* Greek text is *parektos logou porneias* (see *pornography*, below), more or less meaning "apart from an instance (*logos*) of sexual unfaithfulness (*porneia*)," with *porneia* usually meaning "prostitution" (for which see below). The translation of *porneia* as "fornication" descends in English from the first translations of the Bible, with the King James Version quite representative. The learned gathering of scholars who rendered this classic of English literature knew quite well that *fornix* generally meant "vault," "arch," "vaulted opening," or "archway," but as usual these early-seventeenth-century scholars knew their classical texts very well indeed, and they also knew that an alternative meaning for *fornix* in Latin was "brothel," since *fornicatio* (the "vaulting arch" of architects, in Vitruvius, *On Architecture*, VI, 8.3) was characteristic of the basements or cellars of the buildings that housed such establishments (one might call this a Roman "underground profession"). One meets *fornix* as brothel naturally enough in the expected Latin authors (for example, Juvenal, *Satires*, III, 156; Petronius, *Satyricon*, VII, 4; Martial, *Epigrams*, I, 34.6; and Suetonius, *Julius Caesar*, 49.1), but *fornix* as brothel occurs in "proper" writers too, including the admittedly earthy Seneca the Elder in his *Controversiae*, I, 2.21. Medieval Latin gave to Old French and thence to Middle English *fornicacioun*, and the word was standard in our tongue by 1300. In the early seventeenth century, as certainly reflected in the King James Bible of 1611, the word was perfectly suited for educated parlance, and one notes its ordinary use in Shakespeare's day, from a line in *Measure for Measure* (V, 1.105), performed in 1603: "Shee accuses him of Fornication." In Elizabethan English, this meant "adulterous sex," a meaning retained in the language to the present.

Pregnancy derives directly from the Latin *praegnans* ("heavy with young"). The word comes into modern English from Middle English.

Gravid is almost the straight Latin *gravis* ("heavy" or "loaded"). In Latin, the verb *gravidare* normally meant "to make pregnant," as one reads in Cicero, *Nature of the Gods,* II, 83, an author not commonly employing forceful terms on sex. *Gravidus* = "heavy with young" = "pregnant" is illustrated by Celsus, *De medicina,* II, 1.14, and many other writers in classical Latin. One can, of course, speculate with some amusement on the puns that Romans must have made with *gravis* and *gravitas* (whence our "gravity"), the latter a word ordinarily used to point out the "heaviness" and "authority" of an exalted person of senatorial rank in the Roman Republic. To be sure, "strictness," "sternness," and "austerity" are the high school Latin books' translations for *gravitas,* but one cannot escape the delicious image of a rotund senator with a reputation *gravidare* . . .

Parturient comes into English directly from Latin's *parturire* ("to be on the point of giving birth"), as found in several classical Latin texts. Thus medical English also has *parturition* ("childbirth" or "the act of bringing forth young"), ultimately derived from the Latin *partus* ("the act of giving birth"), as exemplified in Vergil, *Georgics,* I, 278. And medical English also sports *parturifacient* (something "inducing or accelerating labor"). The most common parturifacient is called *oxytocin* (Greek *oxus* ["sharp" or "acute"] + *tokas* ["childbirth"]), a hormone (see chap. 12 under *Pituitary*) secreted by the posterior lobe of the pituitary and prepared commercially since the 1930s from bovine and hog pituitary glands.

Insemination comes into English from the Latin *inseminare* ("to implant," "to impregnate," or "to fertilize"), usually in the context of agriculture. Late Latin derived *inseminatus* ("sowed" [as with seeds]). *Semen,* gen. *seminis,* is generally "seed" in Latin, with a variety of contextual meanings: writers on farm life (for example, Cato the Elder, *Agriculture,* 5.3, 48.3, and 151.1) have *semen* as "the seed of plants" or "that which is sown," and the phrase *in semen ire* translates "to go to seed," as describing that phase of the growth cycle of a plant. Sometimes agricultural writers use *semen* to mean specifically the grain of emmer wheat, *Triticum dicoccum* L. (in Columella, *Agriculture,* II, 12.1), and emmer grains were favored in the preparation of helpful pills and pastilles, as one reads in Pliny, *NH,* XVIII, 102, and Scribonius Largus, *Compositiones,* 70. Sometimes *semen* means "semen" or "sperm," a distinction observed in agricultural writers and others who used this nuance for emphasis in poetry (for example, Catullus, 67.26), perhaps reflecting the farmers' lingo recorded by Varro, *Agriculture*, II, 7.8, a gradation of meaning often seen in medical writing (Celsus, *De medicina*, IV, 28.1 and VIII, 13 [in his *Agriculture*, III, 9.12, Varro employs *semen* to mean "a prenatal stage of living creatures," and the word could be extended to indicate "parentage," "descent," "offspring," and even a "race" or "breed"]). If Catullus pointedly borrowed the word to make a sexual emphasis, one perceives that *semen* was a common euphemism in Latin, with shades of meaning ranging from the agricultural to the sexual.

Pollination in modern English almost always is used in connection with botany, that is, the "transfer of pollen from the anther to the stigma" in flowers. *Pollen*, gen. *pollinis*, is classical Latin for "finely ground flour" or "powder," so that Enlightenment botanists borrowed the term and invented the meaning we now have for pollen.

Spermatize is a recent coinage in English borrowed from the dozens of *sperma-* and *spermato-* terms in medical English. *Sperma*, gen. *spermatos*, pl. *spermata*, is "seed" in Greek, with all of the variant shades of meaning observed in Latin. If an uneasy physician wishes to avoid the presumably awkward *semen*, he can learnedly say *spermatic fluid*, the substance with which the male "spermatizes" the female.

Fertilize came into Middle English as *fertilite*, derived from the Latin noun *fertilitas* ("a fruitfulness or fertility of land, crops, and human beings"). *Fructify* descends into English from the Latin *fructus* ("fruits and vegetables," "profits," "the right to enjoy something" [in Roman law this is *usufructus*], "gratification," "satisfaction," and "pleasure.") Not surprisingly, the root verb *frui* (the infinitive of *fruor*) included the refinement "to enjoy someone sexually," as in Ovid, *Metamorphoses*, IX, 724. To be *fecund* in English is to be literally "fruitful," with the Latin *fecunditas* ("fertility" or "productiveness") linked to the verb *fecundare* ("to make fertile or fruitful"), as used by Vergil, *Georgics*, IV, 21. The context of the farm is again paramount, so that one can use *fecund* in English to describe "productive" things in almost any way (as in the "fecund nineteenth century") in a neatly bland manner. Many of these sexual function terms as adapted into medical English have emerged from the ancient Roman farm.

In the 1950s and 1960s, a *prophylactic* was almost always the polite word for "condom," but late-twentieth-century English generally employs the term in its broadest medical meaning, "a defense or protection against disease," usually by means of a drug. One can, of course, assume that a condom will "protect" against any kind of *venereal* disease. *Venereal* derives ultimately from the name given to the Roman goddess of love, beauty, and sexual passion, *Venus,* gen. *Veneris,* an ancient deity of gardens and springs who was later cross-identified by the Romans with the Greek goddess of love and passion, *Aphrodite* (whence our word *aphrodisiac* ["sexual stimulant"]). The old word *venery* ("gratification of sexual desire") is fading out of the language, perhaps because it is often confused with the other English term *venery* ("hunting" or "the chase," derived from Latin's *venari* ["to hunt" or "to chase"]).

Prophylactic is a late-sixteenth-century English creation from the Greek *pro* ("before") + *phylaktikos* ("preservative"), with the adjective *phylaktikos* winnowed from the noun *phylax,* gen. *phylakos* ("watcher," "guard," "sentinel," or "protector"). Common in medicalese is *prophylaxis* (Greek *phylaxis* [a "watching" or "guarding"]), which generally means "prevention of disease." Even among physicians, nurses, and other medical professionals, the term has become fuzzy, since dentists often call the cleaning of teeth a *prophylaxis,* appropriate if one means "prevention" of tooth decay.

Masturbation comes into English directly from the Latin *masturbator,* gen. *masturbatoris,* with the verb *masturbari* ("to masturbate"), words occurring in the *Epigrams* of Martial. Still coyly defined as "sexual self-gratification," masturbation was a disease or human failing throughout the nineteenth century and most of the twentieth century, an opinion vividly typified in the following: "Suppose you are worrying because you have 'wet dreams' or have practiced masturbation once in a while. If it has happened, don't let it scare you. If it's a habit, break it!" (McMillen et al., *Handbook for Boys,* [1948], 412). *Masturbation* came into English in the 1860s, but our Victorian ancestors preferred to say (if they mentioned it at all) *onanism,* a word coined from the name Onan in Genesis, 38.9, a gentleman in the Hebrew traditions who "spilt his seed on the ground every time he slept with his brother's wife, to avoid providing a child for his brother. What he did was offensive to Yahweh, so he brought about his death also" (trans. Jerusalem Bible). Today, *onanism* sometimes is used to mean *coitus interruptus,* but to medical thinking in the nineteenth century, masturbation was not only an evil but also an act subject to divine wrath.

Syphilis is the name invented by Girolamo Fracastoro of Verona (*c.* 1478–1553) for the supposedly "new" disease brought back from the New World by the sailors on Columbus's first voyage (1492). Fracastoro's long poem—modeled after Vergil, but with Lucretius also firmly in mind—was titled *Syphilis, sive morbus Gallicus* (*Syphilis, or the French Disease*) and published in 1530; Fracastoro in good classical manner attempted to weave mythology together with some fresh insights into what we would today call epidemiology. Etymologists continue to debate the origins and derivations of Fracastoro's coinage of *syphilis*, but the best guess is that the name emerges from a medieval corruption of *Sipytus*, the name of a son of Niobe as contained in Ovid, *Metamorphoses*, VI, 146 (Fracastoro's name for a shepherd is Syphilis, the first victim of the disease). Whether this Renaissance plague was "given" to Europe by native Americans, to Spain and thence to Europe as a whole after 1493, also remains hotly disputed among medical historians, but before Paul Ehrlich's (1854–1915) famous "606" (arsphenamine, patented under the name Salvarsan) was first successfully used in 1911 to treat syphilis, this sexually transmitted malady was ultimately fatal.

Syphilis is caused by a *spirochete* (Greek *speira* ["coil"] + *chaitē* ["loose hair," "lion's mane," or "horse's mane"], Latinized into *chaeta* to mean "bristle" by the nineteenth century), a *bacterium* (Greek *baktērion*, pl. *baktēria* ["little staff" or "cane"]) of coiled or twisted appearance, displaying characteristics of both bacteria and a *virus* (Latin *virus* ["slime" or "poison"]). The specific species *Treponema pallidum* (an early-twentieth-century coinage from Greek *trepein* ["to turn"] + *nēma*, gen. *nēmatos* ["thread" or "yard"], + Latin *pallidus* ["pale" or "greenish"]) was not determined until 1905, and Ehrlich's *arsphenamine* as a drug caused very unpleasant side effects, due to its content of arsenic. *Arsphenamine* has a complicated etymology: Greek *arsenikon* ("yellow orpiment" = arsenic trisulfide, whence the modern *arsenic*) is combined with the Greek verb *phainein* ("to appear" or "to show") and then in turn with the Greek *ammōniakon* ("gum and rock salt compound prepared near the shrine of Ammon in Libya" [thus later *sal ammoniac;* Latin *sal,* gen. *salis,* is "salt"]), which is part of eighteenth-century chemistry as *ammonia* obtained from *sal ammoniac,* and by the mid-nineteenth century the derived term *amine* was coined by chemists to designate "a compound derived from ammonia." Syphilis is treated with *penicillin* (Latin *penicillus* ["painter's brush"]), although the bacteria have become more resistant to this antibiotic in recent years.

Gonorrhea (Greek *gonorrhoia* ["involuntary or excessive discharge of semen without copulation" (in males), or "flowing discharge of seed or mucus from the urethra or vagina" (in females)]) was clearly rampant among the Greeks and Romans, much as it is common in modern societies. Recent calculations suggest over 250 million cases of gonorrhea worldwide, and there are annually at least 3 million cases of the disease in the United States (contrasted with world incidence of syphilis of about 50 million; four hundred thousand in the United States). The causative organism of this usually sexually transmitted disease is the kidney-shaped *diplococcus* (Greek *diploos* ["twofold" or "double"] + *kokkos* ["berry"], thus in microbiology "spherical bacteria occurring in pairs"), called *Neisseria gonorrhoeae* (the Latinized form of A.L.S. Neisser [1855–1916], a German doctor, + *gonorrhoia*), generally treatable with penicillin and other antibiotics. Before World War II, gonorrhea was often known as *blennorhea* (Greek *blennos* ["slime"] + *rhoia* ["discharge"]), a term not as sharp as gonorrhea, with its Greek-derived *gonos,* which included among its meanings "procreation," "seed," and "genitals." Greco-Roman medicine had its own clear concepts of *gonorrhoia,* and there is no better account than in the works of Aretaeus of Cappadocia (*fl. c.* A.D. 150), whose extant writings in Greek (openly in imitation of the Ionic Greek in the Hippocratic *corpus*) include sections of *Acute and Chronic Diseases.* In *Causes and Signs of Chronic Diseases,* one reads about how "*gonorrhoia* is not fatal, but disgusting and unpleasant to hear [about]." Aretaeus adds:

> Women can also have this affliction, but their sexual seed [*thorē*] flows out with stimulation and pleasure to the parts, peculiar especially in licentious sexual intercourse with men [the Greek here for "intercourse" is *homiliē*]: for men do not experience the same irritation. For the dribbling fluid in men is thin, cold, without color, and seedless [*agonon*]. Indeed, its nature [*physis*] being cold, how could it send forth life engendering seed? [*zoōgonon sperma*] . . . And the living sexual seed makes us male: hot, strong of limb, hairy, with pleasant voice, cheerful, forceful in thought and action—men make manifest [these characteristics] . . . And any man who would exercise self-control over his sexual seed, he is powerful, courageous, and as strong as wild animals. Instances of moderation and self-control of sex are characteristic of athletes. (Aretaeus of Cappadocia, *Causes and Signs of Chronic Diseases,* II, 5.1–4, in *Works,* IV, 5.1–4, trans. from the Greek text by Hude, *Aretaeus,* 71.)

Note that Aretaeus does not advocate abstinence from sex, but what used to be called *continence*. The Roman doctor has seen a number of prostitutes (for which see below) who exhibited the external symptoms of gonorrhea, but the deep-seated Aristotelian notions of the superiority of men over women may remind a modern of the jokes about preserving the "male essence" in Stanley Kubrick's 1964 motion picture *Dr. Strangelove.* Classical antiquity is the origin of the modern myth that athletes of any type should abstain from sex before a game or competition. Parenthetically, Greco-Roman theories of conception often assumed that the female possessed a "seed" much as did the male, so that Aretaeus's comments would reflect this common notion.

Genital herpes (Latin *genitalis* ["fruitful" or "of birth"], akin to *genitor*, gen. *genitoris* ["father"], + Greek *herpeton* ["creeping thing," "reptile," "snake," and "crawling/creeping"]) is a sexually transmitted infection of the skin and mucosal linings of the genital organs, caused by what is termed the *herpes simplex virus* (Latin *simplex* ["having a single layer"] + *virus* ["slime" or "poison"]), characterized by itchy and sore blisters, which ulcerate and crust before healing, occasionally with heavy scarring. Complications in the nervous system make this somewhat more than an annoying result of sexual promiscuity, so that physicians prescribe *acyclovir* as the drug of choice to eradicate the virus.

Acyclovir is a coined term from the pharmacy of the early 1980s: *a-* ["not"] + Greek *kyklos* ["circle"] + *vir-* [*virus*], but the short form adopted is pulled from an earlier name for the drug, *acycloguanosine + virus*. In biochemistry, *acyclo-* indicates a compound that does not have a closed chain or rings of atoms, and *guanosine* is a nucleotide that has *guanine,* a basic part of DNA and RNA (see chap. 12), with *guanine* a name drived from Spanish American *huano* ("dung"), which becomes in English *guano* (the solid waste of seabirds, found in large amounts on the coasts of Chile and Peru). When physicians prescribe *acyclovir,* they may be unaware that the drug of choice for herpes translates as "non-closed-ring-bird-shit-like-for-slime."

Acquired Immunodeficiency Syndrome has a complicated etymology, suggesting the unhappy entanglements and obscurities of this new entry onto the lists of human physical failings. Latin *ac-* is a variant of *ad-* ("toward"), added to the verb *quaerere* ("to search for," "to earn," among several meanings), giving modern English *acquire*. *Immuno-* derives from *immunity,* coming to us from the Latin *immunitas,* gen. *immunitatis* ("exemption from tax or tribute," with later Roman law narrowing the meaning to "immunity or exemption from an obligation or duty"), + *deficere* ("to be lacking," "to run short," "to fail," among several) + Greek *syndromē* (in the medical Greek of the Roman Empire, quite frequently "concurrence of symptoms," or what today in medical jargon would be "clinical picture," as one reads in Galen, *On a Method of Medicine Addressed to Glaucon,* I, 15 [ed. Kühn, Vol. XI, 59], and Aretaeus of Cappadocia, *Therapeutics for Acute Diseases,* I, 10.19 [ed. Hude,

118], with Aretaeus using *xyndromē* to gather together the various clinical manifestations of *pleuritis*).

Not only is the basic *etiology* (Greek *aitios* ["cause"] + *logos*, thus "study of causes") argued, but the incidence of this almost always fatal affliction (this is being written in late 1989) has engendered its own, sometimes hysterical social response. Moral labels further confuse the basics of *epidemiology* (Greek *epidēmia* [main meaning, "staying at a place" or "visit," with medical meaning "prevalence of a disease," with adj. *epidēmiakos*] + *logos* [the modern medicalese means generally "the study of incidence and prevalence of disease among large groups of people, and the determination of sources and causes of those infectious diseases," and an *epidemic* is a disease affecting many people at the same time, spreading from individual to individual in a place where the disease is not usually or permanently prevalent]). The great majority of cases occur among homosexual or bisexual men, followed by cases among heterosexuals who have shared needles for drug injections. Most tragic are the deaths that occur among *hemophiliacs* (Greek *haima* ["blood"] + *philia* ["affinity" or "friendship," with adj. *philiakos*"]), whose lives sometimes depend on blood transfusions (only 1 percent, however, of the deaths from AIDS are hemophiliacs). As one crusty medical commentator put it, one must "work very hard to get AIDS," so that even the term *epidemic* for this syndrome is rejected by many epidemiologists.

Contraception (Latin *contra* ["against" or "contrary to"] + *cipere* from *concipere* ["to conceive"], whence the participle *conceptum* ["something conceived"]) is easily defined: "the conscious and deliberate prevention of conception by means of drugs, sexual techniques, or mechanical devices," a definition of the term in English since about 1900. But the practice of contraception raises many moral and social issues, especially in the context of traditional religious views on the matter.

Abortion (Latin *abortio*, gen. *abortionis* ["miscarriage"]) raises even more moral, religious, and legal problems, even though modern medical techniques have ensured rather safe conditions as contrasted with the uncertainties of the past. By expelling what some would argue is indeed "human" (at the moment of conception), by definition one is committing murder. On the other hand, that same definition of *human* in both law and common perception often rests on "form and function" (that is does it "look" human and does it "act" human), which means that until a human fetus "looks" human, it is not, and until it "acts" human, it is not. Fuzzy arguments and strongly held opinions lead to uncompromising positions—which suggest why abortion and contraception have spawned vigorous arguments, debates, and occasional violence for thousands of years.

Homosexuality (Latin *homo,* gen. *hominis* ["human being" or "man"]) also raises the irritation levels among some observers, so that careful argument is often impossible. Among women, same-sex preference is frequently called *lesbianism* (from the Greek island of Lesbos, home of the famous and brilliant poet Sappho [*c.* 612 B.C.–?], who preferred relations with women, at least this is what seems to be true from the remnants of her magnificent poetry). Formerly crude terms for homsexual men (*fag, fairy,* and the like) have generally been superseded by *gay.*

Pornography is always culture-bound, even as various state legislatures debate and redebate what it means and how state statutes can constitutionally regulate this sort of literature. As indicated above under *fornication,* the Greek *porneia* usually meant "prostitution," with the practitioner obviously unfaithful to one person with his or her sexual favors. In Greek, there are many terms that reflect the ever common presence of prostitutes, with representative words like *porneion* ("brothel"), *pornoboskos* ("a proprietor of a brothel" [note the masculine gender of the noun]), *pornodidaskalos* ("a teacher of prostitutes' skills"), *pornos* ("a homosexual male" or "a man who practices sodomy" [*sodomy* descends from Middle English as a long-term reflection of God's destruction of Sodom and Gomorrah in Genesis 18 and 19 and usually means "anal or oral copulation" or "anal intercourse as practiced by male homosexuals" and is occasionally synonymous with "bestiality," that is, "copulation practiced by humans with animals"]), *pornokopos* ("one who advertises or sells the skills of prostitutes and call girls"), and *pornotelōnēs* ("a collector of the tax levied on *porneia*" [showing that prostitution was legal—to a point—in ancient Greece: *pornotelōnēs* became a crude way of describing a tax collector of any kind in later Greek]). The literature on such matters was called *pornographos* in Greek ("writing about prostitutes"), and it was a perfectly respectable term labeling a widely popular genre, usually not thought to be obscene but rather uncouth, somewhat beneath the dignity of the gentlemen and ladies of the upper classes (however defined in the various eras of Greek and Roman history). *Pornography* is a late addition in English, with the first printed instance recorded in the 1857 edition of Dunglison's *Medical Dictionary* (the term does not appear in the twelfth edition of 1855); the entry

"Pornography" that appears on page 836 of Dunglison's *Medical Lexicon: A Dictionary of Medical Science* (1874) is identical to that of the 1857 text: "Pornography . . . A description of prostitutes or of prostitution, as a matter of public hygiene." One wonders how Dunglison might define some of the materials commonly proffered in the late twentieth century, ranging from the now tame centerfolds in *Playboy* magazine to the almost starkly anatomical photographs in periodicals aimed at female and male homosexuals.

Prostitution was present in English by the sixteenth century, emerging from the Latin *prostituere* ("to prostitute") and *prostituta* ("a woman who sells sex for pay"), as well as *prostitutus* ("a man who sells sex for pay"). Among the Romans, much more than among the Greeks in the eastern part of the Roman Empire; the *prostituta* was subject to a status of public dishonor, so that one can—depending on the context—translate *prostituta* as "whore" or "strumpet" or, even more Victorianly, "trollop." There is more than mere sex involved, as usual: social status and, in some well-documented instances, religious practices and values have important roles. No, the *prostate* gland does not have etymological kinship with any of these Latin words: *prostate* is invented from two Greek terms that translate as "one who stands before."

SEXUAL ANATOMY: THE "PARTS" (FEMALE)

Vulva: in classical Latin, *vulva* was "the womb," as in Celsus, *De medicina,* IV, 1.2, or "the female sex organ," as the word appears in Juvenal, *Satires,* VI, 129. In modern medical English, it now means "the external female genitalia."

Hymen is Greek *hymēn* (the "thin skin or membrane covering the brain and the heart," according to Aristotle, *HA,* 494b29). In Greek religious observances, *Hymēn* was a god of marriages, and thus a "wedding song" was a *hymēnaios.* In medical English, the hymen is "a fold of mucous membrane partially closing the external orifice of the vagina in a young girl, generally one who has not had sexual experience."

Uterus is a common Latin word for "womb," illustrated in Varro, *Agriculture,* II, 2.14, but sometimes *uterus* was broadened to mean "belly" or "abdomen," as in the street jargon recorded in Juvenal, *Satires,* X, 309. In later Roman law, *uterus* meant "pregnancy" (Paul in Justinian's *Digest,* V, 4.3), and in medical English, the uterus is the portion of the "oviduct in which the fertilized ovum implants and develops prenatal structures." The *cervix* is the "neck" of the uterus, as cervical vertebrae are located in the "neck" (chap. 5, above).

Ovary is a Late Latin to English word from *ovarium,* pulled from the Latin *ovum* ("egg"). The *ovarium* "made" the eggs (pl. *ova*), and thus the *ovary* is now "the female reproductive gland, in which develop the ova and the hormones which regulate female secondary sex characteristics."

Fallopian tube is the oviduct leading to the uterus, bearing the name of Gabriello Fallopio (d. 1562), an Italian anatomist who first described this structure. The Fallopian tubes (a pair) function to transport ova from the ovary to the uterus.

Vagina is ordinary Latin for "the sheath of a sword" or "scabbard," as used by military authors including Julius Caesar in his *Gallic Wars,* V, 44.8. In Roman farming, *vagina* was a "leaf-sheath of an ear of wheat," in Varro, *Agriculture,* I, 32.1. Renaissance anatomists were struck by the analogous shape of this human structure, so that the vagina became "the passage leading from the uterus to the vulva."

SEXUAL ANATOMY: THE "PARTS" (MALE)

Penis: in classical Latin, *penis* meant both "a tail," perhaps a common euphemism suggested by Cicero, *Letters to his Friends,* IX, 22.2, and "the male sexual organ," as one sees in Horace, *Epodes,* XII, 8, and many other texts. Sometimes, an overly randy chap would be nicknamed *Penis*. The modern term is the ancient one.

Testis or *testicle:* in Latin *testis,* gen. *testis,* pl. *testes,* was most often a legal or quasi-legal term meaning "one present at a legal transaction, that is, a witness." A second meaning for *testis* (usually in the plural *testes*) is "testicle," signifying a "witness to one's manhood," suggesting that a male "without balls" was no man at all, perhaps a clear reference to the ancient practice of having eunuchs as favored slaves to serve women. In Greek, *parastatēs* ("witness") also has this second meaning of "testicle," reflecting similar customs in common for the two cultures. Latin's *testiculus,* gen. *testiculi,* pl. *testiculi,* is the diminutive form of *testis,* translated literally as "little witness to one's masculinity," since *testiculus* always means what its English cognate means. The Roman jurisconsults fussed about eunuchs as serviceable slaves and argued the problem under *morbus* ("disease"), with Ulpian pronouncing that a "eunuch (*spado,* gen. *spadonis*) is not diseased, just as one of them who has a single testicle can father children" (Ulpian in Justinian's *Digest,* XI, 1.6.2), arguments that turned in Roman law on the distinction between "faults" or "defects" (*vitia,* sing. *vitium*) and a disease through which the usefulness of a slave might be lessened (Paul in *Digest,* XXI, 1.5). Eunuchs *as* eunuchs in law were suitable slaves for a particular function, even though to ordinary men, they would be "defective." Without *testes,* one could not "bear witness," a sense preserved in English with *testimony* and *testify.* The Latin *spado* is a transliteration of the Greek *spadōn,* gen. *spadōnos* ("eunuch"), which remains as an obscure term in civil law (*spado*) as "someone unable to procreate." English *eunuch* preserves the Greek semi-euphemism *eunouchos* ("chamberlin" or "castrated male who took charge of the women" or, in popular parlance, "bed-watcher"). Greek botanists could describe lettuce as "seedless" (*eunouchos*), which mirrors how the ancient Greeks and Romans would view those males unable to bear witness.

The *epididymis* is exactly as Galen, *On Seed,* I, 15 (ed. Kühn, Vol. IV, 565), used the term, so that this modern medicoanatomical word is the replication of a second-century Roman description. Today's definition is like Galen's, that is, "an elongated organ on the posterior surface of a testis which is the convoluted beginning of the vas deferens." *Vas* is Latin for "vessel," and *deferens* is "carrying," from the Latin verb *deferre*—rather straightforward anatomy, almost completely Latinate adapted from a Greco-Roman source. The "seed" (Galen's *sperma*) would be first "carried" through this structure on its way to the seminal vesicle (= small vessel for semen) and to the prostate gland (see *prostate* under *prostitution* above), which adds a thin, milky, alkaline fluid to the semen in the process called *ejaculation* (the Latin *eiaculatus* is "shot out," in turn derived from *iaculum* ["little spear" or "javelin"]) and in vulgar English called "jacking off" (see *masturbation* above).

The forms of the anatomy of sex and reproduction are easily described; the functions have multiple contexts, reflective of the tangled customs of culture and long observance.

CHAPTER 11

VASCULAR MATTERS: HEART AND BLOOD, "THE LIQUIDS OF LIFE"

> It profits one who is pondering on the movement, pulsation, performance, function, and services of the heart and arteries to read what his predecessors have written, and to note the general trend of opinion handed on by them. For by so doing he can confirm their correct statements, and through anatomical dissection, manifold experiments, and persistent careful observation emend their wrong ones.
>
> . . . blood is continuously passing into the arteries in greater amount than can be supplied from the food ingested, so that, as the whole mass of the blood passes that way in a short space of time, it must make a circuit and return to its starting point.
>
> —WILLIAM HARVEY,
> De motu cordis et sanguinis in animalibus

THESE excerpts from Harvey's booklet describing what we commonly call "closed circulation" have interest for moderns on two counts: first, *De motu cordis* (*Movement of the Heart*) is the early-seventeenth-century work that decisively rejected ancient theories (including those of Galen) of how the heart and blood functioned; second, the text of *De motu cordis* in its early Enlightenment Latin shows the process by which many Latin and Latin-like terms slithered into medical and scientific English. Even some unacquainted with classical Latin could make some accurate guesses about the words in Harvey's text, guesses based on what modern English has preserved, illustrated by the Latin of several lines given above in English (the reader without Latin knowledge should flip from the quoted Latin below to the translation above, and be pleasantly surprised):

De cordis arteriarumque motu, pulsu, actione, usu, et utilitatibus cogitanti, operae pretium est, quae prius ab aliis mandata sunt literis, evolvere; quae vulgo jactata et tradita, animadvertere: ut quae recte dicta, confirmentur; quae falsa, dissectione anatomica, multiplici experientia, diligenti et accurata observatione, emendentur.

Shrewd hunches come immediately for *arteriarumque, pulsu, actione, usu, utilitatibus, cogitanti, operae, mandata, literis, evolvere, vulgo,* and perhaps *animadvertere.* Once past *ut quae* (and filling in the "and" for *et,* as well as "which" for *quae*), a reasonably literate speaker of English could catch the basic gist of all the words in the line *ut quae recte dicta, confirmentur.* Oddly enough, the fundamental term for "heart" in Harvey's Latin (*cor,* gen. *cordis* [here as *de cordis;* the *de* ("on" or "about") calls for the ablative, which means that Franklin must translate "on the movement," *motu,* nom. *motus,* etc.]) might puzzle the normally confident English speaker, unless there is recollection that a "cordial" is a drink that "stimulates the heart" and that a "cordial greeting" comes "from the heart" (Latin's *cordialis* originally meant this or "of the heart"), but with the exception of the infrequently used nineteenth-century terms *cordate* or *cordiform* ("shaped like a heart"), there are a few words descending into English from Latin's "heart," *cor.*

Once it is understood that the *-que* on the tail of *arteriarum* is an enclitic meaning "and," English *artery* springs (correctly) to mind, and *motu* suggests English *motion* (again rightly: Franklin's *movement* is closer to Harvey's intent). *Pulsu* (nom. *pulsus* ["push" or "beat" in Latin]) gives clearly enough *pulsation* (the "beating of the heart and arteries" would be an equally valid translation [*arteriarum* is the genitive plural form of *arteria*]), *actione* (nom. *actio*) yields *action* (Franklin thinks "performance" is the best choice here), *usu* (nom. *usus*) says *use* in English (Franklin chooses "function"), and *utilitatibus* (nom. sing. *utilitas,* gen. *utilitatis* [here in the ablative plural]) suggest *utility* in English (Franklin likes "services," which is a bit less that Latin's firmer "usefulness"). If one *cogitates,* there is thinking or pondering involved (Latin *cogitare* ["to think" or "to ponder"]), and anyone who has sat through a Wagnerian *opera* knows a lot of "work" went into it (Latin *opus,* gen. *operis,* nom. pl. *opera* [our English comes to us from seventeenth-century Italian, which borrowed it from Latin]). *Mandata* suggests *mandate* in English, close but not quite what Harvey's Latin wants to convey: Latin's *mandare* usually means "to commit" or "to command," with Renaissance Latin often using *mandare* as "to set down" or "to give [in writing]," which is why Franklin translates *mandata sunt literis* as he does. If someone is literate, he usually can write (Latin *littera,* gen. *litterae* ["letter of the alphabet" or simply "writing"]). Harvey's *evolvere*

(Latin "to unroll" [as a scroll would be read] or simply "to read," Frankin's translation) is the word that comes into English as *evolve,* with *evolution* derived from the Latin *evolutio,* gen. *evolutionis* ("unrolling a book"), capturing a sense easily approved by Darwinists of all stripes. *Vulgo* here is the Latin adverb "commonly" or "usually" (*vulgus,* gen. *vulgi,* is, one many recall, "the rabble"), so that—again—a "vulgar opinion" would literally mean thoughts held by the rabble; and *animadvertere* is the old-fashioned Latin for "to pay attention to" or "to notice," which becomes Franklin's "to note." The now rare English word *animadversion* (from Latin's *animadversio,* gen. *animadversionis* ["observation" or "censure" or "punishment"]) was a fancily used Victorianism that generally meant an unfavorable comment or criticism, quite in contrast with Renaissance Latin's rather bland meaning of "noting" or "heeding." Latin's *rectus* meant not only "straight" (as in the *rectum*) but also "correct," a sense mirrored when we say someone is a "straight shooter" (someone is honest) or in the prissy term *rectitude,* which says someone is "upright" or has "moral virtue"; when someone *rectifies* something, he "corrects" it or "makes it right." *Dicta* suggests English *dictate, dictation,* and similar words, directly descended from the Latin *dicere* ("to say," "to tell," and other verbs of similar import); the participle is *dictum,* so that *dicta* (those things said) can be translated as "statements." And beginning with *confirmentur,* the reader of modern English will recognize full cognates in all the words that follow, with the exception of *et* (Franklin's translation, however, of the two imperfect subjunctive passive verbs *confirmentur* and *emendentur* ["they may be confirmed" and "they may be corrected," both governed by the preceding *ut* ("so that")] as active verbs is incorrect, even though by making these verbs active in English, Franklin avoids some awkwardness).

Harvey's Latin indicates the manner in which many of these words soon eased into English, especially those terms that demanded precision in the medical sciences. In many respects, those Latin words that provided Harvey with his fundamental arguments for the then revolutionary concept of a closed circuit for the circulation of the blood were also words that often sifted into English as terms carrying single meanings, as contrasted with multiple senses attached to ordinary words. When, for example, we read *motu, usu, et utilitatibus cogitanti,* there is little doubt of the meanings, particularly as Harvey speaks to the basic question of pulsation and its intimate connection with the beating of the heart. *De motu cordis* stands as a splendid document illustrating the transition from a careful employment of ancient Latin for medical descriptions in the European Renaissance and Enlightenment to the equally precise Latinate terms that soon made up "scientific" and "medical" English.

De motu cordis of 1628 is one of the important modern tracts on human physiology, modern in the sense that Harvey signals the beginnings of modern perceptions of how the heart works and how it acts as a pump to keep the blood circulating in the human body throughout life. A key in Harvey's argument is his question of "how much" blood, suggested by the passages in chapter 10 of *De motu cordis,* a question *not* important to physicians in the preceding two millennia. Greek and Roman medicine certainly sought to answer the essential questions of how the living body functions, but until the Renaissance, such questions were generally posed in terms of a theory of "qualities," not the "quantities" so prominent in Harvey's carefully written tract. Yet even as the new understanding of the human body's functioning came to be fundamental in medicine and physiology, many of the pre-Harvey notions survived in terminologies now subsumed within the refurbished science and art of medicine, and it would not be until the early nineteenth century that the Greek notion of elements (four) would be replaced by a fresh theory of elements, founded on the chemistry and physics of the late eighteenth century. Moreover, it would not be until the early twentieth century that the ancient Greco-Roman perceptions of basic "essential liquids" were fully abandoned, and modern medical English still carries the heavy imprint of many of these concepts.

Among the pre-Socratic Greek philosophers, Thales of Miletus (*fl. c.* 585 B.C.) had asserted not only that water was one (if not the only one) of the primordials of the universe but also that water was essential for life itself. Arguments soon raged over "liquids and life," and out of a free-wheeling and long-term debate among philosophers came a general agreement that there were *elements* (Latin *elementum* ["one of the four elements" or "letter of the alphabet" or "first principle"] = Greek *stoicheion*) out of which the universe was made, usually reduced to four: air, earth, fire, and water. By the fifth century B.C., the elements had come to be characterized by their presumed natures, that is, the qualities, also frequently reduced to four: the dry, the cold, the hot, and the wet. Some Greek physicians began to speculate about which of the elements might be dominant in health and disease. Since it was generally agreed that liquids of some sort were also characteristic and necessary for life, the arguments often turned on which liquids (*chymoi* in Greek) were truly necessary and how such *chymoi* could lead to health, and conversely to disease. This debate engendered several humoral theorists (*chymos* means "humor" in the medical context), the most famous of which is the concept of the four humors, most fully explicated in the Hippocratic treatise known as *On the Nature of Man,* of about 350 B.C.:

> The body of man has in itself blood, phlegm, yellow bile and black bile; these make up the nature of the body and through these he feels pain or enjoys health. Now he enjoys the most perfect health when these four are in correct proportion to one another in terms of combination [*krasis*], their respective faculties [*dynameis*] and their quantity [*plēthos*], and when they are mixed most perfectly. Pain results when one of the four is less than it should be, or is in excess of what it should be, or is separated in the body when it should be combined with all the others. (Hippocratic *Nature of Man,* IV, 1–9, trans. from the Greek text by W.H.S. Jones, *Hippocrates,* 4 vols. (London: Heinemann, 1923–31), Vol. IV, 10, 12.)

The Greek text of this famous fourth-century medical tract contains a number of words that have left their marks in modern medical terminologies or related jargons, including *sōma* ("body"), *anthrōpos* ("man"), *haima* ("blood"), *phlegma* ("phlegm"), and *cholē* ("bile"):

> *Sōma,* gen. *sōmatos,* has evolved into English *somatic* ("of the body," "bodily," or "physical"), with derivatives like *somatogenic* (in embryology, "developing from somatic cells," that is, "the cells that take part in the formation of the body to become various tissues, organs, and the like"). In its suffix form the Greek *-soma* or *-some* defines such terms as *chromosome* (Greek "colored-body unit"), which contains *chromatin* (the stainable substance in a cell nucleus, DNA, RNA [see chap. 12, below], and various proteins, which form chromosomes in cell division).

Anthōpos, gen. *anthrōpou*, has bequeathed all sorts of words to English, from the academic specialty called *anthropology* ("the study of humankind") to the fancy and often used *anthropomorphic* (*anthrōpos* + Greek *morphos* ["shape" or "form"]), meaning "shaped like a human being," as when one describes Greek deities as "anthropomorphic gods and goddesses." One can also employ *anthropophagi* in place of "cannibals" (*anthrōpos* + Greek *phagein* ["to eat"], adapted into sixteenth-century Latin as *anthropophagus*, whence the English word).

Phlegma, translated as "phlegm," is the exudate "that issues from the head in cold weather" (common English, simply "snot"). *Phlegm* words remain in English, from *phlegmatic* (someone characterized by phlegm, that is, "apathetic" or "sluggish") to *phlegmatize* (in physical chemistry, this is what one does when "desensitizing" an explosive). In Greek, however, *phlegma*, gen. *phlegmatos*, frequently meant "inflammation," and such a symptom was marked by its hot, angry, or fiery nature. If this is confusing to the modern reader, there is a similar confusion in the Greco-Roman medical texts, even though *phlegma* becomes one of the four canonical humors in the works of Galen (adapted directly from the Hippocratic *Nature of Man*), and at the same time "that which becomes phlegm" is first observed as inflammation or a hot swelling.

Haima, gen. *haimatos*, has come into English (through Latin, which transliterated *haima* into *haema*, later shortened to *hema* as *the* blood word, as in *hematology* ("study of the nature, function, and diseases of the blood"), *hematite* ("iron oxide," Fe_2O_3, with the connotation from the Latin of "bloodstone," since the ore occurs in red, earthy masses), in turn engendering *hematin* (the iron pigment in *hemaglobin* [*hem-* + Latin *globus* ("sphere") + *in* (simply "in")], the "protein coloring-matter of the red blood cells," which conveys oxygen to the tissues). Among the dozens of such words, one can mention *hemophilia* (the "bleeder's disease," literally from the Greek words for "blood" and "lover"). Once the *hem-*, *hema-*, or *hemo-* prefix is understood for what it is, many terms are easily "translated" into ordinary English, for example *hemothorax* ("blood in the pleural cavity") and *hematocrit* (*hemato-* + Greek *kritēs* ["judge"]), which "translates" as a "judgment of blood," not too far from the actual meaning of the modern term, which is "centrifuge for separating the cells of the plasma from those of the blood." And if one says *hematocrit value*, one is indeed expressing a "judgment" in terms of the ratio of the volume of cells to a given volume of blood gained by the *centrifuge* (Latin *centrum* ["center"] + *fugere* ["to flee"], thus "center-fleeing device"), a "judgment" expressed as a percentage.

Cholē—with its two varieties in the Hippocratic text, *melainē-cholē* and *xanthē-cholē* ("black bile" and "yellow bile")—has left its own imprint in medical English. If someone was diagnosed as *melancholic* or suffering from *melancholia* (a perfectly proper and legitimate medical diagnosis by qualified physicians throughout the eighteenth, nineteenth, and early twentieth centuries), that diagnosis was based on the Greco-Roman concept of an "excess of black bile." We still say that someone is *melancholic* (much as did the playwrights of the seventeenth century) when that person is "gloomy" or, in the American idiom, "down in the dumps." Galen and other Greco-Roman physicians postulated excesses of yellow bile as causes of various diseases (the liver and its "jaundice," for example), but a *xanthocholia* did not enter medieval Latin and did not reappear in medical English. One coinage from the nineteenth century, however, has become standard in biochemistry and botany: *xanthophyll,* namely the yellow coloring generally seen in autumn leaves (common in species of *Acer,* the maples), but the substance is more commonly known as *lutein* (from Latin *luteum* ["yellow"]). Another "yellow" word in medical English emerges in *flavo-* (Latin *flavus* ["yellow"], which gives hybrids like *flavonol* (in chemistry, the three-hydroxy derivative of *flavone,* with flavonols [as quercetins] as naturally occurring yellow dyes), *flavobacterium* (self-explanatory), and *riboflavin* (the *-flav-* + *-in* here is the orange-yellow, crystalline compound found in leafy vegetables, eggs, milk, and fresh meat [riboflavin is often called Vitamin B_2]).

The *ribo-* presents a tangled etymology, quite typical of biochemistry. In the 1880s, German chemists obtained a white, crystalline, water-soluble solid from various botanical gums, especially *Acacia* spp., with the gum from this genus traditionally called "gum arabic." Named *arabinose* (*arabin* = the soluble matter + Latin's *-osus* ["full of"]), the substance in German was known as *Ribonsäure* [German *Säure* means acid"] or, shortened in German, as *Ribon,* and *Ribonsäure* were dropped by the turn of the century in favor of the arbitrary coinage *ribose,* which retained the rearranged *rib-* from the letters $r + b + i$ in the original *arabinose,* with the *-ose* suffix as before. Thus *ribose* technically still means "full of the essence of gum arabic," even though the slightly sweet crystals are a pentose sugar usually gained by hydrolysis of RNA (see chap. 12, below). *Riboflavin* = *ribose* + *flav-* + *-in,* which "translates" as "full-of-gum-arabic's-essence-which-is-yellow," rather far from what modern biochemists might be thinking.

The Greco-Roman "four humors" of the body were conceived as liquids, and as liquids they provided the essentials of life. How various liquids got from place to place in the body inspired much ingenious theorizing, with pre-Harvey notions best represented by Galen's concepts as laid out in his *On the Natural Faculties:* substances get to where they are required through body parts' "powers of attraction," and when enough stuff is present to nourish a part (blood via the veins carries the food for each part), then another natural faculty, the "power of repulsion," sets in to get rid of excess and waste. No circulation here.

Once Greek and Roman physicians began to designate the bodily humors not only by their proportions and balances but also by their colors, there emerged a dazzling series of descriptions of various "diseased" states in Greco-Roman pathology, and many of these terms remain in scientific and medical English. An ancient doctor might detect a form of bile as greenish and so call it *chloros;* we have *chlorine* (the gas and liquid that is "greenish"), and a generalized "greenish look" can still be characterized by a physician as *chlorosis.* Botany's *chlorophyll* is literally the short form of the two Greek words that mean "the-green-in-a-leaf," and numerous *chlor-* and *chloro* names and terms in chemistry, mineralogy, and pharmacy ultimately stem from this basic "green" word in Greek.

Ancient eye doctors (if we say *oculists,* then the Latin *oculus* ["eye"] is the source; if *ophthalmologists,* then the Greek *ophthalmos* ["eye"] is the source, with oculist = ophthalmologist in modern medicine) recorded many observations on eye diseases, and they often rendered their diagnoses in color words, including an eye or lens becoming *glaucos* ("grayish-green"), retained in the modern term *glaucoma.* Skin rashes were as common then as now, and Roman doctors might call a bright-red inflammation *rubella* (Latin's *ruber* ["red"]), but Greek-speaking physicians would use their word for "red," *erythros,* whence emerges our word *erythrocyte* ("red blood cell"). A bit less than bright-red was a sort of pink (*roseus* in Latin [literally "rose-colored"]), and doctors today sometimes call a light rash a *roseola.* Homeric and later Greek among the physicians included conditions in which something or someone was *kyanos* ("dark-blue" or "blue-black"), so that when we say *cyanide* (the gas), *cyanotic,* and similar terms, "blue" or "turning blue" is the meaning derived from the Greek. The most common word in Greek for "purple" was *phoinix* (named after the mollusc of the *Murex* spp., which yielded the "royal-purple" dye), but the "purple state" of someone who was poisoned (Greek *ios* ["poison"]) gave medical writers their particular term for "purplish" (*iodēs*), and we have in English *iodine*. As early as the time of Sappho (*fl.* after 600 B.C.) another Greek word for "purple" had cropped up, also designating the "purple" from the Phoenician shellfish among the *Murex* spp.; *porphyra* has likewise descended from the Greek into medical English as *porphyria*, a pathological condition in which *porphyrin* is in excess in the bloodstream (porphyrin is the iron-free product of the decomposition of hematin). One Greek word gives us *iodine* and another *porphyria*. An excess of porphyrin in the blood leads to weird changes in a person's behavior, a kind of "madness" that may have afflicted George III of England, quite possibly an important factor bringing on the American Revolution (see Macalpine and Hunter, *George III and the Mad-Business,* and for the genetic implications, see Dean, *The Porphyrias*).

Liquids and life in Greek, Roman, and Byzantine medicine and pharmacy depended heavily on how physicians and medical theorists described the humors. Blood could be "thick" or "thin" or somewhat in between, with a "bad proportion" (*dyskrasia* in the Greek) of phlegm or the biles. Blood was normally "red," although *dyskrasia* could render it somewhat pallid from too much phlegm or too much yellow bile; oppositely, blood could become too dark from an excess of black bile. This inter-locking theory of what is simply called Humoral Pathology was durable in a manner quite unlike the rapidly changing explanations for health and disease characteristic of modern medicine. If one assumes that the Hippocratic *Nature of Man* was set down sometime in the middle of the fourth century B.C., one then realizes that the theory of four humors was operative in medical thinking for over two millennia; if one merely presumes that it was Galen of Pergamon who ensured that *the* four humors of the Hippocratic *Nature of Man* would become canonical in western medical theory, then one still sees a dominant Humoral Pathology in medical theory for somewhat less than eighteen hundred years.

Heart and blood were recognized in ancient medicine as essential, but though Hellenistic anatomists understood something of the link between the motions of the heart and the pulsing of the arteries, most learned physicians followed the arguments of Aristotle and his students who asserted that the heart was the "seat" in the body for what was long termed "animal heat." Blood, as Galen's *Natural Faculties* argues incisively, was essential to nourish the body, but blood to Galen was merely an altered form of the food taken into the digestive tract. It is striking to reflect that physiologists had little inkling of how, for example, the stomach and its acids actually worked until William Beaumont's 1833 publication of *Experiments and Observations on the Gastric Juice and the Physiology of Digestion,* a pioneering monograph resulting from an unhealed shotgun wound in Alexis St. Martin in 1822 (Dr. Beaumont looked through the hole, recorded what he saw, experimented with the fluids, and made his findings available to the medical world as a whole). Thus one needs also to reflect how different is the medicine of the late twentieth century from that of the early nineteenth, then yet unaware of microorganisms as causative of disease, yet unable to find a reliable anesthetic, and certainly still bound to the theories of a Humoral Pathology proposed two thousand years before in Greek medicine. Harvey's circulation of the blood laid to rest only one aspect of the venerated Greco-Roman medical theories, and doctors remained wedded to their traditional descriptives of health and disease, terminologies that descended directly from Greek and Latin and that almost always presumed some state of liquidity subject to the sense perceptions. Color words formed a single facet of this long-lived vocabulary of the liquids of life and death, fluids everyone understood not in terms of "how much" but "how red" and the like.

Added to colors, ancient physicians liberally employed tastes, textures, and odors in describing how the human body functioned. Treatments and therapies based on painstaking observations of color, taste, touching, and odor were generally logical and precise, even though Greco-Roman physicians widely recognized the fuzzy imperfections resulting from what the doctor could learn from a reddish color, a salty taste, a rough texture of the skin, or a rancid smell—or any of the similar distinctions that enwreathe ancient medical diagnostics and pathological descriptions. How to describe the properties of drugs (*pharmaka,* sing. *pharmakon* [Greek]) also was fraught with difficulty, but ancient physicians did their best, sometimes with admirable precision, as suggested by Aetius of Amida (*fl.* in the reign of Justinian [A.D.

527–65]), who masterfully summarizes the best theories of his own century, culled from a millennium of Greco-Roman experiences with pharmaceuticals:

> The variations of the individual effects of drugs are due to each of them being to a certain degree hot or cold or dry or wet, each having fine or coarse particles. The extent of the degree, however . . . cannot be expressed with truthful accuracy . . . one kind of drugs has the same proportion [*krasis* = the "combination" of humors, etc., as above in the Hippocratic *Nature of Man*] as our bodies . . . four orders [*taxeis*] of drugs can be made: the first is indistinct to the senses, and detecting it necessarily comes through pure reason [*logos*]; the second is distinct and perceivable to the senses; the third is rather hot, but not to the point of burning; the fourth and last is the corrosive or caustic kind of drugs. Likewise also for the cooling kinds of drugs, the first order must come from pure reason in demonstrating its coldness, the second is cooling detectable by the senses, the third is rather cold, and the fourth causes necrosis. Analogous in these definitions are also the wetting and drying drugs . . . One should also use the sense of taste, and retain in the memory the peculiarity of each quality of the juices . . . as for example when unripe wild pears [or] Cornelian cherries are laid on the tongue they greatly dessicate, contract, and deeply roughen . . . every such substance is called sour since it is intensely bitter [*austēron*]. (Aetius of Amida, *Tetrabiblon*, I, preface, trans. from the Greek text by Olivieri, *Aetii Amideni libri medicinales I–IV*, 17–18. See also John Scarborough, "Early Byzantine Pharmacology," *Dumbarton Oaks Papers*, 38 [1984]: 213–32 [esp. 224–26: "Aetius of Amida"]).

Plato, in his work titled *Timaeus* (especially 65B–66B), had some centuries earlier attempted to define what one meant by "taste" and "flavor," and Theophrastus (before 290 B.C.), in his *On Odors*, also tried to define meanings. Both philosophers were forced into comparative terminologies, Plato with what is "less" astringent (*stryphna*, the same term used by Aetius, quoting Galen) or "less" salty (*halyka*), and Theophrastus with perfumes and various spices. Aetius is adapting Galen, who in his turn had tried to classify drugs according to their tastes and textures, and Aetius's streamlining of Galen's pharmacological theories becomes the ultimate origin of the "drugs by degrees" system, used by pharmacists until the middle of the nineteenth century. Even though we no longer depend on the senses of smell, touch, taste, and sight to provide medical terminologies, the impact of Greco-

Roman concepts of elements, qualities, and humors (as perceived by the senses) is still part of medical English as well as other kinds of English. As with the four humors and their derivatives in modern English, so too there are essential terms from classical antiquity's methods of determining substances—the elements and qualities—which remain important in current scientific English.

THE FOUR ELEMENTS

Pyr, gen. *pyros* (Greek "fire"): medical English has inherited many "fire" words from this Greek element, including *pyrosis* ("heartburn"), *pyrophobia* (*pyro-* + Greek *phobos* ["panic" or "fear"], thus an "abnormal fear of fire"), *pyrogen* (an agent or substance "that causes a rise in the body's temperature"), *pyrotic* (a "hot" or "caustic" [that is, "burning"] drug or chemical agent), and the well-known *pyromania* (literally "fire-madness," thus in psychoanalytic jargon a "compulsion to set things on fire"). *Pyrotechnics* is the "art of preparing fireworks."

Gē, gen. *geōn* or *gōn* (Greek "earth"): medical English has derived *geophagy* (*geo-* + *phagos* ["eating"]), the usually abnormal practice of "eating dirt." Most *geo-* words in scientific English are connected to rocks and maps and agriculture, including *geology* (the science dealing with the "physical history of the earth"), *geography* (Greek *geōgraphia* ["description of the earth"], now map making [usually called *cartography,* from the Greek *chartēs* ("sheet of papyrus") + *graphē* ("drawing" or "painting" or sometimes "writing")]) and related studies, and *geoponics* (Byzantine Greek *geōponika* ["a work on agriculture"] now the "science of tillage or agriculture"). Related is the Greek *geōrgos* ("farmer"), so that anyone writing *Georgics* is composing poems on farm life and anyone named *George* is by definition a farmer (Georgia is the feminine form, whence the state name after George, King of England).

Aēr, gen. *aeors,* becomes Latin's *aer* and thence into Middle English as *eir,* cognate with the ancient Greek (air). Most terms in medical English are derived from the Latinate, for example *aerogastria* ("distension of the stomach with gas"), *aeropathy* (any "diseased state induced by large changes in atmospheric pressures, such as 'mountain sickness,' 'caisson disease' and the like"), *aerophagia* ("the swallowing of air"), and the expected psychoanalytic coinage *aerophobia.* The language has not made up its mind how words should be formed from either the Greek or the Latin, since we say *aeronautics* but fly in *airplanes* or (now quaintly) *airships,* and we speak wistfully about lost opportunities in *aerospace* while landing our *aircraft* at *airports*.

Hydōr, gen. *hydatos* (Greek "water"): English and medical English have dozens of *hydro-* words (to be carefully distinguished from *hygro-* words [see "wet" under the four qualities immediately below]), beginning with *hydrotherapy* (loosely "water treatment") and ranging through *hydrogogue* (Greek *hydr-* + *agōgos* ["leading out"], a drug to promote the expulsion of water), *hydremia* (*hydr-* + [*h*]*ema,* an excess of plasma in the blood, *hydrocele* ("accumulation of fluid in a form like a hernia [Greek *kēlē*]," commonly in infants with congenital hydrocele of the tunica vaginalis testis), *hydrorrhea* (*hydro-* + *rhoia* ["a flowing"], the "profuse discharge of watery fluid"), *hydrosalpinx* (*hydro-* + Greek *salpinx* ["war trumpet"], the "accumulation of fluid in the Fallopian tube"), *hydrothionemia* (*hydro-* + Greek *theion* ["sulfur"] + Latinized *hema* ["water" + "sulfur" + "blood"], that is, the presence of hydrogen sulfide in the blood stream), and many other similar hybrids. *Hydrogen* means literally "water-produced" (from the Greek *hydro* + *genēs* ["produced" or "born"]), demonstrated dramatically by Antoine Lavoisier (1743–94) in a public experiment staged on 24 June 1783: Lavoisier burned large quantities of what was then called "inflammable air" and "dephlogisticated air" in a closed vessel; the result was pure water and only water. This was proof that water was *not* an element and signaled the demise of the ancient notion of the four elements. Lavoisier's new chemistry also demonstrated (for example) how a metal dissolved in dilute acid takes oxygen from present water to form a calx (now called an *oxide*); combining with the acid yields a salt, with the hydrogen of the water set free. In 1777, Lavoisier invented the new word *oxygine* (soon becoming *oxygen* in English [Greek *oxys* ("sharp," "keen," and here "acid") + *genēs*]), which along with hydrogen became two of the "new" elements in Lavoisier's *Méthode de nomenclature chimique* (1787) and *Traité élémentaire de chimie* (1789), two books that mark the beginnings of modern chemistry and "elements" as understood in current physics and chemistry.

THE FOUR QUALITIES

Hygra (Greek "wet" or "moist," or with the definite article *hē hygra,* "the wet") was how Greco-Roman physicians characterized water "in" or "dominant" in some manner with body parts or drugs and so on. Thus, this was the "sensory perception" aspect of water, with "the wet" being how one "knew" water. Medical English has preserved a few facets of this notion of "sense perception" in a number of *hygro-* terms, including *hygrostomia* (*hygro-* + *stoma* ["mouth"], which is "excessive salivation or ptyalism"), *hygroblepharic* (*hygro* + *blepharon* ["eyelid"], "moistening of the eyelids," the function of the lacrimal ducts), and *hygroma* ("a cystic swelling with fluid, like a 'housemaid's knee' and similar slowly developing conditions"). *Hygrophilia* is the name of a genus of Asian herbs used as a diuretic, and the modern name means "moisture-loving," as seen from the Greek. Many other technical terms reflect the "sense perception" history: a *hygroscope* measures humidity in the air; a *hygrothermograph* records temperature and relative humidity; and a *hygrometer* measures water vapor in the atmosphere.

Thermos or *thermon* (Greek "hot," or with a definite article in the neuter, *to thermon,* "the hot") sometimes meant simply "heat," as in Aristotle's "Innate Heat," thought to be necessary for activity and intelligence in higher animals. Of course, one is familiar with a *thermos* bottle, which keeps liquids hot (*thermos* was a registered trademark when it was first marketed before 1910), and English *thermal* or *thermic* means "pertaining to or caused by heat or temperature." *Thermotherapy* is "treatment with heat," and if someone has lost the ability to feel heat or cold, he or she is said to suffer from *thermanesthesia. Thermoneurosis* is medicalese for "elevation of the bodily temperatures from emotional factors." The familiar *thermometer* measures temperatures, and the modern science of *thermochemistry* deals with relationships between chemical action and heat. The "hot" to Greek and Roman physicians always characterized fire, sometimes air, rarely water (as steam), but never earth.

Psychros (Greek "cold") has bequeathed *psychroalgia* (*psychr-* + *algos* ["pain"], a painful sensation of cold), and someone who prefers a cold climate is said to be *psychrophilic. Psychrotherapy* is "treatment by cold," and physicians sometimes will say *psychroesthesia* when they mean "chill," that is, a sensation of "cold even though the body is warm." One needs to be wary not to confuse *psychro-* words with *psycho-* terms in medicalese: the telltale *r* (the *rho* in Greek) will not be there when soul words are used, like *psychology.* The "cold" characterizes earth, occasionally water, rarely air (as in a cold mist), but obviously never fire.

Xēros or *xēron* (Greek "dry," or with a definite article in the feminine *hē xēra,* "the dry") has given us the trade name *Xerox* among duplicating machines (this was the first of the "dry" processes back in the early 1960s) and has left its mark in medical English with a number of quasi-perception terms, including *xeroderma* (Greek *xēro-* + *derma* ["skin"], "dry skin"), *xeransis* (direct borrowing of the Greek *xēransis,* "loss of moisture in the tissues," the term used by Galen), *xerophthalmia* ("dry eye" or, more accurately, extreme dryness of the conjunctiva), *xerostomia* ("dry mouth"), and *xerophagia,* an ornate way to say someone is "eating dry food." The "dry" could characterize air and fire and sometimes earth, but never (obviously) water.

Greek and Roman doctors struggled to "explain" taste and odors from the elements and qualities, and Plato's account in *Timaeus,* 65B–66B, had enormous influence on theories of taste and smell well into modern times. Taste, Plato notes, is particular to the tongue: there are small particles denoted as "earthy" that strike the tongue (which is hot) and are "melted" and thereby cause contraction and dessication, perhaps perceived as "astringent" (*stryphna*) or "bitter" or "harsh" (*austēra*), with exceptionally bitter taste perceived as *pikra* ("sharp") and tastes that were a little less sharp perceived as *halyka* ("salty"). *Oxy* described an "acid" taste, *glyky* was "sweet," and *drimea* was "pungent." Plato continues by saying that smells are "thinner" tastes, not too far from modern explanations. *Austēra* has given us *austere,* and someone with a bitter outlook is sometimes described as *austere* or, more pungently (as it would be in classical Greek), "sour." The Greek *pikra* has survived in the name of carbazotic acid, sometimes called *picric* acid, which is a yellow, crystalline, water-soluable, incredibly bitter substance and is quite poisonous (chemical formula $C_6H_2(NO_2)_3OH$, used mostly in the manufacture of explosives). The Greek "salty" turns up in a number of *hals* words (gen. *halos* [usually "salt"]) or words that have *halo-* derived from the genitive form, including *haloid* ("like or resembling common salt"), *halogen* (*halo-* + *genēs* [in chemistry, any of the negative elements chlorine, flourine, iodine, bromine, and astatine, which form binary salts by direct union with metals]), and *halophyte* (a plant that grows in salty or alkaline soil). *Oxy-* terms are common, with *oxygen* heading the list (see above under "The Four Elements": *Hydōr*). In medical English, *oxytocia* (*oxy* + Greek *tokos* ["childbirth"]) is "sharp" or "rapid childbirth," and an *oxytocic* is given to accelerate childbirth (it also helps control postnatal bleeding). In English, an *oxymoron* (*oxy* + Greek *moros* ["foolish"]) is a figure of speech that is apparently self-contradictory, as in "cruel kindness" or in the army's "make haste slowly" (anticipated by the saying among Roman soldiers, *festine lente*). Plato's *glyky* (or *glykys*) is most Greek medical writers' common word for "sweet," and remains very common in medical and biochemical English in words compounded with *gluc-, gluco-,* and *glyk-,* as in the medical *glycosuria,* the excretion of *glucose* (one of the complex sugars) in the urine, an ordinary and ancient "taste test" for diabetes. *Glycerin* (= *glycerol*) is so named because of its sweetish taste.

In English, we occasionally speak of the "nebulous quality" of an argument or a questionable product on the open market, and this too is a survival of that manner of thinking—quite satisfying for two thousand years in medicine—that marked Greek, Roman, and Byzantine concepts of fluids, liquids in the living body, smells, colors, and odors. As Aetius of Amida puts it, one "knows" dung to be dung, and a putrid smell warns against eating something, but "it is not safe to make a judgment of all the properties of simple substances from their smell." And when Greek, Roman, Byzantine, classical Arabic, and early Renaissance physicians and medical theoreticians attempted to explain how the humors and various combinations for the nourishment of the body got from place to place, they fell back on Galen's long-lived concepts of the "powers of attraction and repulsion," specific for each organ and each part as it required food (first turned into blood). At no time was there a demonstration of a closed circulation before Harvey's 1628 *De motu cordis,* which established that the heart was a pump and that the blood circulated in a closed circuit, a concept utterly basic to modern physiology, the science considering the functions of living organisms and their parts. Greco-Roman physiology assuredly studied the "functions of living organisms" (famous were the works on the topic by Aristotle and Galen), but the idea of the closed circulation and "flow" of blood in living mammals eluded everyone before the sixteenth and seventeenth centuries. Part of the problem was the Qualitative Theory of Matter, which did not do much with exact measurements, for example, by asking "how much" blood was involved in a living adult human being.

THE HEART AS MUSCULAR PUMP

Greco-Latinate terminologies appear in modern descriptions of how the heart and vessels "work" as frequently as such terms appear in basic names for anatomical structures of the heart and the circulatory system. Harvey's homely analogy of breathing into a glove as a description of the two parts of a cardiac cycle (relaxation and contraction [*diastole* and *systole*] remains vivid and useful. Or as he writes in a combination of English and Latin: "Actio: thus relaxed receyves blood, contracted scups it over. Universum corpus arteriae respondet as my breth in a glove" (quoted in Whitteridge, *Lectures of William Harvey,* 272). In the medical Greek of the Roman Empire, *diastolē* meant "dilation" (of the heart, as in Galen, *Anatomical Procedures,* VII, 4 [ed. Kühn, Vol. II, 597]), and the term has emerged intact in Harvey's Latin (simply *diastole,* as in *De motu cordis,* pref. [ed. Franklin, 121], and elsewhere). In describing the pumping action of the heart, one should begin with the end of *systolē* (Galen's word means "contraction," exemplified in *Variations among Pulses,* IV, 2 [ed. Kühn, Vol. VIII, 700] and several other works), at which point in the cycle large quantities of blood have come into the *atria,* the two upper chambers of the heart (Latin *atrium,* pl. *atria* ["central room of a house," usually open to the sky at the center], generally preferred by anatomists and cardiologists in place of the traditional *auricles* [Latin *auriculus* ("little ear")], deemed to be confusing). The high pressure of the blood in the upper chambers pushes open the atrioventricular valves, and blood flows rapidly into the *ventricles,* the two lower chambers of the heart (Latin *ventriculum* is "little belly," which does sort of suggest the form of a ventricle). The right atrioventricular valve (*valvae,* gen. *valvarum,* is a Latin plural noun ["leaves of a door"]), is often called the *tricuspid* (Latin *tres, tria* ["three"] + *cuspis* ["point"]), whereas the left atrioventricular valve is termed either the *bicuspid* (Latin *bis* ["two" or twice"] + *cuspis*) or the *mitral* (Greek *mitra* ["headband" or "diadem" or "headdress"]); these two valves function to prevent the backflow of blood from the ventricles into the atria during systole. Sections of the atrioventricular valves (called *vanes* by many anatomists and physiologists) have attached *papillary* muscles (Latin *papilla* ["nipple"]) linked to the walls of the ventricles by *chordae tendineae* (Greek *chordē* ["gut" or "string"] + *tenōn* ["sinew"]), which ensure that the valves do not bulge back during ventricular contraction. In physiological terms, the atrioventricular valves close and open passively, closing when backward pressure *gradient*

(Latin *gradi* ["to step" or "to walk"]) pushes blood back and opening with a pressure gradient going forward.

Systole in the heart begins when the blood pressure in the ventricles reaches a point at which there is enough force to open the *semilunar* valves (Latin *semi* ["half"] + *luna* ["moon"]) leading into the aorta and pulmonary artery. Then the ventricles contract, sending the blood on its way in the dual system of circulation. Physiologists have long understood that the heart's pumping action is a meld of remarkably well-timed and continual adjustments by the heart to varying amounts of blood, coupled with an equally remarkable internal control of cardiac rhythms (Greek *rhythmos* ["a regular recurring motion"]). The amount of blood pumped by the heart depends on amounts returned to the heart through the veins. Since each part of the periphery controls its own amounts of blood flow, there will be different quantities coming back to the heart, and the heart quickly adjusts its action to pump as little as two liters per minute and as much as twenty five liters per minute. This internal ability to adapt to varying amounts of incoming blood is sometimes called the Starling equilibrium (Latin *aequi-* ["equal"] + *librare* ["to balance"]), a clear perception of the physics of blood flow in the balance between intravascular pressure and osmotic force. *Osmosis* is a nineteenth century pseudo Greco-Latinate coinage derived from the Greek *osmos* ("push" or "thust"). In physiology, physical chemistry, cell biology, and many other subspecialties, *osmosis* is a fundamental concept, decribing the tendency of a fluid to pass through a *semipermeable membrane* (Latin *semi* ["half"] + *permeare* ["to pass through"] + *membrana* ["skin" or "parchment" or "membrane"]) into a *solution* (Latin *solutio*, gen. *solutionis* ["a loosening," frequently of a problem, thus problems could thereby "dissolve," giving us the chemical term *solute*]) in which the *solvent* (Latin *solvere* ["to loosen"]) concentration is higher, and thus equalize the concentrations on both sides of the membrane. Ernest Henry Starling (1866–1927) was an English physiologist whose Linacre Lecture of 1915 contained the initial proposals of what came to be known as the Starling equilibrium, which applied to how the heart works in pumping blood. According to the equilibrium, the heart pumps out all the incoming blood, preventing excessive damming of blood in the veins, occasionally termed the heart's *heterometric autoregulation* (Greek *heteros* ["other," "another," or "one or the other of two"] + *metrikos* ["related to measuring," adj. from *metron* ("measure")] + *autos* ["self"] + late Latin *regulare* ["to rule"]).

Cardiac muscle tissue has a special structure, tightly and intricately interlaced bands of fibers, which have special properties of electrical conductivity. Some of these cardiac muscle fibers are even more highly developed for the functions of spontaneous rhythmicity, and these specialized fibers form what anatomists and physiologists call simply the heart's conduction system. The well-known "lub-dub" sound of the heart beating at a rate near seventy two beats per minute originates from the actions of sequential firings and delays of self-excitory impulses by specialized fibers and nodes that have high permeability to sodium ions, then reverse diffusion of potassium ions; high sodium levels thereby engender an electrical action potential, followed in about 0.15 second by rapid increase in potassium conductance going the other way through the membrane. The heart's conduction system has four parts: the *sinoatrial node* Latin *sinus* ["bent or curved surface" or "curve" or "fold"] + *atrium* + *nodus* ["knot" or "knob"]); the *atrioventricular node* (*atrium* + *ventriculus* + *nodus*); the *atrioventricular bundle* (as previous + Middle English *bundel*); and the *terminal conducting fibers* or Fibers of Purkinje (Latin *terminus* ["end"] + *conducere* ["to connect"] + *fibra* ["blade" of grass, "rootlet," and similar meanings]). Johannes Evangelista Purkinje (1787–1869) was a pioneering Czech histologist and physiologist, the first to describe in 1839 the terminal conducting fibers, often still called after his name. Each part receives its name from its location, so that mentally one "sees" what cardiologists term the A–V node near the opening of the coronary sinus in the *septal wall* (Latin *saeptum*, pl. *saepta* ["fence" or "barrier"]) of the right atrium.

Greco-Roman systole and diastole are but the beginnings of modern understandings of how the heart works. Ancient physiologists knew many of the parts, and Renaissance physicians perceived the validity of a closed circulation after Harvey, but modern cardiology almost demands a four-dimensional view. Variations in flow, electrical potentials, and osmotic pressures speak of the heart in motion over time, somewhat more challenging than the static, three-dimensional perception of heart and vessels so commonly offered to students of anatomy and physiology. As always, the "parts" are simple, but the "functions" defy easy analysis.

HEART AND VASCULAR ANATOMY

After the complicated theories and their heritages, connected to blood and the other humors, the elements, qualities and derivative notions of perception—in addition to the marvelously complex understandings of pressure gradients, electrochemistry, and the biophysics of blood flow—the basic anatomical parts of heart and vascular anatomy are easily and quickly described:

Our word *heart* descends from the Middle English *herte*. In Greek, the usual word was *kardia,* and in Latin, *cor,* gen. *cordis.* Most medicalese heart words are those compounded with the Latinized Greek *cardi-,* as in *cardiology* and *cardiovascular;* "translated" *carditis* means "inflammation of the *pericardium* or *myocardium* or *endocardium*" (note combinations of *cardium* with *peri-* [Greek "around"], *myo-* [Greek *mys,* ("muscle")], and *endo-* ["within"], using classical adaptations met previously). The very common *coronary* derives not from *cor* but from the Latin *corona* ("crown"), a seventeenth-century coinage that reflected the "crownlike" or "garlandlike" appearance of the *coronary arteries* that originate in the *aorta* (see below) and supply the muscle of the heart with blood. The major parts of the heart (atria, ventricles, valves, etc.) are given above under "The Heart as Muscular Pump."

Aorta is Greek for "great artery," which it is, and literally in Greek means "something hung" or "something carried." The aorta, which describes a loop as it ascends from the aortic opening of the left ventricle, is the main trunk of the arterial vessels and conveys oxygenated blood to the entire body with the exception of the lungs. At the top of the loop (often termed the aortic arch), the aorta gives off three branches: the *brachiocephalic* trunk (sometimes called the *innominate* artery); the left common *carotid* artery; and the left *subclavian* artery. The *brachiocephalic* (Greek *brachiōn,* gen. *brachionos* ["arm" or "shoulder"], + *kephalos* ["head"]) is the largest branch of the aorta and is the major supplier of arterial blood to the head and right arm (it is unknown why some mid-nineteenth-century anatomists should have labeled this branch the *innominate* [Late Latin *innominatus* ("unnamed"), sometimes also *arteria anonyma*]). The left common *carotid* is one of two major vessels by this name (the right common *carotid* artery begins at the bifurcation [medieval Latin *bifurcare* ("to fork"), stemming from Latin's *bifurcus* ("having two prongs")] of the brachiocephalic trunk), each with branches (external and internal carotids); the term descends directly from a mid-seventeenth-century adaptation of Galen's description of these important arteries. In his *Use of Parts,* XVI, 12, Galen clearly acknowledges the name for these vessels, "which since ancient times have been called carotids (*karōtidēs*) and which buried deep in the neck, go straight up into the head" (ed. Helmreich, Vol. II, 427; trans. May, Vol. II, 718), but he does not like the name, since the term in Greek is coined from *karōdēs* ("drowsy" or "causing stupor"), and his own dissections have proved this assumption about these arteries quite wrong. Rather semisarcastic is Galen's comment that "the nerves running with the arteries they term the so-called carotids (*karōtidēs*) were also known by my teachers" (*Anatomical Procedures,* VIII, 5 [ed. Kühn, Vo. II, 675]), but it is in his involuted arguments on earlier theories on sensations carried from the heart that Galen reveals both why he thinks the name *carotid* is a bad one and why the name had stuck:

> "The heart and brain are connected by three kinds of vessels that are common to the whole body, veins, arteries, and nerves: the veins are the so-called jugular veins, the arteries, the carotid arteries, and the nerves the ones that lie beside these arteries . . . When the arteries have been intercepted by ligatures or cut . . . the animal will not be voiceless or stupified (*karōdēs*), as the majority of Hippocrates' successors have written because of their faulty dissection . . . The animal does not become stupified even after you cut the nerves, much less the arteries . . . But most physicians and philosophers, who intercepted the nerves along with the arteries and then saw the animal become immediately voiceless, thought that the effect was the work of the arteries and called it stupor (*karos* [often "heavy sleep" or "torpor"])—wrongly in my opinion, unless they mean to give the name stupor to voicelessnesss. In that case their error here would be only in the name; but they would be mistaken about the reality itself if they should suppose that the animal becomes voiceless when the arteries are intercepted. (Galen, *Doctrines of Hippocrates and Plato,* II, 6.4–17, ed. and trans.—lightly adapted—by De Lacy in *CMG* V 4, 1, 2, Vol. I, 148–53.)

Terminologies were heatedly debated in Roman antiquity, and Galen presumed that the "wrong name" for these arteries would be the one that survived. And it has, but why seventeenth-century anatomists would choose this badly misleading name that becomes our *carotid* is something of a mystery.

The carotids and their branches and subdivisions supply blood to numerous structures in the neck and head, suggested by their names, normally quite easily "translated" from Greco-Latinate terms met previously, for example the *superior thyroid,* the *lingual,* the *facial,* the *occipital,* the *ascending pharyngeal,* the *superficial temporal,* the *maxillary,* the *hyoid,* the *sternocleidomastoid,* the *su-*

perior laryngeal, the *cricothyroid*, the *sublingual*, and so on. Arterial names usually specify "where" according to muscle terms or names for particular anatomical parts. Thus the third major branch from the aortic arch, the *subclavian*, tells one instantly that the artery is important for parts "below the collarbone," with its branches having names indicating "where," including the *vertebral*, the *thyrocervical*, the *internal mammary*, the *costocervical*, the *posterior inferior cerebellar*, the *medullary*, the *pontine*, the *internal auditory*, etc. And as one follows the arterial system throughout the body, one will find names that suggest what bone, organ, or muscle (for example, arteries with names *radial, ulnar, left gastric, common hepatic, retroduodenal, sigmoid, inferior gluteal, femoral, popliteal, anterior tibial, first dorsal metatarsal,* and so on signal exactly "where they are" and "what they supply").

The *pulmonary artery* carries blood from the right ventricle to the lungs, conveying blood that has given up its oxygen into the lungs for the all-important exchange of carbon dioxide for fresh oxygen. The pulmonary artery has two major branches, the right and the left, sometimes labeled the *ramus dexter* and *ramus sinister* (Latin *ramus* ["branch"] + *dexter* ["right" or "right-handed"] and *sinister* ["left" or "perverse" or "unfavorable"]).

Veins (Latin *vena* ["blood vessel" and often "artery"]) make up the structures of the return circuit of deoxygenated blood to the heart from all the body parts. The *vena cava* was (and is) the great "trunk vein," and like the arteries, most veins receive their names from where they are or what structures they drain. Linking the veins with the arteries are microscopic *capillaries* (Latin *capillus* ["hair"]), which appear like tiny hairs under the microscope. Sometimes, when physiologists and hematologists want to specify the smallest branches of the arterial circulation, which merge into the capillaries, they will write *arterioles* (the derivation remains *arterion* [Greek for "windpipe"] with the added Latin suffix *-olus* [a variant of *-ulus* ("small" or "tiny")]); occasionally, *venule* or *veinule* (Latin *vena* + *-ulus* designates the tiniest veins that emerge from the capillaries). Important, of course, are the *pulmonary veins*, which return oxygenated blood from the lungs to the left atrium of the heart. Each lung has two major veins, which join to form the pulmonary vein entering the left atrium. In a simplified manner, the blood in motion—the "closed circulation" demonstrated in its basic patterns by Harvey—venous blood from the body to right atrium, then to right ventricle, then to pulmonary artery to lung and capillaries (CO_2 for O_2 exchange), then to pulmonary vein into left atrium, to left ventricle, into aorta, and thence into the *systemic* circulation (Greek *systēma,* gen. *systēmatos,* with adj. *systēmatikos* ["the whole compounded of several parts or members"]). The central pumping organ is the heart.

CHAPTER 12

SOME MORE FLUIDS: THE ENDOCRINE GLANDS, HORMONES, AND LYMPH

An austere view of the ultimate purpose of sex is that it is a way of ensuring that a particular fragile pattern of hydrogen bonds survives in the world . . . this is the DNA molecule that inhabits the nucleus of every cell and propagates genetic information from generation to generation. That molecule, the famous double helix, is held in shape largely by the hydrogen bonds between its components, and its replication depends on the sequence of components acting as a template for the construction of a copy . . . From this point of view, evolution is the consequence of the competition between patterns of hydrogen bonds . . . The testosterone molecule is a shortened version of the cholesterol molecule . . . Testosterone is the male sex hormone. Its secretion from the Cells of Leydig in the testes is initiated at puberty and controls the development of the secondary sexual characteristics, including differences in the skeleton, the voice, the pattern of body hair, patterns of behavior, and the organs of reproduction themselves. Testosterone molecules also induce the retention of nitrogen and hence encourage protein formation (anabolism), which leads to enhanced musculature. Testosterone is a member of the class of compounds called steroids, of which cholesterol is both a member and a metabolic precursor.

—P. W. ATKINS, *Molecules* (1987)

IN 1953, James D. Watson and F.C.H. Crick published the now famous "double helix," the celebrated model of DNA (deoxyribonucleic acid), and since the early 1960s, almost all notions of how the human body works and exists have shifted from the macroscopic to submicroscopic concepts. Replacing the venerated humors are hormones that necessarily exist in the living human body in pecisely regulated and timed amounts, not too disimilar to the "balances" (*kraseis*) assumed by physicians for humors until the late nineteenth century. Yet the differences in concepts are enormously greater than the similarities, since molecular biology and physiology form the foundations for this new medicine of the late twentieth century. Pharmacy and resultant therapeutics likewise are part of this new and strikingly revolutionary approach to disease and health, and even though Greco-Latinate terminologies remain essential, the modern terms suggest form or function occasionally rather distant from their Greek or Latin originals. Some knowledge, however, about why scientists have chosen the terms that now litter medical journals generally serves to demystify the jargons of medical physiology, molecular biology, endocrinology, and the dozens of kindred subspecialities. And in its new guise, modern medicine continues to phrase old questions and essential ideas within the contexts of a living, ongoing molecular biology—questions as old as humankind: "What is aging?" "What is death?" "How do drugs work?" "How does the body defend itself against disease or foreign intrusions?" "How are babies made?" "Why do people become gloomy in the winter?" And hosts of similar queries.

A lucid illustration of how recently the new biochemistry and molecular biology have revolutionized medicine is gained by comparing basic texts, those fundamental guides to "what is known and acceptable" that are fed to medical students and graduate students in biochemistry. In 1959, a leading summary of biochemistry included the following: "Some insight into the mechanism of self-duplication is at hand. The Watson-Crick formulation of DNA structure states that each DNA molecule is a double-stranded helix in which the two strands are bound by hydrogen bonds between amino and keto groups on adjacent bases, adenine to thymine or guanine to cytosine" (White et al., *Principles of Biochemistry*, 2d ed., 614). Slightly less than decades later, the seventh edition of this widely employed text (now expanded to two volumes of 1,646 pages, compared with the single-volume second edition of 1,149 pages) flatly begins a twenty-page summary, fully subheaded with "Double-Helical Structure of DNA," by stating, "DNA is a right-handed double helix in which two polynucleotide strands are wound around each other so that there are 10 base pairs for each turn" (Smith et al., *Principles of Biochemistry*, 7th ed., Vol. I, 136). Thirty years is a microsecond in the history of medicine, and without doubt, the pace of change will quicken in the decades to come.

238   MEDICAL TERMINOLOGIES

Atkins's summation of sex as survival of hydrogen bonds makes liberal use of a number of terms firmly based in Greek and Latin etymologies, and one can choose a few of the important words to illustrate how even the new molecular biology rests on terminologies from the classical languages:

Molecule is a Late Latin coinage from Latin's *moles,* gen. *molis* ("mass" or "bulk"), with the addition of the diminutive suffix *-culus* becoming *-cula,* thus "small mass." There are two basic meanings in scientific English: (1) the smallest physical unit of an element or compound, consisting of one or more like atoms and two or more different atoms in compound; and (2) a quantity of a substance, the weight of which, measured in any chosen unit, is numerically equal to the molecular weight, also expressed as *gram molecule.* In common speech, a *molecule* is any very small particle.

Hormone is a twentieth-century invention based on the Greek *hormōn,* the present participle of *hormaiein* ("to impel"). The word was first used in print by Ernest Henry Starling in the British medical journal *Lancet* 5 (August 1905): 340, "These chemical messengers . . . or 'hormones' . . . as we might call them." Defined in biochemistry, medical physiology, and similar specialties, a hormone is any of various internally secreted compounds formed in endocrine organs that affect the functions of specifically receptive organs or tissues when transported to them by the bodily fluids (for example, insulin and thyroxin [for which see below under "The Endocrine Glands"]). Knowing what *hormone* means saves an enormous number of words.

Helix is straight Latin (gen. *helicis*) for "spiral," a name applied by the Romans to an ivy, a particularly winding kind of willow, and a type of shellfish displaying similar spirals, as well as to a volute (the spiral or scroll shape atop a Corinthian capital). The Romans borrowed the term directly from the Greek *helix* ("anything twisted"), derived from the Greek verb *helissein* ("to turn" or "to twist" or "to roll").

Nucleus is Latin for "kernel" (*Nucula* ["little nut"] = *nux* ["nut"] + *-ula* + *-eus*). In modern English, a *nucleus* is the "center" or "heart" of something, a meaning replicated in physics, cytology, chemistry, and biochemistry.

Genetic—now a common word in English—is derived from the Greek *genesis,* which meant "origin" or "source." Thus the science of *genetics* is the science of heredity, and any term with the suffixal

-*genetic* says immediately that the word describes something to do with "birth," "origins," or "early development." How characteristics are passed from generation to generation is central to genetics. Parenthetically, a Roman epithet for Venus was *Genetrix* ("mother").

Anabolism usually is defined as "constructive *metabolism*" (for which see below), the opposite of *catabolism*. The root for all such terms is the Greek verb *ballein* ("to throw" [with an alternative form *bolein*]), so that -*bol*- with prefixes and/or suffixes indicates some sort of "change" taking place. Thus the Greek *ana*- ("up") + -*bol*- + -*ism* (from the Greek -*ismos,* a suffix to form action nouns from verbs [for example, *baptismos* from *baptein*]) "translates" as "thrown-up-in-action," or as the usual definition in medical physiology might read, "the synthesis in living organisms of more complex substances from simpler ones." Thereby *catabolism* (Greek *kata* ["down," "back," "through," "against," and other similar meanings]) would be "destructive metabolism," that is, the breaking down, in living organisms, of more complex substances into simpler ones, with the release of energy.

Deoxyribonucleic acid has a complicated mix of derivations, again typical in the hisory of chemical nomenclatures. Latin's *de* ("from," "away from," "of," and "out of") is the initial prefix here, and its position in the term—before the -*oxy*- part—would suggest that this substance is partially named from its molecular intensity or "deprivation" of the Greek-sounding *oxys* ("sharp" or, in chemical lingo, "acid"). The -*ribo*- root is the same as that contained in *ribo*flavin (above, chap. 11, under *cholē* ["bile"]), even though the "essence of gum-arabic" is far from modern biochemists' thoughts when DNA is considered; and the *nucleic* comes from the same "little nut" derivation as *nucleus* above. What all this actually means to chemists is clarified as follows: "The deoxyribonucleic acids (DNA's) differ from ribonucleic acids (RNA's) in that the ribose rings have hydrogen atoms in DNA in place of the hydroxl group that is present in RNA" (Maciel, Traficante, and Lavallee, *Chemistry,* 377). Thus the *deoxy*- is treated as a prefix in its own right, with hydrogen atoms in place of hydroxyl groups reflected in that doubled prefix.

Cholesterol instantly signals the "bile" word from Greek, *cholē,* quite important in Greco-Roman humoral pathology, so that something akin to bile must be involved. There is, as one might expect, far more: *stereos,* with an alternative form *sterros,* was a Greek adjective that meant "firm" or "solid," so that when nineteenth-century chemists began to isolate a number of substances from living tissues that seemed to be not quite solid, they invented the word *steroid*. The *ol* suffix in chemistry generally means a "chemical derivative with alcohol or phenol," which is unhelpful unless one has a clear notion of the substance and its molecular structure. Thus *cholesterol* is self-defined as a *sterol* (steroid + alcohol), or a hydroxy acid, written in simplified fashion as $C_{27}H_{45}OH$, or if an author gives a diagram (as does Atkins, *Molecules,* (56), he can write the following: "This molecule has an elaborate, rigid, hydrocarbon framework, its business end (more formally its functional group) is primarily the -OH group. In other words, cholesterol is chemically an elaborate alcohol (hence the *-ol* in its name)." Itself, *cholesterol* "translates" as "bile solid," but that rendition fails to account for the multiple properties now understood by biochemists for this substance. *Alcohol* is derived from the Arabic *al-kuḥūl*, originally meaning "distillate" or "powered antimony," indicating that "distillation" was discovered sometime in the Middle Ages by Arabic alchemists and technologists.

Testosterone incorporates the Latin *testis* ("testicle"), as well as the Greek root *-ster-*, as immediately above, along with the suffixal *-one*. This suffix is confined to chemistry and is derived from feminine patronymics in *-one,* and always means something is a *ketone,* in turn defined as an organic compound having the carbonyl group $>C=O$, to which other carbon atoms are attached. The term *ketone* is a short form of *acetone,* derived in turn from the Latin *acetum* ("vinegar" or "sour wine"). Chemists in the nineteenth century were reminded of vinegar's pungent odor when they first isolated acetone.

Cell comes straight from Latin's *cella* ("room" or "storeroom").

Microscopic and *macroscopic:* Greek *mikros* ("small") and *makros* ("large," "long," "great") + *skopos* ("looking," "seeing" "aiming," and similar meanings from the verb *skopein* ["to behold," "to see," "to contemplate," "to inspect," etc.]) have bequeathed our *microscope,* by which we perceive *microorganisms,* sometimes called *microbes* (*mikros* + *bios* ["life"]), as we do *microbiology.* When something is even smaller, we add *sub-* (Latin for "under") as a prefix to *microscopic.* In an odd twist, biochemists speak of *macromolecules,* that is, those of proteins, colloids, and polymers, which may have thousands of atoms. Philosophers like to speak of the *macrocosm* (*makros* + Greek *cosmos* ["universe"]), which is, indeed, "large." *Micro-* and *macro-* words in English suggest opposite ends of the scale of size—but this is always relative to the size of the observer:

a maggot hungrily devouring dead tissue attached to living organisms probably views the meal of dead cells as "macroscopic."

Metabolism: for *-bol-* + *-ism,* see *anabolism,* above. Add *meta-* (Greek for "with), and the Greek *metabolē* becomes "transition," "change," "turnover." In its modern guise, *metabolism* means "all the physical and chemical functions in a living organism through which protoplasm is made, maintained, and destroyed, and through which energy is produced to ensure living function."

THE ENDOCRINE GLANDS

When anatomists searched for classical words analogous to the shapes and sizes of these small structures, they returned to "nut" terms, and thus our *endocrine glands* is a compound of Greek *endon* ("within") + *krinein* ("to separate") + Latin *glans,* gen. *glandis* ("acorn" or "nut"). These structures secrete their hormones into the bloodstream, as contrasted with the *exocrine glands* (for example, the salivary glands, the *sebaceous* glands [Latin *sebum* ("tallow" or "grease")], and the *lachrymal* glands [Latin *lacrima* ("tear")], which give saliva directly into the mouth, oil to the skin, and tears for the eyes, respectively). Although the glands themselves are parts of the gross structures demonstrated anatomically, their secretions (as hormones) are within the submicroscopic world of medical physiology, biochemistry, and molecular biology. And as the nature of hormones has become increasingly understood, this clear definition of an *endocrine secretion* has undergone important refinements:

As time progresses, our understanding of what a hormone is must be redefined. A growing realization is that classical endocrine hormones and neurotransmitters may be more similar than different. Thus we treat epinephrine as a hormone of the adrenal medulla and norepinephrine as a major neurotransmitter . . . The hormones with nervous activity which operate across synapses may be defined as paracrine hormones, those substances which are secreted like traditional endocrine hormones, but which operate over a shorter, defined distance . . . we must recognize a newer class of hormones which can be gathered under the heading of autocrine hormones. These are hormones that are synthesized and released by the same cell upon which the hormones act. They may also act on neighboring cells . . . we conceive of three major groups of hormones based not on their structures or on the nature of their receptors as much as on the extent of their radius of action: endocrine, paracrine, and autocrine in the order of decreasing effective distances. (Norman and Litwack, *Hormones* 2–3.)

As research proceeds, there will probably be greater refinements of definition among endocrinologists, and there may well be literally thousands of such substances in our bodies to regulate the millions of physiological functions and actions we call "life."

Norman and Litwack's "traditional endocrine hormones" are those secreted by demonstrable anatomic structures, and these glands produce some very important hormones, reasonably well understood. Some of the major glands and their hormones include the following:

> The *pituitary* is the so-called master gland of the body and is labeled from the Latin *pituitarius* ("phlegm-producing"), in turn derived from the Greek *pitua* (= *putia* = *tamisos* = *puetia* ["curdled milk obtained from an animal's stomach and used as rennet," in Aristotle, *HA*, 522b5]). The following are among the hormones secreted by the pituitary:
>
>> *Melanocyte-stimulating* hormone (MSH): authorities differ as to whether this hormone comes from the posterior or anterior pituitary; MSH has the function of darkening the skin, thus the name from Greek *melas* ("black") + *kytos* ("body," "container," or "receptacle"): in modern medical physiology, *kytos* is used to mean "cell," as in *cytology*.
>>
>> *Somatotropic* hormone (STH): from the anterior lobe of the pituitary, this is the "growth hormone." STH stimulates hard and soft tissue growth; the name is derived from the Greek *sōma* ("body") + *trophein* ("to nourish").
>>
>> *Thyroid Stimulating* hormone (TSH): from the anterior lobe of the pituitary, TSH is the "trigger" for a number of thyroid hormones (see below) that are essential in the metabolism of iodine, glucose, amino acids, and several other functions.
>>
>> *Adrenocorticotropic* hormone (ACTH): from the anterior lobe of the pituitary, ACTH is another "trigger" hormone, this one to the *cortex* (Latin for "rind") of the adrenal glands (see below).
>>
>> *Follicle stimulating* hormone (FSH): from the anterior lobe, FSH stimulates the production of eggs and the secretion of estrogen by the

ovaries in the female and sperm development and testosterone secretion in the testes of the male. *Folliculus* is Latin for "pod," "small bag," or "shell."

Luteinizing hormone (LH): from the anterior lobe of the pituitary, LH triggers progesterone secretion by the ovaries, prepares the uterus for the fertilized egg, and stimulates the development of the breasts. The Latin adjective *luteus* means "the yellow color of egg yolk" (= Greek *xanthos*), which is why older texts of obstetrics describe the process as "producing corpora lutea" or "undergoing transformation into corpora lutea."

Prolactin is produced in the anterior lobe of the pituitary and triggers the production of milk by the breasts or "mammary glands." *Pro-* is Greek for "before," and *lac*, gen. *lactis*, is Latin for "milk."

Oxytocin is manufactured in the posterior lobe of the pituitary; it triggers uterine contraction during birth and stimulates the ejection of milk from the mammary glands. *Oxytocin* is derived from the two Greek words meaning "sharp" or "rapid" (*oxys*) and "birth" (*tokos*).

The *thyroid* gland (so named by late-seventeenth-century anatomists from its presumed resemblance to a shield [Greek *thyreoeidēs* ("shaped like a shield")]) lies in two lobes, connected by an *isthmus* (Greek *isthmos* ["neck of land"]), atop the lower part of the larynx and the upper part of the trachea. Weighing up to twenty grams, the thyroid gland has thirty million follicles (Latin *folliculus*, as above under FSH) involved in its endocrine functions. The major hormone produced by the thyroid is called *thyroxin* (labeled T_4 because it has four organically bound atoms of iodine), and this hormone is responsible for the metabolism of iodine as taken in through the human diet (small amounts of iodine are essential for human beings). Iodine deficiency in the diet causes *goiter* (a seventeenth-century coinage from the Latin *guttur*, gen. *gutturis* ["throat"]), which is the enlargement of the thyroid gland on the front and sides of the neck.

The *parathyroid* glands secrete a *parathyroid* hormone (PTH), which increases the calcium level in the blood and decreases the level of phosphorus. *Para* is Greek for "beside," suggesting imperfectly these four small glands lying on the thyroid on its lateral lobes, measuring about six millimeters in length and three to four millimeters in breadth. *Calcitonin* is a second hormone secreted by the parathyroids (as well as the thyroid), and this substance inhibits the withdrawal of calcium from bone.

The *adrenal* glands "sit like hats on the upper poles of the kidneys and consist of a central *medulla* within a *cortex* or outer bark. The cortex is essential to life" (Greene, *Human Hormones,* 46). *Adrenal* is a combination of Latin *ad* ("on" or "near" or "toward") with *ren,* pl. *renes* ("kidney"), which is why endocrinologists sometimes prefer *suprarenal* as the name of the gland, since it describes more accurately the placement of the glands "atop" the kidneys (*supra* is Latin for "above"). The adrenals secrete as least thirty hormones, among them:

Aldosterone is produced by the adrenal cortex and causes sodium retention and potassium depletion, essential for salt metabolism; this hormone is independent of any pituitary triggers. Tumors of the zona glomerulosa (a single layer of cells, from which comes aldosterone) are life-threatening. The name *aldosterone* is coined from *aldo-* + *-ster-* + *-one,* with the *ald-* signaling that this substance is an *aldehyde* (= modern Latin *al*[cohol] *dehyd*[rogenatum], "dehydrogenated alcohol") + a *sterol.*

Hydrocortisone or *cortisol* also comes from the adrenal cortex and regulates the metabolism of fats, carbohydrates, and proteins; this hormone has a fundamental role in anti-inflammation. The chemical name fuses *hydr-* + *-cort-* + *-one* (hydrogen + cortex + steroid). Synthetic products that act like the cortisones are sometimes labeled *corticoids.*

Adenaline or *epinephrine* is a vasodilator, increasing blood pressure as it dilates the arteries, and is often called the "fight-or-flight" hormone. The adrenal medulla produces adrenaline. *Adrenaline* as a name is *adrenal-* + *-ine* (Latin *-inus* ["made of" or "from"]), and *epinephrine* is equally noncommittal: *epi-* (Greek for "on") + *-nephr-* (Greek *nephros* ["kidney"]) + *-ine* (Latin *-inus,* as above). *Adrenalin*—note the absence of the final *e*—is a trade name (Parke-Davis). Adrenaline was one of the first adrenal hormones to be isolated and synthesized, and it has chemically varied functions, from being a vasoconstrictor in the skin to a vasodilator in skeletal muscle. *Noradrenaline* (or *norepinephrine*)—which along with adrenaline raises levels of blood sugar by mobilizing glycogen from the liver—is probably a "parent" compound (*nor-* is a chemical short form for *normal*).

The *pancreas* (see chap. 9 above for a brief etymology) secretes at least two major hormones directly into the bloodstream and functions both as an exocrine and as an endocrine gland. The hormone *in-*

sulin is deservedly famous; *glucagon* is not as well-known outside circles of endocrinologists:

Insulin is so named because the hormone is produced in the "islets" of Langerhans (Latin *insula* ["island"]), named after Paul Langerhans (1847–88), who demonstrated the presence of these specialized cells in his inaugural M.D. dissertation at Berlin in 1869. Insulin functions to decrease blood sugar levels, to promote storage of glucose, and to decrease blood potassium and phosphate levels. If insulin production is damaged, the condition known as *diabetes mellitus* results (Greek *diabainein* ["to pass over"], from which was derived *diabētēs* as the name of the disease characterized by excessive urination [by Aretaeus of Cappadocia in his *Causes and Signs of Chronic Diseases,* II, 2], + Greek *melitta* = *meli* ["honey"], suggesting the sweet taste of the urine of a patient so affected). This disease generally brings death, since the body is unable to utilize blood sugars effectively. The tale of the research on the pancreas by F. G. Banting (1891–1941) and C. H. Best (1899–1978) in Toronto—with the first clinical trials of insulin conducted in 1922—makes for fascinating reading, both in terms of the oddly haphazard methods that engendered success and in terms of the seemingly normal, vicious state of academic politics among pioneers in twentieth-century medicine.

Glucagon is named from the Greek roots *glyk-* ("sweet") + *-gon* (from *gōnon* ["angled"]), and this hormone increases the levels of blood sugar, converts fats and proteins into glucose, and increases blood levels of potassium and phosphates.

The *ovaries* in the female produce at least two major hormones:

Estrogen is a name coined from the Latin *oestrus* ("wild desire," "passion," or "frenzy"), which has become *estrus* in modern scientific Latinated English. *Estrus* as used by zoologists means "the time of heat or rut, or the time of maximum sexual receptivity by the female of the species." The *-gen* comes from the same Greek roots giving us *genesis,* here meaning "engendering." The hormone indeed engenders sexual receptivity in the human female: estrogen is responsible for the maturation of the female sex organs as well as for the development of female sexual characteristics; the hormone "clicks in" during puberty.

Progesterone as a label exploits *pro-* (Greek for "before") + the *-ster-* root from the Greek *sterros* ("solid") + the *-one* met repeatedly above: the inserted *-ge-* says that something is being prepared to grow (the Latin verb *gestare,* participle *gestatum,* meant "to carry in the womb," in Pliny, *NH,* X, 175). Progesterone is essential for preparing the uterus for the implantations of the egg (the agricultural metaphors are carried through from Aristotle), as well as for the development of the breasts for their functions of suckling the newborn.

The *testes* in the male produce *testosterone* (above, under the words described from Atkins, *Molecules*)

The *thymus* derives its name from the Greek *thymos* ("warty excrescence" in Dioscorides, *Materia medica,* II, 28, and "gland in the neck or breast of young animals," in Rufus of Ephesus [*fl. c.* A.D. 100], *Names of the Parts of the Body,* 168, and Galen, *Use of Parts,* VI, 4). This gland is very prominent as a mass of tissue in the fetus and newborn, a large gland lying in the upper mediastinum and beneath the sternum—but in the adult it is completely vestigal. Endocrinologists have recognized the fundamental importance of the thymus gland in the biochemistry and physiology of the immune system in human beings, and there are at least six "hormones" from the thymus (all peptides), called *thymosins,* which control the development of the thymus-dependent lymphic system (see "The Lymphatic System," below) as the thymus participates in immune regulation. There is some evidence that the thymus "hormones" regulate the timing of the release of other hormones from other endocrine glands (for example, of *prolactin* from the anterior pituitary [for which see above, under *pituitary*]), but the greatest interest currently rests on the thymosins' potential as crucial agents for treatment of immunodeficiency diseases as well as some cancers.

The *pineal* gland (seventeenth-century Latin *pinealis* ["like a pinecone"] from Latin's *pinea* ["pinecone"]) is the Third Eye of science fiction writers, a notion not too far from the findings of comparative physiology (especially studies of fish, amphibians, and reptiles). This small gland is flat and cone-shaped in structure (about eight millimeters long by five millimeters wide) and is located between the thalamus and mesencephalon (see chap. 6 above, under "The Brain and Its Parts"), at the posterior border of the third ventricle above the roof of the diencephalon. The pineal secretes *melatonin* (Greek *melas* ["black"] + English *tone* [here used in artists' jargon, "to make a hue or color less intense," since melatonin in amphibians lightens the skin] + *in* [simply "in"]) and probably *serotonin* (Latin *serum* ["whey," which by the seventeenth century has become our *serum* of the blood] + *tone* + *in* [as above]. Melatonin secretion is a response to the sensitivity of the pineal to light, and melatonin is a key hormone in biorhythms of mammals, with a special role in seasonal sexual cycles governed by amounts of daylight according to season; serotonin is also a neurotransmitter and is involved in patterns of sleep, of depression and elation, and perhaps in memory itself.

THE LYMPHATIC SYSTEM

The *lymphatic system* was generally unnoticed until the brilliant demonstration of its existence by John Hunter (1728–93) as a separate system of vessels and nodes, distinguished from arteries and veins. Hunter believed that the lymphatics "absorbed" foreign substances from the tissues, a "concept that has since been extended to apply also to the absorption of bacteria" (Qvist, *John Hunter,* 113). Lymph nodes and vessels (some having paired valves) are distributed throughout the body, and the main "organs" of the system are the *spleen* (Greek *splēn*) and the *thymus,* the latter especially in babies and children.

Lymph was coined in the eighteenth century from a pseudo-Latin word then in common use, *lympha* (taken to mean "water"), a word pulled from the Greek *nymphē* ("water nymph"). The Latin adjective *limpidus* ("clear" or "transparent") also seemed to fit what Hunter and others found in these vessels: a clear, yellowish fluid, quite distinct from the contents of either veins or arteries. *Lymphocytes* are thus white blood corpuscles, *leukocytes* (Greek *leukos* ["white" or "bright"]) made in the lymphatic system, and the "white cells" produced in lymphatic tissues are normally about 35 percent of the total number of white blood cells circulating in the body. Lymphocytes and other leukocytes are, of course, fundamental in our immune systems and fight intrusions by microorganisms or other foreign matter into the body. Lymph *nodes* (Latin *nodus* ["knot"]) are also distributed everywhere in our bodies, but they are particularly concentrated around the stomach, pancreas, the kneecap, and in profusion in the groin; in addition, a band of nodes runs from the mandible to the armpits (the *axillary* nodes)—they "collect" unwanted bacteria and viruses, as well as dead white cells.

Clearly there are intimate links between the body's autoimmune systems and the lymphatics, coupled with the hormonal actions promoted by the thymus (which slowly shrinks as children mature into adults). Endocrinologists are reformulating a number of fundamental theories on the operation of our immune systems, and it is probable that future solutions to current questions about immune-deficiency diseases will emerge from research on the biochemistry of the lymphatics and their functions interlocking with those of the thymus.

CHAPTER 13

THE HUMAN CONTEXT: SIGHT, SOUND, VOICE, AND TOUCH

THE sense organs allow us to perceive the world, and even though modern physics teaches us that our five senses are very limited in their abilities, those senses engender wonder, accompanied by puzzlement. The cerebral cortex of the brain (see chap. 6, above) "translates" sights, sounds, tastes (for the tongue, see chap. 9, above), smells, and what is meant by *touch*. The eyes "record" colors and aid mental computations of space, shapes, and distance but have nothing to say about heat or cold or any of the sensations classed as *tactile* (Latin *tactilis* ["tangible"]). Transmissions of sounds through the ear to the brain provide grass that rustles in the wind, a clap of thunder after the flash of raw flame we term *lightning,* and a wondrous meld of counterpointed sounds making up music in any culture, but how such translation by the brain takes place evokes quandary among physicists and musicians alike. Explaining the senses often involves circular logic:

Why do things look as they do? . . . the answer to this question [is found in three theories]: [in] the inference theory, things look as they do because of the inferences we make about what given stimuli (or sensations) must likely represent in the world; [in] the Gestalt theory, because of the spontaneous interactions in the brain to which the components of the stimulus give rise; [in] the stimulus (or psychophysical) theory, because of the sufficient information we receive from the stimulus. (Rock, *Perception,* 221.)

Physics yields other explanations, typified by the following:

The first of the two major transformations accomplished by the visual cortex is the rearrangement of incoming information so that most of its cells respond not to spots of light, but to specifically oriented line segments. (David E. Hubel and Torsten N. Wiesel, "Brain Mechanisms of Vision," in Wolfe, *The Mind's Eye,* 44.)

Greco-Roman philosophy long pondered the problem of vision and how it worked, and Galen's compacted theory fuses much he had inherited from earlier thinkers:

> A body that is seen does one of two things: either it sends something from itself to us and thereby gives an indication of its peculiar character, or if it does not itself send something, it waits for some sensory power to come to it from us. Which of these alternatives is the more correct may best be judged in the following way: we see through the perforation at the pupil; if this perforation waited for some portion or power or image or quality of the external bodies underlying our perceptions to come to it, we would not discern the size of the objects seen, which might be, for example, a very large mountain. An image the size of the mountain would have come from the mountain and entered our eyes, which is utterly absurd; it is also absurd that at one moment of time the image should reach every viewer, even though they are countless [*myrioi*]. And the optic pneuma cannot extend itself and acquire such a stream as to envelop the whole object being viewed . . . [thus] the surrounding air becomes for us the kind of instrument that the nerve in the body is at all times . . . the effect produced on the air around us by the emission of the pneuma is of the same sort as the effect produced on it by the light of the sun. For sunlight, touching the upper limit of the air, transmits its power to the whole and the vision that is carried through the optic nerves has a substance of the nature of pneuma, and when it strikes the surrounding air it produces by its first impact an alteration that is transmitted to the furthest distance . . . (Galen, *On the Doctrines of Hippocrates and Plato,* VII, 5. 1–7, trans. by De Lacy in *CMG* V 4, 1, 2, Vol. II, 453, 455.)

Gritty logic leads Galen to his conclusions, a line of reasoning that indicates both the nature of the eye and its connections to the brain; the nature of any "surrounding medium" (Galen uses air), coupled with the role of sunlight, must be accounted for in any theory of vision. And if we return to Hubel and Wiesel, we can discern almost exactly the same assumptions, equipped with the vocabularies of modern optics and physics:

> To sum up, the retinal ganglion cells and the cells of the lateral geniculate—the cells supplying the input to the visual cortex—are cells with concentric, center-surrounded receptive fields. They are primarily concerned not with assessing levels of illumination but rather with making a comparison between the light level in one small area of the visual scene

and the average illumination of the immediate surround. (Hubel and Wiesel, "Brain Mechanisms of Vision," 44.)

As human beings, we continue to see things in relation to other things, and we also speak to one another about what we see (or hear, or smell, or touch) through what we treasure as "the arts," whether sculpture, painting, poetry, music, the weaving of rugs, or any of the countless (Galen's *myrioi*) variations of how we enjoy the use of our senses. Viewing Orion's belt stars in the crisp and glittering night sky of a Wisconsin winter is comparable to the sense experienced in a museum displaying the enormous bones of a woolly mammoth. The human mind insists on connections, links, contexts. Our senses translate those contexts, and we become embedded in the time-stream of thought, interpretations of sight and sound, touch and smell, familiar and unfamiliar, as our contexts expand. Anatomically, the parts of eye and ear can be taught as finite structures, but "how they work" to give birth to our sense of wonder at the stars, or at great art that stretches our intellects and emotions, remains defiant of scientific analysis.

THE EYE AND ITS PARTS

Greek and Latin terms provide most of the names for the structures making up the eye, and many of these labels have lengthy histories, a few reaching back into Alexandrian anatomy. Our Greek and Roman ancestors were as curious and intrigued about how vision "worked" as we are, so their dissections occasionally were painstaking as they sought answers through forms as discovered in actual cadavers. (The six extraocular muscles are considered above in Chap. 7, "Muscles").

> The *retina* is derived from the Latin word for "net" (*rete*, gen. *retis*), suggesting its physical appearance under a low-power microscope. The retina contains *rods* and *cones*, cells that are sensitive to light, and their shapes are indicated by their names: the cones function in color vision, and the rods allow vision in dim light.
>
> The vascular tunic of the eye is called the *uvea* (medieval Latin, derived from Latin's *uva* ["the fruit of the vine" = "grape"]) and is made up of three parts:
>
>> The *iris*: Iris in Greek mythology was the messenger of the gods among themselves (Homer, *Iliad*, VIII, 398, and Hesiod, *The-*

ogony, 780), but *iris* in Greek carried several other meanings, including "rainbow" (Homer, *Iliad*, XI, 27), "brightly-colored circle surrounding another body" (the "lunar rainbow" of Aristotle, *Meteorologica*, 375a18), the "iris" flower and its medically useful rhizome (Theophrastus, *HP,* I, 7.2, and Dioscorides, *Materia medica,* I, 1), and "the iris of the eye" (Rufus of Ephesus, *Names of the Parts of the Body,* 24). The *iris* of the eye is its "color" in common speech, as in "she has dark brown eyes."

The *choroid* is so named because it resembles a "membrane" (Greek *choroeidēs*), supposedly similar to the *chorion* (Greek), the outermost of the extraembryonic membranes in the developing fetus.

The *ciliary* body that part of the uvea between the choroid and the iris) is named from the Latin *cilia* (neuter plural of *cilium* ["eyelash" or "eyelid"] and consists mostly of the ciliary muscle.

The *sclera* and *cornea*: Greek *sklēra* means "hard," and this portion of the external covering of the eyeball is a dense, white, and fibrous membrane. Medieval Latin's *cornea* presumably described the "horny web" of the eye, a misleading label (which has stuck, nevertheless) for the transparent anterior part of the external coat of the eye covering the iris and *pupil* (Latin *pupilla* ["little doll," which is what one seemed to see when looking into the dark aperture of someone else's eye—one saw one's own reflection in miniature]), and the cornea is continuous with the sclera.

The terms *aqueous humor* and *vitreous humor* are two more instances in which the Greco-Roman "humoral" vocabulary remains in modern medicine. The *aqueous humor* (Latin *aqua* ["water"]) is the anterior chamber in front of the lens, and the *vitreous humor* (Latin *vitrum* ["glass"]) is the transparent, gelatinous substance filling the eyeball behind the crystalline lens.

The *conjunctiva* (Latin *coniunctus* ["joined" or "connected"]) is the mucous membrane that lines the inner surface of the eyelids.

The label *lens* is Latin (gen. *lentis*) for "lentil," the seeds of which are flattened and biconvex, quite like the shape of the crystalline lens of the eye; the lens is that part of the eye that focuses the rays of light entering the eye, the process described as *optics* (Greek *optikos* ["of sight"]).

Impulses of images (however they might actually work) are conveyed from each eye by means of an *optic* nerve (Greek *optikos*, as above), which crosses with its opposite number at the *optic chiasma* (that is, the Greek letter *X* or *chi*). Then the impulses continue—at least partially—in the *optic tract* (Latin *tractus* [a "stretch" of space, or a "drawing out"]) through what is called the lateral *geniculate* body (Latin *geniculatus* ["knotted"]) and thence into the visual *cortex* (Latin for "bark," "rind," or "husk"), located in the occipital lobe of the brain.

THE EAR AND ITS PARTS

Anatomically, the ear comprises the *external auditory meatus* (Latin *meatus* is "channel"), the *tympanic membrane* (Greek *tympanon* ["drum"]), usually called simply the *eardrum,* three small bones or *ossicles* called by their Latin names *malleus, incus,* and *stapes* ("hammer," "anvil," and "stirrup" [see above, chap. 7, "Muscles," under "Three Muscles and Their Names: Gastrocnemius, Sartorius, Stapedius"]), and the *cochlea* (Greek *kochlias* ["snail with a spiral shell," related to *konchē,* ("conch shell")]), which is continuous with the *labyrinth* (Greek *labyrinthos* ["maze," famed from the complex palaces of Minoan Crete and the Egypt of Herodotus's day]). "Hearing" is conveyed by the *vestibular* and *cochlear* nerves in a manner not well understood; von Buddenbrock, *Die Welt der Sinne* (1953), translated into English as *The Senses* (Ann Arbor: University of Michigan Press, 1958), gives as judicious an account of the problems in understanding the physiology of hearing as one can find, even after almost forty years (see especially "The Sense of Hearing," 93–106, of the English translation).

The inner ear contains an amazing set of small structures, essential for balance and equilibrium. The cochlea and vestibule are concerned with the process of hearing (the base of the tiny stapes bone is the "foot plate" of the stirrup and attaches to the margin of the *fenestra vestibuli* [*fenestra* is Latin for "window"], and impulses of sound waves are transmitted into the ultimate distribution of the auditory nerve), but the whole labyrinth with its three semicircular canals is hollowed out of the bone of the skull in an intricate pattern exactly suited for its three-dimensional functions. The labyrinth is filled with *endolymph* (Greek *endo-* ["within"] + *lymph* [chap. 12, above, under "The Lymphatic System"]), and the membranous labyrinth is separated from the bone by a thin cushion of *perilymph* (Greek *peri* ["around"] + lymph). Occupying the upper and back part of the vestibule is the membranous sac called the *utricle* (Latin *utriculus,* diminutive of *uter,* gen. *utris* ["bag"], thus "little bag"), which communicates behind by five openings with the semicircular ducts or canals. The three semicircular canals (called *superior, posterior,* and *horizontal* or *external*) are at right angles to each other and thus occupy all three planes in space (if one bends the head forward at about thirty degrees, the two horizontal canals are roughly horizontal to the earth's surface, and then the superior canals are in vertical planes projecting forward and forty-five degrees outward, along with the posterior ducts, which are likewise vertical projecting backward and forty-five degrees outward. Each canal has an *ampulla* (Latin for "two-handled flask") as it abuts the utricle, and each ampulla has a *crista ampullaris* (Latin *crista* ["rooster's comb" or "crest"]) equipped with ciliated cells (often termed simply "hair cells"—the utricle is similarly endowed), which send impulses along the vestibular nerve to indicate the body's position relative to the surface of the earth, as well as gravitational pull. All these activities take place within structures occupying somewhat less than thirty millimeters by fifteen millimeters (the superior semicircular canal—the largest of the three—is about twenty millimeters long in its loop).

SPEAKING

Humans proudly communicate with one another in the thousands of languages that separate us even while uniting us in our ability as a species to articulate, to vocalize, to express our deepest feelings in the form of words. Like vision and hearing, speech encompasses more than mere parts "working"; in many ways, our speech reflects our very souls, our words delineating the highest emotions of love or the depths of hatred. All are within that unique human context, and—as far as can be determined in the last decade of the twentieth century—we are the only species having the enormous range of expressed communion in speech and writing. Language teachers often say, "Hear the new words you read, then speak them." Inner sounds become words spoken, concepts beyond simple parts of the respiratory system functioning to bring impulses into particular speech-control centers of the cerebral cortex.

One way of "explaining" the voice is certainly through anatomy, physiology, and physics: we know something about breathing centers resting in the brain stem, and we also know that speech results from the action of specific structures in the mouth and nasal cavities producing *articulation* and *resonance*. Moreover, there are clearly two separate mechanical operations that produce speech, the first called *phonation* (from the larynx) and the second termed *articulation* (from the structures of the mouth). Anatomically, the larynx is equipped with *vocal cords,* acting as a *vibrator,* and each vocal cord stretches between the thyroid cartilage and an *arytenoid* cartilage. From the view of physiology, contraction of the *posterior cricoarytenoid* muscles pulls the arytenoid away from "the thyroid cartilage and thereby stretches the vocal cords. The *transverse arytenoid* muscle pulls the arytenoid cartilages together and . . . approximates the two vocal cords . . . [to] vibrate in a stream of expired air." Continuing Guyton's masterly summary of the process:

Conversely, contraction of the *lateral cricoarytenoid* muscles pulls the arytenoid cartilages forward and apart to allow normal respiration . . . the vocal cords [do not] vibrate in the direction of the flowing air . . . they vibrate laterally. [Cord vibration results] when the vocal cords are approximated and air is expired, [and] pressure of the air from below first pushes the vocal cords apart, which allows rapid flow of air between their margins. The rapid flow of air then immediately creates a partial *vacuum* between the vocal cords, which pulls them once again toward each other, [stopping air flow, with] pressure building up behind the cords, and the cords open once more . . . continuing a vibratory pattern . . . The pitch of the sound emitted by the larynx can be changed in two difference ways . . . A change can be achieved by stretching or relaxing the vocal cords . . . in addition to the effects of the *intrinsic* muscles, the muscles attached to the external surfaces of the larynx can also pull against the cartilages . . . the entire larynx is moved upward by the external laryngeal muscles . . . when one emits a very high *frequency* sound, and the larynx is moved downward, with corresponding loosening of the vocal cords, when one emits a very bass sound . . . The second means for changing the sound frequency is to change the shape and mass of the vocal cord edges. [In high frequencies], different slips of the *thyroarytenoid* muscles contract [so that] the edges of the vocal cords are sharpened and thinned [and in] bass frequencies . . . the thyroarytenoid muscles contract in a different pattern so that broad edges with a large mass are approximated . . . The three major organs of articulation are the lips, the tongue, and the soft *palate* . . . The resonators include the mouth, the nose and associated nasal sinuses, the pharynx, and even the chest cavity itself. (Guyton, *Physiology,* 466–67.)

Greek and Latin provide terminologies for labeling this multi-staged process, the production of sounds we call "the voice." Some of the more important include the following:

Vocal- words all emerge from the Latin *vox,* gen. *vocis* ("voice," "sound," "cry," "word," "saying," and so on).

The *-ation* suffixes are almost always derived from Latin words, generally ending in *-tio* (for example *vocatio,* gen. *vocationis* ["invitation" or "summons"]), used to form abstract nouns from verbs or stems not identical with verbs, to express action (again, for example, *lucubratio,* gen. *lucubrationis* ["work by lamplight" or "nocturnal study"], from which we gain English's *lucubration* ["laborius work, especially during the night," which has acquired the modern nuance of "a literary effort of a pretentious or solemn kind"]), or to express a state (for example *distractio,* gen. *distractionis* ["variance"], which becomes the English *distraction* ["the state of diversion or drawing away"]). In English, the Latin *-tio* can also become *-cion, -ion, -sion,* and *-xion.*

Phonation combines Greek *phōnē* ("voice") with Latinated *-ation* and is a technical term in the specialty called *phonetics,* the definition of which suggests why phoneticists would use *phonation* instead of the following: "rapid, periodic opening and closing of the glottis through separation and apposition of the vocal cords, which, accompanied by breath under lung pressure, constitutes a source of vocal sound." *Phonation* says all of this . . .

Articulation is tricky, and technical use always depends on context. In English, it has two basic technical meanings: (1) in phonetics, the act or process of articulating speech or the adjustments and movements of speech organs involved in producing a particular sound, taken as a whole; (2) in anatomy and zoology, a joint, as in the joining or juncture of bones or of the movable parts of an arthropod. Among dentists, an *articulation* would mean the positioning of teeth in a denture, most often on an *articulator,* for correct occlusion. *Articulatio* is a coinage by Renaissance anatomists, derived from the Latin verb *articulare* ("to divide into distinct parts"), although in classical Latin *articulatio,* gen. *articulationis,* meant "jointed structure" (Pliny, *NH,* XVI, 101, and XVII, 163), as well as "a disease affecting the joints of vines" (Pliny, *NH,* XVII, 226).

SIGHT, SOUND, VOICE, AND TOUCH 257

Vibrate, vibro-, and *vibra-* words are derived from the Latin verb *vibrare* ("to shake" or "to move to and fro" [participle *vibratum*]). *Vibratio* is a Renaissance Latin creation from the verb root and gives us *vibration* and similar terms.

Thyroid- words: see above, chap. 8, "Breathing and How It Works," under *Larynx.*

Arytenoid is a term derived in Renaissance Latin from the Greek *arytainoeidēs* ("shaped like a ladle"), related to the Greek *arytaina* ("pitcher," "funnel," or "ladle"). The two small cartilages do resemble flattened miniature ladles.

Crico- words: see above, chap. 8, "Breathing and How It Works," under *Larynx.*

Vacuum is a direct borrowing of the Latin adjective *vacuum* (the neuter form of *vacuus*), meaning "empty." *Vacua* is the plural form.

Intrinsic is another of those tricky words, with at least two basic meanings in scientific and ordinary English: (1) in anatomy, an *intrinsic* muscle, nerve, vessel, and so on is one that belongs or lies within a given part; (2) in nontechnical English, *intrinsic* is an adjective used to describe something that belongs to a thing by its very nature, or as we would say, "intrinsic quality." *Intrinsecus* is a medieval Latin adjective meaning "inward," derived from classical Latin's *intrin-* (= *inter* + *in* ["inside"]) + *-secus* ("according to" or "following"). If one knows what *intrinsic* means, one also knows what *extrinsic* means.

Frequency comes from the Latin *frequentia* ("crowd," "multitude," or "throng") and its adjective *frequens* ("crowded," "numerous," "regular," or "repeated"), and the Latin has bequeathed to English the many words with *frequen-* roots. We say *frequent* when we mean "repeated many times," and technical English (usually derived from the basic meaning in physics) uses *frequency* to describe a rate of recurrence or, more formally, the number of periods or regularly occurring events of any given kind in a unit of time, usually in one second. Thus sound waves have *frequencies.*

Palatum is Latin for "roof of the mouth," and in modern anatomy, the roof of the mouth is divided into the anterior bony portion (the hard palate) and the posterior, muscular portion (the soft palate), which separates the nasal cavity from the oral cavity.

Resonator is one of several English words with a *reson-* root, derived from the Latin verb *resonare* ("to reecho" or "to resound"), and the

Latin *resonantia* (as used by Vitruvius, *On Architecture,* V, 3.7) meant "reverberation" or "tendency to return sounds." Thus in English anything that *resonates* will reflect sounds or will "amplify" sounds, as do the *resonators* in Guyton's description of vocalization.

The essentials of anatomy, physiology, and physics still do not explain how and why the voice is produced, a puzzle often probed by ancient and modern physiologists, philosophers, and anatomists. Among many accomplishments, Galen of Pergamon performed specific vivisections and dissections in attempts to answer the problems of voice production, and it was he who first demonstrated that particular nerves (the recurrent laryngeal, branches of the tenth cranial nerve, the vagus) were fundamental in the production of the voice. Galen showed both structure and function through vivisection of pigs in public demonstrations in Rome, and not only were his great skills in anatomy brilliantly displayed, but he also focused on the basic, philosophic questions. His approaches in dissection, as well as the methodology of logic as applied to the problem of the origin of the voice, are neatly illustrative of the long history of this special question for humans and their faculty of speech. Analogy through comparative anatomy is (as always) Galen's foundation:

I promised a demonstration of the minutest nerves, and to show how there is a hairlike pair implanted in the muscles of the larynx, on both left and right, which if ligated or cut render the animal speechless without damaging either its life or its functional activity . . . I showed that an intake of breath is produced by the dilation of the thorax, an exhalation by its contraction, and displayed the muscles by which it is dilated and contracted, and also the nerves branching to them which have their origin in the spinal cord. (Galen, *On Prognosis,* V, 14, 18; trans. [with Greek text, edited] by Nutton, *Galen on Prognosis* [*CMG* V 8, 1], 97, 99.)

Now of the nerve, of which I said that it comes from the thorax, proceeding along the neck until it reaches the larynx . . . It adjoins that part of the larynx, and enters it where the lower border of each of the two muscles . . . terminates, and at just that spot are also the [right and left] joints between the two large laryngeal cartilages. I call these two nerves the "recurrent nerves" and "those that come upwards and backwards," on account of a special characteristic of theirs which is not shared by any of the other nerves that descend from the brain. For there is amongst the nerve pairs that spring from the brain one that descends to

SIGHT, SOUND, VOICE, AND TOUCH 259

the thorax, travelling in the neck, and that is the sixth pair [vagus].*
When the nerves of this pair reach the thorax, from each there arises
another pair, and these are two small nerves which mount upwards,
travelling in the neck to the side of the trachae, and, at the place I have
described, they enter the larynx. (Galen, *On Anatomical Procedures*, XI,
4, ed. [Arabic text] and trans. by Duckworth, as rev. by Lyons and Towers,
Galen on Anatomical Procedures, 81–82.)

*Galen's "sixth pair" of cranial nerves consisted of our vagus, glossopharyngeal, and spinal accessory; the branches described here are, of course, from the vagus.

. . . for a demonstration it is better to place threads under all the nerves without tying them. Then you can show that the animal cries out when struck, but that it suddenly becomes silent after the nerves have been tied. The spectators are astonished. They think it wonderful that phonation is destroyed when small nerves in the back are tied . . . if you want to loosen [the ligatures] to show how the animal recovers its voice—for this surprises the spectators even more—do not bind the loops too tightly. (Galen, *On Anatomical Procedures*, VIII, 4, trans. by Singer, *Galen on Anatomical Procedures*, 208–9.)

Let us now speak of those parts for the sake of which primarily nerves come down from the brain, and let us begin with those concerned with the voice . . . I have shown that the usefulness of a part cannot be determined before the action is known. Since, then, the larynx is the principal and most important instrument of the voice, and since it is composed of three cartilages and has the epiglottis within it and nearly twenty muscles to serve it, it is your task to consider how Nature has distributed nerves from the brain to all these muscles. (Galen, *Use of Parts*, XVI, 4, slightly altered from the translation by May, *Galen on the Usefulness of the Parts*, Vol. II, 688–89.)

Galen's "explanation" of why the voice functions as it does is almost—but not quite—as satisfying as the modern "explanation" of vocal functions that originate in rather vaguely defined areas of the medial geniculate aspects of the brain, or perhaps in cerebral matter slightly lateral and posterior. Of course, as Galen demonstrated in the second century A.D., knowledge of the basic anatomy of the vagus and the branches of that cranial nerve called the recurrent laryngeals allowed a physician to diagnose correctly the voice loss resulting from back injuries, as Galen recounts in his *On the Affected Parts*, I, 6:

And one fellow fell and struck the ground in the middle of his back, and by the third day could only speak very weakly; by the fourth day, he was speechless and he had become without feeling in his legs although his hands remained normal. He had no difficulty, however, in breathing. Even though he had no sensation from the cervical parts of the spinal column downwards, it turned out that the thorax would continue to be moved by the diaphragm and the six upper thoracic muscles, because the nerves to these muscles are from the cervical portions of the spinal column. But the nerves of the muscles between the ribs [intercostals] were affected, and as I have shown, these nerves engender exhalation. The doctors wished vainly to give harmful treatment to the legs as well as to the larynx because of the disturbance to the voice, but I prevented this, and I treated only the injured area. The swelling of the spinal column went down after seven days, and speech and movement of his legs were restored to the young fellow. (trans. from the Greek text, ed. Kühn, Vol. VIII, 50–51.)

Vocalization involves words, memory, the syntax of language, hearing, and responding—all parts of the human context and all as intriguing and enigmatic to modern neurophysiologists and psychiatrists and phoneticists as such were to our clever ancestors.

TOUCHING

The human skin is what we see every day, that outermost covering that is the first sentinel and guard of all the biochemical and physiological activities that are essential for the living system we call "the body." What we do not see—but what we know from the moment of birth (if not before)—is how incredibly sensitive skin is to touch and pressure, as well as to variations of heat and cold. That sensitivity is now recognized as fundamental for survival among newborns, since babies not held and fondled by parents do very poorly, and the earliest "bonding" among humans is through the sense of touch.

Even in its basic structures, the skin is not simple:

> The *epidermis* (Greek *epi* + *derma,* thus "upper skin") is the surface layer, with dead cells continually flaking off in the millions. "Try scraping off a little of the dust from under one of the buttons of your mattress and look at it under a low-powered microscope . . . you will find it well populated with the dust mite patiently devour-

ing the flakes of your shed skin which drop through the sheets" (Andrews, *The Life That Lives on Man*, 11).

The *dermis* (Greek *derma* ["skin"] has living cells, slowly forced toward the surface in a continuous replacement process that serves to keep the "covering" intact.

Hairs in hair *follicles* (Latin *folliculus* ["pod," "small bag," or "shell"]) occur over most of the surface of the body and are usually accompanied by *sebaceous* glands (Latin *sebum* ["grease" or "tallow"]) and sweat glands (any substance or drug that induces sweating is termed *sudorific*, from the Latin verb *sudare* ["to sweat"]); most hairs are equipped with tiny *arrector pili* muscles (Latin *adrigere* ["to raise"] + *pilus* ["hair"]), which give the familiar "goose bumps" on the skin. Our idiom "hair-raising experience" (in terror or when becoming chilled) preserves this inner sense of tactility for the skin, much as the Romans might have said *pilos arrexit*. Each hair also has a tiny nerve fiber entwining its base (sometimes labeled a "hair end-organ"), one of six different touch receptors in human beings (the hair-end organ can detect the movement of tiny critters as they crawl from place to place on the surface of our skin, and when we feel something we cannot see, it is this extremely sensitive organ of touch in operation).

Our sense of touch is exquisitely developed, and simple free nerve endings are almost everywhere in the skin, recording touch and pressure. Of particular sensitivity are the large numbers of *Meissner's corpuscles* (Georg Meissner [1829–1905], a German anatomist who first described these sense organs in 1853, + Latin *corpusculum*, diminutive of *corpus*, thus "little body") in the tips of the fingers and toes, as well as in the lips. Meissner's corpuscles allow us to determine spatial characteristics of touch and to discern precisely what point on the body is touched and the texture of that touch. Extremely hairy surfaces on our bodies have few Meissner's corpuscles but do have what the physiologists call expanded tip tactile receptors (also common in fingertips and tips of the toes), and these allow us to sense continual or repeated touching. *Pacinian corpuscles* (Filippo Pacini [1812–83], who first described these onionlike bodies wrapped around nerve endings, + *corpusculum*, as above) are distributed widely beneath the skin, and through them we detect tissue vibrations both in surface structures and in deeper tissues like tendons (Pacinian corpuscles are also very sensitive to pressure). And there are millions of *Ruffini's corpuscles* or end organs (named for the Italian anatomist Angelo Ruffini [1874–1929], who discovered these branching sensory neurons in 1898, neurons generally parallel to the skin), which enable us to detect and respond to heavy or steady pressure to the skin or to distortions occurring in deeper structures in the body.

Touch is perhaps the most human of all our senses, since it connects us instantly with other human beings, much as it links us to the wider world as a whole. Running one's finger over a finely woven Turkish rug speaks immediately of the care and sensitivity invested in that work of art, much as cradling children in our arms will speak of our finest qualities as human beings. Touching is an essential facet of the human context.

APPENDICES

1. GREEK AND ROMAN NUMBERS

The following might appear in a textbook of anatomy:

> Uniformly, the hemispheres display triplicate surface structures, but occasionally, there may occur examples that show tetrahedral shapes and others that are heptagonal, but these are not common.

If that seems like nonsense, this is even more so:

> A quart of polysaccharides may equivilate a semicubic meter, but if one began accounting for the enneads, there would be at least a myriad of semiconcepts that could multiply into quintuplicate kilograms, suggesting how a researcher could set down results in hectaliters, hexameters, or triginal pentameters.

If a reader is suspicious of the "anatomy" sentence, instincts of how English functions are well developed, since the combination of two-dimensional with three-dimensional terms makes a jumble of the meaning. Yet the sentence itself is quite proper in regard to grammar and syntax, stuffed as it is with half-understood number-words. The second sentence is complete nonsense, quite in keeping with the pseudo-language employed by modern practitioners of alchemy, astrology, and other purported "sciences" (whose data can never be verified); sometimes the unhappily jargon-prone "social sciences" unwittingly slip into these sorts of slippery sentences. Reading such literature, one must always be on guard when number-words are proffered, since they "support" what can be called "soft data," giving the patina of "hard data." The second sentence above is "correct" as far as "good English" is concerned; still it is pure gobbledegook, even though it looks and feels "scientific" with its numerology.

Medical and scientific English is replete with Greco-Latinate number-terms, and a reader can detect fraud only by knowing what the numbers really are. Numbers are either *cardinal* (for example, "one") or *ordinal* ("first"), so that in English, we might say that if something is "sixth" (ordinal), it would be number "six" (cardinal) behind five others. Greek and Latin have bequeathed both cardinals and ordinals to modern medical and scientific English, with the more common derivatives coming from Latin:

I	*unus* (masc.)	*una* (fem.)	*unum* (neuter)	one
	primus	*prima*	*primum*	first

APPENDIX 1

II	*duo*	*duae*	*duo*	two
	secundus	*secunda*	*secundum*	second
	(or) *alter*	*altera*	*alterum*	second
III	*tres*	*tres*	*tria*	three
	tertius	*tertia*	*tertium*	third
IV	*quat[t]uor*			four
	quartus	*quarta*	*quartum*	fourth
V	*quinque*			five
	quintus	*quinta*	*quintum*	fifth
VI	*sex*			six
	sextus	*sexta*	*sextum*	sixth
VII	*septem*			seven
	septimus	*septima*	*septimum*	seventh
VIII	*octo*			eight
	octavus	*octava*	*octavum*	eighth
IX	*novem*			nine
	nonus	*nona*	*nonum*	ninth
X	*decem*			ten
	decimus	*decima*	*decimum*	tenth

Latin cardinal and ordinal numbers follow a pattern, so that one can assume ordinal formations (as adjectives):

11	XI	*undecim* (cardinal)	*undecimus* (ordinal)
12	XII	*duodecim*	*duodecimus*
13	XIII	*tredecim*	*tertius decimus*
14	XIV	*quattuordecim*	*quartus decimus*
15	XV	*quindecim*	*quintus decimus*
16	XVI	*sedecim*	*sextus decimus*
17	XVII	*septendecim*	*septimus decimus*
18	XVIII	*duodeviginti*	*duodevicesimus*
19	XIX	*undeviginti*	*undevicesimus*
20	XX	*viginti*	*vicesimus*
21	XXI	*viginti unus*	*vicesimus primus*
30	XXX	*triginta*	*tricesimus*
40	XL	*quadraginta*	*quadragesimus*
50	L	*quinquaginta*	*quinquagesimus*
60	LX	*sexaginta*	*sexagemimus*
70	LXX	*septuaginta*	*septuagesimus*
80	LXXX	*octoginta*	*octogesimus*
90	XC	*nonaginta*	*nonagesimus*
100	C	*centum*	*centisimus*
101	CI	*centum et unus*	*centesimus primus*
121	CXXI	*centum viginti unus*	*centesimus vicesimus primus*

200	CC	ducenti (masc.), -ae (fem.), -a (neuter)			ducentesimus
300	CCC	tricenti			trecentesimus
400	CCCC	quadrigenti			quadrigentesimus
500	D	quingenti			quingentesimus
600	DC	sescenti			sescentesimus
1000	M	mille			millesimus
1100	MC	mille centum			millesimus centesimus
2000	MM	duo milia			bis ("twice") millesimus

The Latinate numerology enables one to figure out *uniformly, quart, quintuplicate,* and *trigintal,* in the nonsense sentences, but the rest of the number-words in scientific English in those sentences come from Greek roots, as observed from the following (note how Greek letters, standing alone, with acute accents, are numbers):

1	α'	eis (masc.)	mia (fem.)	hen (neuter)	one
		prōtos	prōtē	prōton	first
		hapax			once
2	β'	duo			two
		deuteros	deutera	deuteron	second
		dis			twice
3	γ'	treis	treis	tria	three
		tritos	trita	triton	third
		tris			thrice
4	δ'	tettares	tettares	tettara	four
		tetartos	tetarte	tetarton	fourth
		tetrakis			four times
5	ε'	pente			five
		pemptos	pempta	pempton	fifth
		pentakis			five times
6	ς'	hex			six
		hektos	hekta	hekton	sixth
		hexakis			six times
7	ζ'	hepta			seven
		hebdomos	hebdoma	hebdomon	seventh
		heptakis			seven times
8	η'	octō			eight
		ogdoos		ogdoon	eighth
		oktakis			eight times

9	θ'	ennea			nine
		enatos	enata	enaton	ninth
		enakis			nine times
10	ι'	deka			ten
		dekatos	dekatē	dekaton	tenth
		dekakis			ten times
11	ια'	hendeka			eleven
		hendekatos	hendekatē	hendekaton	eleventh
		hendekakis			eleven times
12	ιβ'	dodeka			twelve
		dōdekatos	dōdekatē	dōdekaton	twelfth
		dōdekakis			twelve times

Formation of Greek cardinals and ordinals follows a clear pattern, as the following examples illustrate:

13	ιγ'	treiskaideka	thirteen
		tritos kai dekatos [etc.]	thirteen
		treiskaidekakis	thirteen times
14	ιδ'	tettares [or tettara] kai deka	fourteen
		tetartos kai dekatos	fourteenth
15	ιε'	pentakaideka	fifteen
		pemptos kai dekatos	fifteenth
20	κ'	eikosi	twenty
		eikostos eikostē eikoston	twentieth
		eikosakis	twenty times
21	κα'	eis kai eikosi	twenty-one
		prōtos kai eikostos	twenty-first
30	λ'	triakonta	thirty
		triakostos	thirtieth
40	μ'	tettrakonta	forty
		tettrakostos	fortieth
50	ν'	pentēkonta	fifty
		pentēkostos	fiftieth
60	ζ'	hexekonta	sixty
		hexekostos	sixtieth
70	ο'	hebdomēkonta	seventy
		hebdomēkostos	seventieth
80	π'	ogdoēkonta	eighty
		ogdoēkostos	eightieth

90 ϟ	enenēkonta		ninety
	enenēkostos		ninetieth
100 ρ'	hekaton		one hundred
	hekatostos		hundredth
200 σ'	diakosioi		two hundred
	diakosiostos		two hundredth
500 φ'	pentakosioi		five hundred
	pentakosiostos		five hundredth
600 χ'	hexakosioi		six hundred
	hexakosiostos		six hundredth
1000 ,α	chilioi chiliai chilia		one thousand
	chiliostos		one thousandth
	chiliakis		a thousand times
2000 ,β	dischilioi dischiliai dischilia		two thousand
	dischiliostos		two thousandth
10,000 ,ι	myrioi myriai myria		ten thousand
	myriostos		ten thousandth
	myriakis		ten thousand times
20,000 ,κ	duo myriades [or] dismyrioi		twenty thousand
100,000 ,ρ	dekahismyrioi		one hundred thousand

From the Greek, one can discern the meanings of *tetrahedral, heptagonal, enneads, myriad, kilograms, hectaliters, hexameters,* and *pentameters.* The sentence is patently utter nonsense, even though it might feel scientific. Yet there are many instances in which number-words can be legitimately derived from these Greek roots, so that if one wanted to multiply something by thirty, one could *triakontate* it (Latinized as *triacontate*). The *decades* we know are "ten-year periods," the ancient Greek warship with fifty oars is a *pentekonter* (literally "fifty-er"), a *hebdomad* is a "week" (that is, seven successive days), and *hectaliter* and *hectometer* (one hundred liters and one hundred meters, respectively) are common terms within the metric system. A reader, however, must be wary if number-words turn up in contexts that do not seem to "fit." Mixing two-dimensional with three-dimensional things should cause unease, unless an author makes clear the reasons for such mingling, and if a would-be writer describes something in terms of *hexameters* or *pentameters,* a perceptive reader should ask why some physical object is being given labels normally designating "six-beat" or "five-beat" lines in poetry. Of course, advertising experts know all too well the power of numbers, however meaningless they might be: if "50 percent more doctors recommend one kind of acetosalicylate" than another, what does this mean?

2. THE GREEK ALPHABET AND THE TRANSLITERATION OF GREEK INTO ROMAN LETTERS

The Greek alphabet, seen in part above as used for writing numbers, has twenty-four letters, and most have near equivalents in the Roman alphabet (the one I am using). Greek, however, has two "long vowels," *eta* (η) and *omega* (ω), which are transliterated as $\bar{e}$ and $\bar{o}$ respectively, whereas the *epsilon* (ε) and *omicron* (o) receive their equivalents in the Roman alphabet. *Chi* (χ) becomes *ch*; *xi* (ξ) is *x*; *rho* (ρ) is *r* or *rh*; *theta* (θ) becomes *th*; *phi* (ϕ) is *ph*; and *psi* (ψ) is transliterated as *ps*. Greek has no letter for *h* (as in English "heavy"), but the sound is represented by a "rough breathing" mark (‛), so that the Greek for "six" is written ἕζ and transliterated as *hex*. Two letters (borrowed from the Phoenician alphabet) had dropped out of written Greek by the classical period but were retained in the number system: the *digamma* (ϛ), which stood for "six," and the *koppa* (ϙ), which remained as "ninety." The vowel *upsilon* (v) most frequently is Latinated as *y* but sometimes as *u*, depending on pronunciation or the choice of modern inventors of scientific terms; if, for example, a borrowed term from the Greek has a diphthong αv, the transliteration can be either *au* or *ay*, but vi usually comes into the Roman alphabet as *ui* (the two vowels pronounced separately as "yew-ee" or "yew-eye"). Two gammas in a Greek word, as in διφθογγος, will appear transliterated as *ng*, so that the word is *diphthongos* ("having two sounds") in its Romanized version. Most written Greek words carry accents, so that "eleventh" is written ἑνδέκατος and transliterated as *hendekatos,* and "first" is πρῶτος and transliterated as *prōtos*.

3. PRONUNCIATION OF GRECO-LATIN TERMS

Students rightly ask, "How do we say those multisyllable terms?" Hearing them pronounced carefully by a teacher is one way to learn pronunciation and where to place stress in a word drawn from Greek or Latin into English, but there are a few tricks that are useful in gaining a sense of correct pronunciation from the printed form on its own.

Grammarians have given names to the last three syllables of multisyllabic words, and one should always chop a word into syllables when first meeting a new term: the last syllable is the *ultima* (Latin for "last" or "farthest"); the next-to-last syllable is called the *penult* (from Latin *paen ultima* ["almost the last"]); and the syllable before the penult is the *antepenult* (Latin *ante* ["before"], thus "before almost the last"). A great many of the multisyllabic terms can be puzzled out in pronunciation by remembering the "antepenult rule": put stress on the third-from-the-last syllable. For example, three names of ancient figures in medicine and science—(Erasistratus, Asclepiades, and Agatharcides)—often baffle beginning students in courses on Greek and Roman medicine, until they realize the pronunciations are Era*SI*stratus, Asclep*Ia*des, and Aga*THAR*cides. Now it is clear why we say Ari*STO*phanes, not Aristo*FANES*, a wonderful barbarism I chanced to hear recently. Scientific terminologies can thereby be broken down: *diplopoda* is pronounced di*PLO*poda (I am misplacing word divisions intentionally), *formaldehyde* becomes in speech for*MAL*deehide, and *enterostomy* is enter*OS*tomee. There are reverse tricks too, since terms like *foramen* have stress on the penult (for*A*men) syllable, as does *diplococcus* (diplo*KAW*kus); and one senses what the grammarians call a "long vowel sound," much as is common in English with the addition of a silent *e* to make a previous vowel long (*mate* as contrasted to *mat*). To be sure, the best way to determine pronunciation is to use the accent indications given in any good dictionary or to pay close attention to these accents provided in the listings of the better medical dictionaries.

4. SOME ABBREVIATED PARADIGMS

Through the book, I have normally provided two forms of a word in the Greek or Latin (usually nouns): the *nom.* stands for "nominative," and *gen.* means "genitive." Greek and Latin contain many more inflections than does English, although one can illustrate inflections through English by noting the alteration in a word's form, which shows grammatical relationships within a sentence. One says "who," or "whose," or "whom" depending on how one wishes to express the relationship in English, and these limited inflections show the nominative ("who"), the gentive or possessive ("whose"), and the accusative or objective ("whom"), the last form swiftly falling out of use in speech. One can illustrate the same principles with "he," "his," and "him," but English inflections are small in number when compared with Greek and Latin, languages rich in grammatical precision through the use of word endings indicating not merely grammatical relationships (nominative, genitive, and accusative are three of six cases in Latin) but also gender (masculine, feminine, and neuter) and number (singular or plural [abbreviated as *sing.* and *pl.*]). Also common in the formation of terms from Latin and Latinized Greek are participles (usually the perfect passive forms), verbal adjectives ordinarily given in Latin primers as the "fourth principle part" of verbs (thus *amatus* ["loved"] is the participle of the verb *amare* ["to love"]). Participles are declined like nouns and adjectives; in addition to tense and voice (properties of verbs), they have case, gender, and number. Sometimes scientific or medical terms emerge from present participles (for example, *amans* ["loving"]); these mostly are brought into technical terminologies without alteration and can easily be recognized for what they are. Coinages from the Latin dative or ablative cases are relatively rare in the modern sciences, and the vocative case has no role at all, so the following paradigms will indicate inflections for nouns and adjectives in the nominative, genitive, and accusative cases (participles are declined similarly, but very uncommon are terms derived from other than the nominative singular masculine [*amatus*] or neuter [*amatum*]). The following are examples drawn from Latin alone, but similar rules apply to the five cases in Greek, so that forms displayed in scientific words reflect both languages even as they descend generally through or from Latin.

Latin Declensions: Nouns

1st Declension

	sing.	sing.
Nom.	*medicina* ("medicine")	*rosa* ("rose" or "rose tree")
Gen.	*medicinae*	*rosae*
Acc.	*medicinam*	*rosam*
	pl.	pl.
Nom.	*medicinae*	*rosae*
Gen.	*medicinarum*	*rosarum*
Acc.	*medicinas*	*rosas*

In spite of the most common gender in the first declension—the feminine signified by the -*a* in the nominative singular—there are a number of nouns in Latin with -*us* (normally masculine) endings that are feminine, especially the names for trees (for example, *prunus* [nom.], *pruni* [gen.], the plum tree, or *quercus* [nom.], *quercus* [gen.], the oak [a fourth-declension noun]). If one is uncertain about the gender of a noun (this becomes important in terms of adjectival derivatives, which must "agree" with the gender of the noun), one should look it up in a good Latin dictionary.

2nd Declension

	masculine	neuter
	sing.	sing.
Nom.	*radius* ("stick," "rod,"	*bacillum* ("stick" or "lictor's
Gen.	*radii* "ray," "spoke")	*bacilli* staff")
Acc.	*radium*	*bacillum*
	pl.	pl.
Nom.	*radii*	*bacilla*
Gen.	*radiorum*	*bacillorum*
Acc.	*radios*	*bacilla*

SOME ABBREVIATED PARADIGMS

	masculine sing.	neuter sing.
Nom.	*liber* ("book")	*collum* ("neck")
Gen.	*libri*	*colli*
Acc.	*librum*	*collum*
	pl.	pl.
Nom.	*libri*	*colla*
Gen.	*librorum*	*collorum*
Acc.	*libros*	*colla*

3rd Declension

	masculine sing.	feminine sing.	neuter sing.
Nom.	*carbo* ("charcoal")	*nox* ("night,")	*caput* ("head")
Gen.	*carbonis*	*noctis* "darkness")	*capitis*
Acc.	*carbonem*	*noctem*	*caput*
	pl.	pl.	pl.
Nom.	*carbones*	*noctes*	*capita*
Gen.	*carbonum*	*noctium*	*capitum*
Acc.	*carbones*	*noctes*	*capita*
	sing.	sing.	sing.
Nom.	*homo* ("human being")	*pars* ("part")	*corpus* ("body")
Gen.	*hominis*	*partis*	*corporis*
Acc.	*hominem*	*partem*	*corpus*
	pl.	pl.	pl.
Nom.	*homines*	*partes*	*corpora*
Gen.	*hominum*	*partium*	*corporum*
Acc.	*homines*	*partes*	*corpora*
	sing.	sing.	sing.
Nom.	*dens* ("tooth")	*vis* ("force")	*animal* ("animal")
Gen.	*dentis*	*vis*	*animalis*
Acc.	*dentem*	*vim*	*animal*
	pl.	pl.	pl.
Nom.	*dentes*	*vires*	*animalia*
Gen.	*dentium*	*virium*	*animalium*
Acc.	*dentes*	*vires*	*animalia*

4th Declension

	masculine sing.	feminine sing.	neuter sing.
Nom.	*versus* ("row," "line")	*manus* ("hand")	*cornu* ("horn")
Gen.	*versus*	*manus*	*cornus*
Acc.	*versum*	*manum*	*cornu*

	pl.	pl.	pl.
Nom.	versus	manus	cornua
Gen.	versuum	manuum	cornuum
Acc.	versus	manus	cornua

5th Declension

	sing.	sing.	sing.
Nom.	dies ("day")	res ("thing")	facies ("appearance")
Gen.	diei	rei	faciei
Acc.	diem	rem	faciem
	pl.	pl.	pl.
Nom.	dies	res	facies
Gen.	dierum	rerum	facierum
Acc.	dies	res	facies

Latin Declensions: Adjectives

1st and 2nd Declensions

	masculine	feminine	neuter
	sing.		
Nom.	bonus ("good")	bona	bonum
Gen.	boni	bonae	boni
Acc.	bonum	bonam	bonum
	pl.		
Nom.	boni	bonae	bona
Gen.	bonorum	bonarum	bonorum
Acc.	bonos	bonas	bona

3rd Declension

	sing.		
Nom.	acer ("sharp")	acris	acre
Gen.	acris	acris	acris
Acc.	acrem	acrem	acre
	pl.		
Nom.	acres	acres	acria
Gen.	acrium	acrium	acrium
Acc.	acres	acres	acria

	masculine	feminine	neuter
	sing.		
Nom.	celer ("swift")	celeris	celere
Gen.	celeris	celeris	celeris
Acc.	celerem	celerem	celere
	pl.		
Nom.	celeres	celeres	celeria
Gen.	celerium	celerium	celerium
Acc.	celeres	celeres	celeria

	masculine & feminine	neuter
	sing.	
Nom.	*omnis* ("all," "every," "any")	*omne*
Gen.	*omnis*	*omnis*
Acc.	*omnem*	*omne*
	pl.	
Nom.	*omnes*	*omnia*
Gen.	*omnium*	*omnium*
Acc.	*omnes*	*omnia*
	sing.	
Nom.	*dulcis* ("sweet")	*dulce*
Gen.	*dulcis*	*dulcis*
Acc.	*dulcem*	*dulce*
	pl.	
Nom.	*dulces*	*dulcia*
Gen.	*dulcium*	*dulcium*
Acc.	*dulces*	*dulcia*
	sing.	
Nom.	*felix* ("fruitful," "fortunate")	*felix*
Gen.	*felicis*	*felicis*
Acc.	*felicem*	*felix*
	pl.	
Nom.	*felices*	*felicia*
Gen.	*felicium*	*felicium*
Acc.	*felices*	*felicia*
	masculine & feminine	neuter
	sing.	
Nom.	*sapiens* ("wise")	*sapiens*
Gen.	*sapientis*	*sapientis*
Acc.	*sapientem*	*sapiens*
	pl.	
Nom.	*sapientes*	*sapientia*
Gen.	*sapientium*	*sapientium*
Acc.	*sapientes*	*sapientia*

As in English, adjectives have comparative forms in Latin (English: good, better, best; Latin: *bonus, melior, optimus*), and many of these comparatives (called *positive* [good], *comparative* [better], and *superlative* [best]) emerge in the terminologies of medicine and the zoological and botanical sciences. Frequent is the appearance of the superlative forms, which can be rendered by "very" or "most" in the usual contexts of scientific words (for example, *latissimus* ["very wide" or "most wide"] from *latus* ["broad" or "wide"]). Some common derivations include:

positive	comparative	superlative
latus, -a, -um ("wide," "broad")	latior, latius	latissimus, -a, -um
longus, -a, -um ("long")	longior, longius	longissimus, -a, -um
fortis, -e ("strong")	fortior, fortius	fortissimus, -a, -um
levis, -e ("light," "easy")	levior, levius	levissimus, -a, -um
bonus, -a, -um ("good")	melior, melius	optimus, -a, -um
malus, -a, -um ("bad")	peior, peius	pessimus, -a, -um
magnus, -a, -um ("great")	maior, maius	maximus, -a, -um
multus, -a, -um ("many")	—— plus	plurimus, -a, -um
parvus, -a, -um ("small")	minor, minus	minimus, -a, -um

More extensive paradigms are usually incorporated as appendices at the ends of Latin textbooks intended for use in classes. Of the more recent texts (one that is also good for self-study) is *Latin for People: Latina pro Populo* by Alexander Humez and Nicholas Humez (Boston: Little, Brown & Co., Parvula Fuscaque Societas, 1976), which maintains a welcome sense of humor even as it conducts the reader through the intricacies of grammar and syntax. There are, of course, many such texts, and one can choose the textbook that suits one's own tastes according to need or objective. Among Latin grammars, one of the best remains Charles E. Bennet, *New Latin Grammar*, 2d ed. (Boston: Allyn & Bacon, 1918; reprint, 1957). A reader will find nuances explained simply and clearly, and there are paradigms included throughout according to specific considerations.

Among Greek textbooks and grammars, I have my own favorites, especially two that have worn well over the decades of the twentieth century. James Turney Allen, *The First Year of Greek*, rev. ed. (New York: Macmillan, 1931; reprint, 1963), is succinct, and Allen's treatment of beginning Greek takes into account English speakers' familiarity with some aspects of syntax to introduce them into the delicious manners in which Greek can "say" so much. Allen incorporates paradigms of nouns, adjectives, verbs, pronouns, and the rest within the text, so that someone seeking to learn Greek on his or her own can master specifics, step by step, much as one would do in formal classroom instruction. Herbert Weir Smyth, *Greek Grammar*, rev. Gordon M. Messing (Cambridge, Mass.: Harvard University Press, 1956; reprint, 1972), is probably the best of its kind in English. Somewhere within Smyth's 784 pages, one is likely to find an answer to almost any question about how Greek "works," and there are multiple paradigms neatly illustrating variations in verb forms and many of the more troublesome facets of Greek; including the always infamous particles, so essential in comprehending what most writers in classical Greek are trying to say.

BIBLIOGRAPHY

ON GAINING MORE INFORMATION

MEDICAL and scientific etymology is a grand melding of several separate aspects of scholarship, ranging from Greek, Roman, and Byzantine history and biography to specific research into the histories of words in botany, chemistry, zoology, or any of the other discrete subjects within the broadest rubric of "science." I am suggesting the following titles to indicate avenues for further pursuit of particular subjects and interests as they might occur; the references contain their own bibliographies, so that a well-researched volume will always lead to many others in several languages. Full bibliographical data on all the following titles will be found below.

Probably the best single-volume compaction of information in English on almost all aspects of classical antiquity is Hammond and Scullard, *The Oxford Classical Dictionary*. Most articles are brief snippets, but many (on Aristotle, Plato, and the major figures in Greco-Roman philosophy, as well as the famous writers like Vergil, Tacitus, Homer, and so on) are important and lengthy in their own right; each essay has a bibliography, sometimes useful in tracking down English translations not found in the Loeb Classical Library. Excellent introductory essays, characterized by the latest and most up-to-date scholarship, are in Grant and Kitzinger, *Civilization of the Ancient Mediterranean* (1988). These are lucid accounts of agriculture, various technologies, law, Greek and Roman warfare, athletics, medicine, marriage, and philosophy, among many subjects; each essay has its own bibliography (some more extensive and lengthy than others). *The Oxford Dictionary of Byzantium*, edited by Kazhdan, is a welcome addition to reference works on this fundamental culture and civilization, from which we derive so much. Unlike earlier summaries of Byzantine life and history, Kazhdan's volumes include all the sciences (botany, zoology, ornithology, medicine, the veterinary arts), so that one can now gain a clear focus on these subjects for the millennium of Byzantine civilization, in addition to the usual consideration of religion, art history, and military events; bibliographies attached to the essays in these volumes list basic texts as well as important secondary works in a number of modern languages.

For almost all biographical particulars in the history of science (including the history of medicine), the best place to begin is the multivolume *Dictionary of Scientific Biography*, as edited by Gillispie. Here one will find Harvey, Pasteur, and Vesalius, along with the host of twentieth-century scientists who so completely changed our view of what "science" is, as well as the many individuals in the history of science and medicine from all eras, from antiquity through the nineteenth century; bibliographies are extensive. Ancient medicine has received much attention from scholars in the past thirty years, and Galen's influence in medical theory and "anatomy-by-analogy" is now widely recognized. *Galenism,* by Temkin, stands as the best account of this long-term authority, which remained weighty indeed down through the eighteenth century. Nutton's *From Democedes to Harvey* has several fundamental articles that not only redate Galen but also improve our comprehension of Galen's medical practice in its intellectual context of the Second Sophistic in the second-century Roman Empire. Smith's *The Hippocratic Tradition* shows how Galen adapted Hippocrates—or the writings known as "Hippocratic"—into a form that ensured humoral pathology's place in Western medicine well into the nineteenth century. Lloyd's books have revised our notions of how science and medicine "worked" among the Greeks and Romans, and I recommend highly his *Magic, Reason and Experience, Science, Folklore, and Ideology,* and *The Revolutions of Wisdom.* Epidemiology—ancient and modern—gains meticulous analysis in Grmek's *Diseases in the Ancient Greek World;* my own *Roman Medicine* is a summary of materials from the Etruscans through the time of Galen; and Jackson's *Doctors and Diseases in the Roman Empire* is a fine collection of data, best drawn from archaeology, that augments all previous scholarship. *Dioscorides on Pharmacy and Medicine,* by Riddle, is the only good book available on this most important figure in ancient medicine and drug lore, whereas for most aspects of Byzantine medicine, one can now consult the essays in my *Symposium on Byzantine Medicine.*

In pharmacy and its quirky history, chock-full of information on words and substances (not too good, however, for earlier eras) is Mann, *Modern Drug Use.* A kind of encyclopedia for ancient, medieval, and modern pharmacology and pharmocognosy is Schneider's *Lexikon zur Arzneimittelgeschichte;* Schneider carefully traces the "ancient-to-modern" terminologies in plants and plant-derived drugs, and there are frequent references to ancient texts in Greek and Latin as they impinge on pharmacy's history in modern times. In chemistry, one happily enjoys the fun and puns—and the splendid research—in Nickon and Silversmith's *Organic Chemistry: The Name Game,* and there is good information on this topic in *Organic Chemical Nomenclature,* by Fresenius. Davis's *The Chemical Elements* remains one of the better accounts of how the "new" elements got their names, and *Historical Studies in the Language of Chemistry,* by Crosland, reveals much that is "alchemical" in chemical names.

I found many leads (to be verified in *OED,* or *LSJ,* or *OLD*) in two rather amazing compilations of etymologies of zoology and general science: Jaeger's *Source-Book of Biological Names and Terms* and Brown's *Composition of Scientific Words*. And, of course, there are numerous books in many languages of medical etymologies, some of which are based on the long history of such studies in Europe, going back to the Renaissance. One of the most recent of these traditional-format treatments (that is, lists of roots, medical derivations by tables, and the like) is the very competent *Introduzione alla terminologia medica,* by Mazzini, with its bibliographical listings of previous works in English, German, French, and Italian. Quite enlightening in how Greek medicine attempted its own precision is Skoda's *Médecine ancienne et métaphore.* Perhaps the best of the German etymology texts is *Einführung in die medizinische Fachsprache,* by Michler and Benedum; the authors both control the texts of ancient medicine in their Greek and Latin originals, and their *Einführung* is thereby quietly enriched. Beginners will appreciate the clarity of the still useful *Everyday Greek,* by Hoffman, and Muldoon's *Lessons in Pharmaceutical Latin* shows how Latin coinages—some "real" Latin, some not—were essential in pharmacy before World War II. Specialized meanings of Greek and Latin words, sometimes carrying through into modern medicine and science, also were characteristic of ancient philosophy, and for this aspect one can consult Peters's *Greek Philosophical Terms* and, more fully, *Philosophical Greek,* by Fobes. Since euphemisms abounded in classical antiquity, much as they do today, readers will find two books especially helpful in teasing out puns and jokes (occasionally with medical contexts) in Latin and Greek: *The Latin Sexual Vocabulary,* by Adams, and *The Maculate Muse,* by Henderson.

One slim volume on "roots" is so much better than any of the others I have used that I will recommend it without hesitation: Borror's *Dictionary of Word Roots and Combining Forms* is by the same individual who authored one of the standard texts of entomology, and Borror's care and precision in his *Dictionary* match the clarity of descriptions in the deservedly definitive *Introduction to the Study of Insects.* The subtitle of the *Dictionary* says modestly "Compiled from the Greek, Latin, and other languages, with special references to biological terms and scientific names"; anyone curious about medical or biological nomenclatures should have this book, which remains in print.

TEXTS AND SOURCES

Greek and Latin

With the exception of the specific editions listed below, texts and translations of Greek and Latin authors (Aelian, Aristotle, Celsus, Homer, Cicero, Tacitus, Plato, Suetonius, etc.) are in the Loeb Classical Library series (published in Cambridge, Massachusetts, by Harvard University Press). Medical and scientific works form only a small portion of the over 450 volumes in the Loeb series (if one excepts Aristotle): Celsus (ed. and trans. by W. G. Spencer) is in three volumes; Galen is represented by a single volume, *On the Natural Faculties,* edited and translated by Arthur John Brock; the Hippocratic works have six volumes, edited with translations by W.H.S. Jones, Paul Potter, and E. T. Withington; and Theophrastus (in addition to the works cited under "Abbreviations") has three volumes recently completed, *De causis plantarum,* edited with translations by Benedict Einarson and G.K.K. Link. Pliny the Elder's *Natural History* (also listed under "Abbreviations") occupies ten volumes in the Loeb series. Harvard University Press (which has become the sole publisher of the Loeb volumes, since William Heinemann of London no longer is the copublisher) keeps volumes of the Loeb Classical Library continuously in print, so that (for example) volumes first published in the series early in the twentieth century (Brock's *Galen on the Natural Faculties* appeared in 1916) remain available.

Aetius of Amida:
    Olivieri, Alexander, ed. (Greek text only). *Aetii Amideni libri medicinales I–IV.* Leipzig: B. G. Teubner, 1935 (*CMG* VIII 1).
    Olivieri, Alexander, ed. (Greek text only). *Aetii Amideni libri medicinales V–VIII.* Berlin: Akademie-Verlag, 1950 (*CMG* VIII 2).

Antyllus: see Oribasius below

Aretaeus of Cappadocia:
    Adams, Francis, ed. and trans. *The Extant Works of Aretaeus, the Cappadocian.* London: Sydenham Society, 1856. The English translation is rendered from the Greek text, as available in the early nineteenth century.
    Hude, Carolus, ed. (Greek text only). *Aretaeus.* 2d ed. Berlin: Akademie-Verlag, 1958 (*CMG* II). This is the best-edited Greek text of Aretaeus's works.

Dioscorides:
    Berendes, J., trans. with commentary. *Des Pedanios Dioskurides aus Anazarbos Arzneimittellehre.* Stuttgart: Ferdinand Enke, 1902. Reprint. Schaan (Liechtenstein): Sändig Reprint Verlag, 1983. Berendes' German translation remains useful, even though rendered from unevenly edited Greek texts of the early nineteenth century.
    Wellmann, Max, ed. (Greek text only). *Pedanii Dioscuridis Anazarbei De materia medica.* 3 vols. Berlin: Weidmann, 1906–14. Reprint. 1958. This is the best-edited Greek text. There is no reliable English translation.

Festus:
- Lindsay, Wallace M., ed. (Latin text only). *Sexti Pompei Festi De verborum significatu quae supersunt cum Pauli epitome.* Leipzig: B. G. Teubner, 1913. Reprint. Hildesheim: Georg Olms, 1965.

Galen:
- De Lacy, Phillip, ed. with English translation. *Galen on the Doctrines of Hippocrates and Plato.* 3 vols. Berlin: Akademie-Verlag, 1978–84 (*CMG* V 4, 1, 2).
- Furley, David J., and Wilkie, J. S., eds. and trans. *Galen on Respiration and the Arteries.* Princeton: Princeton University Press, 1984. Greek texts (with occasional Arabic fill-ins of lacunae) and English translations of Galen's *Use of Breathing, Blood in the Arteries, On the Use of the Pulse,* and *On the Causes of Breathing.*
- Helmreich, Georg., ed. (Greek text). *Galeni De usu partium.* 2 vols. Leipzig: B. G. Teubner, 1907–9. Reprint. Amsterdam: A. Hakkert, 1968. English translation (from the Helmreich text): Margaret Tallmadge May, trans., *Galen on the Usefulness of the Parts of the Body.* 2 vols. Ithaca, N.Y.: Cornell University Press, 1968.
- Kühn, C. G., ed. (Greek texts with Latin renditions). *Claudii Galeni Opera omnia.* 20 vols. in 22 parts. Leipzig: Cnoblichius, 1821–33. Reprint. Hildesheim: Georg Olms, 1964–65. In spite of its numerous faults, this edition of Galen's works remains most frequently cited.
- Moore, Michael Garrett, ed. and trans. *Galen: Introduction to the Bones.* Ph.D. diss., University of Michigan, 1969.
- Nutton, Vivian, ed. with English trans. and comm. *Galen on Prognosis.* Berlin: Akademie-Verlag, 1979 (*CMG* V 8, 1).
- Singer, Charles, trans. (from the Kühn ed. text as above). *Galen on Anatomical Procedures.* London: Oxford University Press for the Wellcome Historical Medical Museum, 1956. A translation—not completely trustworthy—of the surviving books (I–VIII) in Greek. W. L. H. Duckworth, trans. (from the Arabic), M. C. Lyons and B. Towers, eds., *Galen on Anatomical Procedures: The Later Books.* Cambridge: University Press, 1962. Books IX–XV of Galen's *Anatomical Procedures* have reached us only in an Arabic translation, made from the Greek in the ninth century.

Herophilus:
- Von Staden, Heinrich, ed., trans., and comm. *Herophilus: The Art of Medicine in Early Alexandria.* Cambridge: Cambridge University Press, 1989.

Isidore of Seville:
  Lindsay, Wallace Martin, ed. (Latin text only). *Isidori Hispalensis Etymologiarum.* 2 vols. Oxford: Clarendon Press, 1911.
Justinian, *Digest:*
  Krueger, P., and Mommsen, T., eds. *Corpus Iuris civilis.* 15th ed. Vol. I: *Institutiones* (ed. Krueger); *Digesta* (ed. Mommsen). Berlin: Weidmann, 1928. English translation: Alan Watson, ed., *The Digest of Justinian.* 4 vols. Philadelphia: University of Pennsylvania Press, 1985.
Nicander of Colophon:
  Gow, A.S.F., and Scholfield, A. F., eds., with translation and notes. *Nicander: The Poems and Poetical Fragments.* Cambridge: Cambridge University Press, 1953. Here one will find the *Theriaca* and *Alexipharmaca* in both Greek and English, accompanied with helpful notes and references, somewhat limited by the format.
Oribasius:
  Raeder, Johannes, ed. (Greek text only). *Oribasii Collectionum medicarum reliquiae.* 4 vols. Leipzig: B. G. Teubner, 1928–33. Reprint. Amsterdam: A. Hakkert, 1964.
Philumenus:
  Wellmann, Max, ed. (Greek text only). *Philumeni De venenatis animalibus eorumque remediis.* Leipzig: B. G. Teubner, 1908 (*CMG* X 1, 1).
Pollux:
  Bethe, Eric, ed. (Greek text only). *Pollucis Onomasticon e codicibus ab ipso collatis.* 3 vols. Leipzig: B. G. Teubner, 1900–1937. Reprint. Stuttgart: B. G. Teubner, 1967.
Rufus of Ephesus:
  Daremberg, C., and Ruelle, C. E., eds. and French translations. *Oeuvres de Rufus d'Éphèse.* Paris: J.-B. Baillière, 1879. Reprint. Amsterdam: A. Hakkert, 1963.
Scribonius Largus:
  Sconocchia, Sergio, ed. (Latin text only). *Scribonii Largi Compositiones.* Leipzig: B. G. Teubner, 1983.
Soranus:
  Ilberg, J., ed. (Greek text only). *Sorani Gynaeciorum libri IV. De signis fracturarum. De fasciis. Vita Hippocratis secundum Soranum.* Leipzig: B. G. Teubner, 1927 (*CMG* IV). English translation (from the Ilberg text): Owsei Temkin, trans., *Soranus' Gynecology.* Baltimore: Johns Hopkins Press, 1956.
Theophrastus (in addition to works cited under "Abbreviations Used" and the description of the Loeb Classical Library, above):

Eichholz, D. E., ed., trans., and comm. *Theophrastus De lapidibus.* Oxford: Clarendon Press, 1965.

Ross, W. D., and Forbes, F. H., eds. and trans. *Theophrastus Metaphysics.* Oxford: Clarendon Press, 1929.

Stratton, George Malcolm, ed., trans., and comm. *Theophrastus and the Greek Physiological Psychology before Aristotle [Theophrastus On the Senses].* London: Allen & Unwin, 1917. Reprint. Amsterdam: Bonset, 1964.

Wimmer, F., ed. (Greek texts with Latin translations). *Theophrasti Eresii Opera, quae supersunt, omnia.* Paris: Didot, 1866. Reprint. Frankfurt: Minerva, 1964. This edition of Theophrastus's works remains the most complete and includes numerous "fragments" embedded in later writings that quote Theophrastus.

Renaissance and Enlightenment

Dobell, Clifford, ed. and trans. (from the Dutch). *Antony van Leeuwenhoek and His "Little Animals."* London: John Bale, Sons & Danielsson, 1932. Reprint. New York: Dover Books, 1960.

Linnaeus, Carl. *Species Plantarum.* 2 vols. Facsimile of the first edition (1753), introduction and appendices by J. L. Heller and W. F. Stearn. London: Ray Society, 1957–59.

Whitteridge, Gweneth, ed. *The Anatomical Lectures of William Harvey.* Edinburgh: Livingston, 1964. William Harvey, *De motu cordis et sanguinis in animalibus.* Frankfurt: W. Fitzer, 1628. English translation: Kenneth J. Franklin, trans., *Movement of the Heart and Blood in Animals . . . by William Harvey.* Oxford: Blackwell, 1957.

Ancient Egyptian

Breasted, James Henry, ed., trans., and comm. *The Edwin Smith Surgical Papyrus.* 2 vols. Chicago: University of Chicago Press, 1930.

SECONDARY WORKS

Adams, J. N. "Anatomical Terminology in Latin Epic." *Bulletin of the Institute of Classical Studies* (London) 27 (1980): 50–62.

———. *The Latin Sexual Vocabulary.* Baltimore: John Hopkins University Press, 1982.

Allen, James Turney. *The First Year of Greek.* Rev. ed. New York: Macmillan, 1931. Reprint. 1963.

Andrews, Michael. *The Life That Lives on Man.* London: Faber & Faber, 1976.

Atkins, P. W. *Molecules.* New York: W. H. Freeman, 1987.

Bailey, L. H. *How Plants Get Their Names.* London: Macmillan, 1933. Reprint. New York: Dover Books, 1963.
Beavis, Ian C. *Insects and Other Invertebrates in Classical Antiquity.* Exeter: University of Exeter, 1988.
Bennett, Charles E. *New Latin Grammar.* 2d ed. Boston: Allyn & Bacon, 1918. Reprint. 1957.
Bergquist, Patricia R. *Sponges.* Berkeley: University of California Press, 1978.
Berkow, Robert, and Fletcher, Andrew J., eds. *The Merck Manual.* 15th ed. Rahway, N.J.: Merck, Sharp and Dohme, 1987.
Borradaile, L. A., and Potts, F. A., with chapters by Eastham, L. E. S., and Saunders, J. T. *The Invertebrata.* 4th ed., rev. G. A. Kerkut. Cambridge: Cambridge University Press, 1961.
Borror, Donald J. *Dictionary of Word Roots and Combining Forms.* Mountain View, Calif.: Mayfield Publishing Co., 1960. Reprint. 1971.
Borror, Donald J.; Triplehorn, Charles A.; and Johnson, Norman F. *An Introduction to the Study of Insects.* 6th ed. Philadelphia: Saunders, 1989.
Borror, Donald J., and DeLong, Dwight M. *An Introduction to the Study of Insects.* Rev. ed. New York: Holt, Reinhart and Winston, 1964.
Bright, Donald E. "Two New Species of *Phloeosinus* Chapuis from Mount Kinabalu, Borneo, with Taxonomic Notes." *Coleopterists Bulletin* 43 (1989): 79–82.
Brimble, L.J.F. *Intermediate Botany.* Rev. 4th ed., S. Williams and G. Bond. London: Macmillan, 1980.
Brown, Roland Wilbur. *Composition of Scientific Words.* Rev. ed. Washington, D.C.: Smithsonian Institution Press, 1956. Reprint. 1985.
Buchsbaum, Ralph. *Animals without Backbones.* 2d ed. Chicago: University of Chicago Press, 1976.
Buchsbaum, Ralph; Buchsbaum, Mildred; Pearse, John; and Pearse, Vicki. *Animals without Backbones.* 3d ed. Chicago: University of Chicago Press, 1987.
Busvine, J. R. "The 'Head' and 'Body' Races of *Pediculus humanus* L." *Parasitology* 39 (1948): 1–16.
———. *Insects, Hygiene, and History.* London: University of London, Athlone Press, 1976.
Cain, A. J. *Animal Species and Their Evolution.* 3d ed. London: Hutchinson, 1971.
Cartmill, Matt; Hylander, William L.; and Shafland, James. *Human Structure.* Cambridge, Mass.: Harvard University Press, 1987.
Christianson, E. H. "The Search for Diagnostic and Therapeutic Authority in the Early American Healer's Encounter with 'The Animals which Inhabit the Human Stomach and Intestine.'" In John Scar-

borough, ed., *Folklore and Folk Medicines,* 62–85. Madison, Wis.: American Institute of the History of Pharmacy, 1987.

Clarke, Edwin, and Dewhurst, Kenneth. *An Illustrated History of Brain Function.* Berkeley: University of California Press, 1974.

Cloudsley-Thompson, J. L. *Spiders, Scorpions, Centipedes, and Mites.* Oxford: Pergamon Press, 1968.

Crosland, M. P. *Historical Studies in the Language of Chemistry.* London: William Heinemann, 1962. Reprint. New York: Dover Books, 1978.

Crowson, R. A. *Classification and Biology.* New York: Atherton Press, 1970.

Dales, R. Phillips. *Annelids.* 2d ed. London: Hutchinson, 1970.

Davidson, Stanley. *The Principles and Practice of Medicine.* 8th ed. Edinburgh: E. S. Livingston, 1966.

Davis, Helen Miles. *The Chemical Elements.* New York: Ballantine Books, 1959.

Dean, Geoffrey. *The Porphyrias: A Story of Inheritance and Environment.* 2d ed. London: Pitman Medical, 1971.

Du Cange, D. *Glossarium mediae et infimae Latinitatis.* New ed., 10 vols., ed. L. Favre. Niort (France): Favre, 1883–87.

Dunglison, Robley. *Medical Lexicon: A Dictionary of Medical Science.* 12th ed., rev. 8th ed. Philadelphia: Blanchard and Lea, 1855.

———. *Medical Lexicon: A Dictionary of Medical Science.* Rev. and augmented. Philadelphia: Lea, 1868.

———. *Medical Lexicon: A Dictionary of Medical Science.* New ed., rev. Richard J. Dunglison. Philadelphia: Lea, 1874.

Easton, W. H. *Invertebrate Paleontology.* New York: Harper & Row, 1960.

Essig, E. O. *College Entomology.* New York: Macmillan, 1947.

Evans, Glyn. *The Life of Beetles.* London: Allen & Unwin, 1975.

Faust, Ernest Carroll, and Russell, Paul Farr. *Craig and Faust's Clinical Parasitology.* 7th ed. Philadelphia: Lea & Febiger, 1964.

Fernald, Merritt Lyndon. *Gray's Manual of Botany.* 8th ed. Cambridge, Mass.: Harvard University Press, 1950. Reprint. Portland, Oreg.: Dioscorides Press, 1987.

Fobes, Francis H. *Philosophical Greek.* Chicago: University of Chicago Press, 1957.

Fresenius, Philipp. *Organic Chemical Nomenclature.* Trans. from the second German ed. (1983) by A. J. Dunsdon. New York: John Wiley, 1989.

Gibson, Ray. *Nemerteans.* London: Hutchinson, 1972.

Gillispie, C. C., ed. *Dictionary of Scientific Biography.* 16 vols. + 2 supplement vols. New York: Charles Scribner's Sons, 1970–90.

Gledhill, D. *The Names of Plants.* 2d ed. Cambridge: Cambridge University Press, 1989.

Gleick, James. *Chaos.* New York: Viking Penguin, 1987.
Goss, Charles Mayo. *A Brief Account of Henry Gray F.R.S. and His Anatomy, Descriptive and Surgical, during a Century of Its Publication in America.* Philadelphia: Lea & Febiger, 1959.
Grant, Michael, and Kitzinger, Rachel, eds. *Civilization of the Ancient Mediterranean: Greece and Rome.* 3 vols. New York: Charles Scribner's Sons, 1988.
Gray, Henry. *Anatomy of the Human Body.* 27th ed., ed. Charles Mayo Goss. Philadelphia: Lea & Febiger, 1959.
Greene, Edward Lee. *Landmarks of Botanical History.* Rev. ed., 2 vols., ed. Frank N. Egerton. Stanford, Calif.: Stanford University Press, 1983.
Greene, Raymond. *Human Hormones.* New York: McGraw-Hill, 1970.
Grmek, Mirko D. *Diseases in the Ancient Greek World.* Baltimore: Johns Hopkins University Press, 1989.
Guyton, Arthur C. *Textbook of Medical Physiology.* 4th ed. Philadelphia: Saunders, 1971.
Hammond, N.G.L., and Scullard, H. H., eds. *The Oxford Classical Dictionary.* 2d ed. Oxford: Clarendon Press, 1970.
Heller, John Lewis. *Studies in Linnaean Method and Nomenclature.* Frankfurt: Verlag Peter Lang, 1983 (*Marburger Schriften zur Medizingeschichte* 7).
Henderson, Jeffrey. *The Maculate Muse: Obscene Language in Attic Comedy.* New Haven: Yale University Press, 1975.
Hickey, M., and King, C. J. *100 Families of Flowering Plants.* Cambridge: Cambridge University Press, 1981.
Hoeppli, R. *Parasites and Parasitic Infections in Early Medicine and Science.* Singapore: University of Malaya Press, 1959.
Hoffman, Horace Addison. *Everyday Greek: Greek Words in English, Including Scientific Terms.* Chicago: University of Chicago Press, 1919.
Howse, P. E. *Termites.* London: Hutchinson, 1970.
Humez, Alexander, and Humez, Nicholas. *Latin for People: Latina pro Populo.* Boston: Little, Brown & Co., Parvula Fuscaque Societas, 1976.
Huxley, Thomas Henry. *The Crayfish: An Introduction to the Study of Zoology.* London, 1880. Reprint. Cambridge, Mass.: MIT Press, 1979.
Imms, A. D. *A General Textbook of Entomology.* 9th ed., rev. O. W. Richards and R. G. Davies. London: Methuen, 1957.
Jackson, Benjamin Daydon. *A Glossary of Botanic Terms.* New York: Hafner, 1950.
Jackson, Ralph. *Doctors and Diseases in the Roman Empire.* Norman: University of Oklahoma Press, 1988.
Jaeger, Edmund C. *A Source-Book of Biological Names and Terms.* 3d ed. Springfield, Ill.: Charles C. Thomas, 1955.
Kazhdan, Alexander P., and Talbot, Alice-Mary, eds. *The Oxford Dictio-*

nary of Byzantium. 3 vols. New York and Oxford: Oxford University Press, 1991.

Kingsbury, John M. *Poisonous Plants of the United States and Canada.* Englewood Cliffs, N. J.: Prentice-Hall, 1964.

Levi-Setti, Riccardo. *Trilobites.* Chicago: University of Chicago Press, 1975.

Lloyd, G.E.R. *Magic, Reason, and Experience: Studies in the Origins of Greek Science.* Cambridge: Univesity Press, 1979.

———. *The Revolutions of Wisdom: Studies in the Claims and Practice of Ancient Greek Science.* Berkeley: University of California Press, 1987.

———. *Science, Folklore, and Ideology: Studies in the Life Sciences in Ancient Greece:* Cambridge: Cambridge University Press, 1983.

Longrigg, James. "Anatomy in Alexandria in the Third Century B.C." *British Journal of the History of Science* 21 (1988): 455–88.

Mabberley, D. J. *The Plant-Book.* Cambridge: Cambridge University Press, 1987.

Macalpine, Ida, and Hunter, Richard. *George III and the Mad-Business.* London: Allen Lane, 1969.

Maciel, G. E.; Traficante, D. D.; and Lavallee, D. *Chemistry.* Lexington, Mass.: D. C. Heath, 1978.

Mackinnon, Doris L., and Hawes, R.S.J. *An Introduction to the Study of Protozoa.* Oxford: Clarendon Press, 1961.

McMillen, Wheeler, and Lucas, Lex R., eds. *Handbook for Boys.* 5th ed. New York: Boy Scouts of America, 1948.

Majno, Guido. *The Healing Hand: Man and Wound in the Ancient World.* Cambridge, Mass.: Harvard University Press, 1975.

Mann, R. D. *Modern Drug Use: An Enquiry on Historical Principles.* Boston: MTP Press, Kluwer, 1984.

Manton, S. M. *The Arthropoda.* Oxford: Clarendon Press, 1977.

Mazzini, Innocenzo. *Introduzione alla terminologia medica.* Bologna: Patron Editore, 1989.

Mencken, H. L. *The American Language: Supplement I.* New York: Knopf, 1945.

Michler, M., and Benedum, J. *Einführung in die medizinische Fachsprache.* Berlin: Springer-Verlag, 1981.

Miner, Roy Waldo. *Field Book of Seashore Life.* New York: Putnam's, 1950.

Morton, A. G. *History of Botanical Science.* London: Academic Press, 1981.

Morton, J. E. *Molluscs.* 4th ed. London: Hutchinson, 1971.

Muldoon, Hugh C. *Lessons in Pharmaceutical Latin.* 3d ed. New York: John Wiley, 1937.

Nickon, Alex, and Silversmith, Ernest F. *Organic Chemistry, The Name Game: Modern Coined Terms and Their Origins.* Oxford: Pergamon Press, 1987.

Norman, Anthony W., and Litwack, Gerald. *Hormones*. Orlando, Fla.: Academic Press, 1987.
Nutton, Vivian. *From Democedes to Harvey*. London: Variorum Reprints, 1988.
Partridge, Eric. *Origins: A Short Etymological Dictionary of Modern English*. 4th ed. London: William Heinemann, 1966.
Pennak, Robert W. *Fresh-Water Invertebrates of the United States*. New York: Ronald Press, 1953. 3d ed., New York: John Wiley, 1989.
Peters, F. E. *Greek Philosophical Terms: A Historical Lexicon*. New York: New York University Press, 1967.
Qvist, George. *John Hunter*. London: William Heinemann, 1981.
Restak, Richard. *The Brain*. New York: Bantam Books, 1984.
Richards, O. W., and Davies, R. G. *Imms' General Textbook of Entomology*. 10th ed. 2 vols. London: Chapman & Hall, 1977.
Riddle, John M. *Dioscorides on Pharmacy and Medicine*. Austin: University of Texas Press, 1985.
Rock, Irvin. *Perception*. New York: W. H. Freeman, 1984.
Romer, Alfred Sherwood. *Vertebrate Paleontology*. 3d ed. Chicago: University of Chicago Press, 1966.
Rudwick, M.J.S. *Living and Fossil Brachiopods*. London: Hutchinson, 1970.
Ryland, J. S. *Bryozoans*. London: Hutchinson, 1970.
Scarborough, John. "Nicander's Toxicology, II: Spiders, Scorpions, Insects and Myriapods." *Pharmacy in History* 21 (1979): 3–34, 73–92.
———. *Roman Medicine*. Ithaca, N. Y.: Cornell University Press, 1969. Reprint. 1976.
———, ed. *Symposium on Byzantine Medicine*. Washington, D.C.: Dumbarton Oaks, 1985 (*Dumbarton Oaks Papers* 38 [1984]).
Schmitt, Waldo L. *Crustaceans*. Ann Arbor: University of Michigan Press, 1965.
Schneider, Wolfgang. *Lexikon zur Arzneimittelgeschichte*. 7 vols. in 9 parts. Frankfurt: Govi-Verlag, 1968–75.
Service, M. W. *A Guide to Medical Entomology*. London: Macmillan, 1980.
Simak, Clifford D. *Mastodonia*. New York: Ballantine Books, 1978.
Simpson, George Gaylord. *Principles of Animal Taxonomy*. New York: Columbia University Press, 1961.
———. "The Principles of Classification and a Classification of Mammals." *Bulletin of the American Museum of Natural History* 85 (1945): 1–350.
Skeat, W. *A Concise Etymological Dictionary of the English Language*. Rev. ed. Oxford: Clarendon Press, 1927.
Skoda, Françoise. *Médecine ancienne et métaphore*. Paris: Peeters, Selaf, 1988.

Smith, Emil L.; Hill, Robert L.; Lehman, I. Robert; Lefkowitz, Robert J.; Handler, Philip; and White, Abraham. *Principles of Biochemistry.* 7th ed. New York: McGraw-Hill, 1983.

Smith, Wesley D. *The Hippocratic Tradition.* Ithaca. N. Y.: Cornell University Press, 1979.

Smyth, Herbert Weir. *Greek Grammar.* Rev. Gordon R. Messing. Cambridge, Mass.: Harvard University Press, 1956. Reprint. 1972.

Stearn, William T. *Botanical Latin.* 2d ed. Newton Abbott: David & Charles, 1973.

Sugar, Oscar. "How the Sacrum Got Its Name." *Journal of the American Medical Association* 257 (1987): 2061–63.

Temkin, Owsei. *Galenism.* Ithaca, N. Y.: Cornell University Press, 1973.

Thompson, D'Arcy Wentworth. *A Glossary of Greek Birds.* London: Oxford University Press, 1936. Reprint. Hildesheim: Georg Olms, 1966.

———. *A Glossary of Greek Fishes.* London: Oxford University Press, 1947.

Thorne, Gerald. *Principles of Nematology.* New York: McGraw-Hill, 1961.

Thorson, Gunnar. *Life in the Sea.* Translated from the Danish by M. C. Meilgaard and A. Laurie. New York: McGraw-Hill, 1971.

Von Buddenbrock, Wolfgang. *Die Welt der Sinne.* Berlin: Springer Verlag, 1953.

White, Abraham; Handler, Philip; Smith, Emil L.; and Stetten, DeWitt, Jr. *Principles of Biochemistry.* 2d ed. New York: McGraw-Hill, 1959.

White, Lynn, Jr. *Medieval Technology and Social Change.* Oxford: Clarendon Press, 1962.

Wilcocks, Charles, and Manson-Behr, P.E.C. *Manson's Tropical Diseases.* 17th ed. London: Bailliere Tindal, 1978.

Winsor, Mary P. *Starfish, Jellyfish, and the Order of Life.* New Haven: Yale University Press, 1976.

Wolfe, Jeremy M., ed. *The Mind's Eye.* New York: Freeman, 1986.

Wright, C. A. *Flukes and Snails.* London: Allen & Unwin, 1971.

Zimmermann, W. J.; Hubbard, E. D.; Schwarte, L. H.; and Biester, H. E. "*Trichinella spiralis* in Iowa Wildlife during the Years 1953–1961." *Journal of Parasitology* 48 (1962): 429–32.

See also "Abbreviations" for references frequently cited and not included in the previous bibliography.

Index

Asterisk (*) indicates that entry includes brief etymology.

*Abortion, 208–209
Abstractions, chemical names, 3
*Acanthocephala (phylum), 52
*Acarina (arthropod order, mites), 122–23
Acetabulum. See Bones
*Acetone, 240
*Acetylcholine, 164
Achilles tendon. See Tendo calcaneus
*Acyclovir (drug for herpes), 207
Adams, J. N., on sexual euphemisms in Latin, 197–98
Adjectives, comparative and superlative forms, 273
Aelian: on gills, 57; on termites, 98
*Aerogastria, 224
*Aeropathy, 224
*Aerophagia, 224
*Aetiology, 68
Aetius of Amida, on drug properties, 222–23
Agassiz, Louis, 42
Agassiz, Louis (son), 42
Agriculture, Roman, 158
*AIDS (Acquired Immunodeficiency Syndrome), 207–208
Air, as element, 216
Aitiai ("causes"), according to Aristotle, 25
Albertus Magnus, on plant names, 22
*Alcohol, 240
Alexander the Great, 143–44
Alexandria, Egypt, 144; museum and library, 144
*Algae, 27
"Amazon" ants, 116–17
*Amine, 12
Amino acid (*hirudin), lacking tryptophan, arginine, methionine, 59
*Amoeba proteus, 37
*Ampulla, inner ear, 254
*Amygdala, 148
*Amylase pancreatic enzyme, 194
*Anabolism, 239
*Anaphylaxis, 115
Anatomy, comparative, and dissection, 160–62

*Ancient, 6
*Ancylostoma spp. (hookworms), 49–50
Anemones, sea, 41
*Angiospermae, 28–29
*Annelida (phylum), 56–59
Anoplura (insect order), 101–102
Antenna(e): in ancient Latin, 86; of butterflies and moths, 113
Antepenult rule in pronunciation, 268–69
*Anther, 26
*Anthozoa (sea anemones), 41
*Anthrax, 111
*Anthromorphic, 218
*Anthropology, 218
*Anthropopagus, 218
Anticoagulant, leeches and *hirudin, 59
Ant lions (insects), 105
Ants, 115–17
Antyllus, on leeches, 59
*Anus, 194
*Aorta, 8, 232
Apes, Barbary, and Galen's dissections, 160
*Aphasmidia (class of Nematodes), 48–49
*Aphrodisiac, 204
*Aplacophora (class of Molluscs), 61
*Apoidea (superfamily of bees), 117
*Aponeurosis, 162–63
*Appear, 8
*Appendicitis, 193–94
Apuleius, *Golden Ass*: on breathing, 180; on feces as scum, 185
*Aqueous humor of eyeball, 252
Arabic: derivation for *alcohol, 240; origin of Latin dura and pia mater, 146–47; ultimate origin of "sugar," 190
*Arachnida (class of Arthropods: spiders), 119–21
*Arachnoid membrane, 146–47
*Arches, 8
Aretaeus of Cappadocia: *Acute Diseases,* on the bronchus, 178; *Chronic Diseases,* on diabetes, on gonorrhea, 206
*Arginine (amino acid), 59
Aristotle: on animal classes, 32–34, 35;

on animal lungs, 174; on classification, 24–26; on gills, 57; on meninges, 146; on numbers of insects, 73; works, 25. *HA,* on antennae of crustaceans, 62; on barnacles, 77; on calf of a leg, 165; on a chrysalis, 87; on coverings for the wings of a flying insect, 106; on earth wasps, 118; on *entoma,* 72; on fish scales, 113; on intestinal worms, 44; on knuckles, 135; on limpets, 61; on mayflies, 122; on mites, 122; on a moth chrysalis, 79; on the *olekranon,* 132 (*see also* Bones); on the "paper nautilus," 68; on roundworms and flatworms 50; on small crustaceans, 80; on the thorax, 128; on wood lice, 78–79. *Meteorlogica,* on stones colored dark red (anthrax), 111
*Arms, 5
Arrector pili muscles, 261
Arrow worms, 54–55
*Arsenic, 205
*Arsphenamine (to treat syphilis), 205
Arteries: *brachiocephalic, 232; *carotids, 232–33; pulmonary and branches, 234
*Arterioles, 234
*Arthropoda, 72
*Articulation, 163; in speaking, 256
*Arytenoid cartilages, 257
*Ascaris spp. (roundworms), 50
Assassin bugs, 103
Athenaeus, *Deipnosophistae,* on rock-boring shellfish, 66
-ation (suffix), 256
*Atrioventricular node, heart, 231
*Atrium, heart, 229
Aulus Gellus, *Attic Nights,* on "sitting bones," 131
*Auricle, heart, 229
*Austere, 227
Autry, Gene, 20
Azalea. *See* Rhododendron

Bacon, Nat, and Bacon's Rebellion, 20
*Bacterium, 205
Bancroft, Joseph, 51
Banting, F. G., 245
Barnacles, 77–78
Baseball, jargon, 8
Beaumont, William, 222
Bedbugs, 103
Bees, 117
Beeswax, 117–18

Beetles, 105–108; nematode parasites of, 51–52; numbers of, 34
Best, C. H., 245
Bicuspids. *See* Teeth
*Bicuspid valve, heart, 229
*Bifurcation, 232
Big toe bone. *See* Bones, hallux
*Bile, 194
Bird lice, 100–101
*Bivalvia. *See* *Pelycypoda (class of Molluscs)
Black bile as humor, 217
Black Death, 109–10
Black widow spider, 119–20
Blood as humor, 217
*Bombinae (subfamily of bumblebees), 117
Bones: *acetabulum, 130; *acromion, 131; *Atlas, 127; auditory ossicles, 167, 253; *axis, 127–28; *calcaneus, 137–38; *caput femoris, 134; *cervical vertebrae, 127–28; *clavicle, 131; *coccyx, 129; *condyles of femur, 135; *coracoid process, 131; *coronoid process of ulna, 132; *coxa, 130; *femur, 134; *fibula, 136–37; *foramina in, 127; *frontal, 126; *gladiolus, 131; *hallux, 138–40; hip, 129–30; *humerus, 132; *hyoid, 177; *ilium, 130; *incus (*see* Bones, auditory ossicles); inner ear (*see* Bones, auditory ossicles); *ischium, 130; *lumbar vertebrae, 128; *malleus (*see* Bones, auditory ossicles); *mandible, 127; *manubrium, 131; *maxilla, 127; *metacarpals, 133; *metatarsals, 138; *nasal, 126–27; *occipital, 126; *olecranon, 132; *os coxae, 129; *os pubis, 130–31; *ossa carpi, 132–33; *os sacrum, 128–29; *parietal, 126; *patella, 135; *phalanges, 134; *pollex, 134; *radius, 132; *scapula, 131; *semilunar notch of ulna, 132; *sesamoid, 126; skull, 126–27; *sphenoid, 126; *stapes (*see* Bones, auditory ossicles); *sternum, 131; *synovial membrane, 163; *tarsal, 137–38; *temporal, 126; *thoracic vertebrae, 128; *tibia, 136; *trochanter of femur, 134; *ulna, 132; *xiphisternum, 131; *zygomatic, 126
Book lice, 100
*Borax, 96
*Boubōn (Greek), 109–10

INDEX

*Brachiocephalic artery, 232
*Brachiopoda (phylum), 56
*Branches, 8
*Branchiopoda (subclass in Arthropoda), 75–76
*Branchiura (subclass in Crustacea), 76–77
*Bread, 184
Bright, Donald E, on new beetle species from Borneo, 88
Bristletails (insects), 91
*Bronchi, 178
Brothels (*fornices* in Latin), 201
*Bryophyta, 28. See also Mosses
*Bryozoa (phylum), 55–56
Bubonic plague, 109–10
Buchsbaum, Ralph, on mygalomorphs, 121
"Bugs," 103–104
Bumblebees, nematode parasites of, 51
Busvine, J. R., on human lice, 101–102
Butterflies, 112–14
Byzantine Greek: adapted names for scabies mite, 122; on bedbugs, 103; *enzyme, 189; on *geōponika*, 224; on *sinai* for "Chinese," 97

Caestus, as "Venus girdle," or Roman boxing glove, 42
Caisson disease, 224
Calculus, renal, 195
*Cambrian period, 74
*Cancer (genus of crabs), 81
*Canines. See Teeth
*Capillaries, 234
*Capsicum spp., red peppers among nightshades, 21
*Car, 5
*Carbohydrate, 189–90
*Carbon, 189
*Carcinology, 75
Cardiac cycle, systole and diastole, 229
*Cardiac orifice, 191
Cardinal numbers, 263
*Cardiology, 232
*Cardiovascular, 232
*Cardium (genus of cockles), 64–65
*Carnal, 184–85
*Carotid arteries, 232–33
*Cartilage, 163; *arytenoid, 257; *thyroid and *cricoid, 177
*Cartography, 224
*Catabolism, 239
Caterpillars, 112–13

Cato the Elder, on Triticum (wheat), 15
Catullus, on homosexual lovers, 200
"Causes," according to Aristotle, 25
Cecropia moths, 113–14
*Cecum, 193
*Cell, 240
*Cellulose, 99, 190
*Celom, 9
Celsus, Cornelius: on ilia as "flanks," 130; on pelvis, 129; on pubes, 131
*Centipedes, 83–84
*Centrifuge, 218–19
*Cephalopoda (class of Molluscs), 66–68
*Cera, 117
*Cerebellum, 146
*Cerebrum, 146
*Cestoda (class of Platyhelminthes), 45–46
*Chaetognatha (phylum), 54–55
Change as *metabolē* (Greek), 25
Chaos, as science, 31
Chapuis, M. F., 88
Chaucer, Geoffrey, on Socrates' wife, 188
*Chelicera, 122
Chiggers, 122
*Chilopoda (centipedes), 83–84
*Chitin (insects' exoskeleton), 60
*Chiton (genus in Polyplacophora), 60
*Chlorine, 220
*Chlorophyll, 27, 200
*Cholesterol, 239–40
*Chordae tendineae of heart, 229
*Choroid of eye, 252. See also Uvea
Christianson, Eric, on length of extruded tapeworms in seventeenth and eighteenth centuries in Colonial America and England, 45
*Chromosome, 217
*Chyme, 192
*Chymoi as humors, 217
Cicadas, 104
Cicero, Marcus Tullius, *Nature of the Gods*, on mice, 156
*Ciliary body of eye, 252. See also Uvea
*Ciliated columnar epithelium, 178
*Cilophora (class in Protozoa), 37–38
*Cirripedia (subclass in Crustacea [barnacles]), 77–78
Clam, giant sea, 64
Clams, 64
Clam shrimps, 76
Clam worms, 57
Club mosses. See Pteridophyta
Cobb, N. A., on nematodes, 47

*Coccidia (parasitic order in phylum Protozoa), 37
*Cochlea of inner ear, 253
Cockles, 64–65
Cockroaches, 95–96
*Cocoon, 87
*Coelenterata, 39–41
*Coition, 200–201
Cold (quality), 217
*Coleoptera (insect order), 105–108
Collarbone, 131
*Collembola (order of insects), 91
*Colon, 194
Columella, Lucius Junius, *Agriculture,* on *capreolus* ("weeding fork"), 108
"Comb jellies," 41–42. *See also* Ctenophora
Comparative forms, adjectives, 273
*Compositae (plant family), 19
Comstock, Anthony, 196
*Concubine, 200
Conifers. *See* Gymnospermae
*Conjunctiva of eye, 252
*Connection, 8
Continence, 206
*Contraception, 208
*Convolutions of cerebrum, 147
*Copepoda (subclass in Crustacea), 76
*Coprolagnia, 187
*Coprolite, 187
*Copulation, 200
Cordus, Valerius, on plant names, 22
*Corn (American), 16–17
Corn (British for wheat), 14–16
*Cornea of eye, 252
*Coronary, 232
*Corpuscle, 261
*Cortex, cerebral, 141, 249; cranial, visual centers, 253. *See also* *Geniculate body
*Cowrie shells, 63
Crabs, 80–84
Cranial nerves: *abducens, 150; *acoustic, 150–51; *facial, 150; *glossopharyngeal, 151; *hypoglossal, 151; *oculomotor, 149; *olfactory, 149; *optic, 149; *spinal accessory, 151; *trigeminal, 150; *trochlear, 149–50; *vagus, 151
*Cranium, 9
Crayfish, 80
*Creosote, 65–66
*Cretaceous era, 68

Crick, F. C. H., 236
Crickets, 93–94
*Cricoid cartilage, 177
*Crista ampullaris of inner ear, 254
Cro-Magnon cave art, 31
*Crown, 9
*Ctenophora, 41–42
*Crustacea (class of Arthropods), 75–81
Cuttlefish, 67
Cuvier, Georges, on nemerteans, 46
*Cyanide, 220
*Cyanotic, 220
Cycads. *See* Gymnospermae

Damselflies, 92
*Dandelion, 17, 18
Darwin, Charles, and *Origin of Species* (1859), 42
Datura stramonium L., 20–21. *See also* Jimsonweed; Thornapple
*Decades, 6, 267
*Decapoda (order in Crustacea), 79–81
Deerflies, 111
de Lamarck, Jean-Baptiste, 16
"Dental" words, 188–89
*Dentifrice, 188–89
*Dermaptera (insect order), 97–98
*Dermestidae (beetle family), 89
*Dermis, 261. *See also* Skin
de Saussure, Henry Louis Frederic, 97
Desfontaines, R. L., 15
*Dextrin. *See* Salivary glands
*Dextrorotatory, 190
*Diabetes mellitus, 245. *See also* Hormones, insulin
*Diaphragm, 179
Diastole of heart, 229
Dicotyledons. *See* Angiospermae
*Dictyoptera (insect order), 95–96
*Diminutives, 159
*Dinoflagellata (class of Protozoa), 36–37
Dioscorides: on anemone, 41; on copper flakes, 113; on *eczema, 102; on the navelwort, 28
*Diplopoda (millipedes), 82–83
*Diptera (insect order), 110–12
*Diphthong, 268
Dissections, human, at Ptolemaic Alexandria, 144–45
Distillation, Arab discovery of, 240
*DNA (deoxyribonucleic acid), 236–37, 239

INDEX 293

Dobsonflies, 105
Doodlebugs (antlions), 105
Double helix, DNA, 236–37
*Dracunculus spp. (guinea worms), 51
Dragonflies, 92
Drug properties, Aetius of Amida on, 222–23
"Drugs by Degrees" system, 223
Dry (quality), 217
*Dung, 185
Dung beetles, 108
*Duodenum, 193
*Dura mater, 146
Dust lice, 100
*Dynamis (Greek), 143

Eardrum, 253. See also Tympanic membrane
Earth, as element, 217
Earthworms, 57–58
Earwigs, 97–98
*Eczema, 102
Edwin Smith Surgical Papyrus, on bonesetting, 124
*Eggplant, 21
Egypt, ancient, and Edwin Smith Surgical Papyrus, 124
Ehrlich, Paul, and *arsphenamine (Salvarsan, or 606), 205
Eimer, Gustav Heinrich Theodor, 37
*Ejaculation, 212
*Elements (ancient, four), 216–17; air, 224–25; earth, 224; fire, 224; water, 225
*Elephantiasis, 50
*Elongate, 9
*Elytron (beetle wing cover), 106
*Embioptera (insect order), 99
*Embryo, 8
Empedocles, 181; on breathing, 173–74
*Emulsification, 194
*Endocrine glands and *hormones, 241; *adrenals and hormones, 244; *ovaries and hormones, 245–46; *pancreas and hormones, 244–45; *parathyroids and hormones, 243; *pineal and hormones, 246–47; *pituitary and hormones, 242–43; *thymus and hormones, 246; *thyroid and hormones, 243
*Endolymph of inner ear, 253
*Endoprocta (phylum), 54
Ennius, Quintus, on triticum (wheat), 15

*Enterobius spp. (pinworms), 50
*Entomology, 70, 72–73
*Enzyme, 66, 189; enzymes of Teredo spp., 66
Ephedra. See Gymnospermae
*Ephemeroptera (insect order), 91
*Epidemiology, 208
*Epidermis, 260–61. See also Skin
*Epididymus, 212
*Epiglottis, 177
*Equate, 6
*Equilibrium, 230
Erasistratus, 144; on pneuma, 175
*Ericaceae (plant family), 20
*Erythrocyte, 220
*Esophagus, 191
Estrus. See Hormones, estrogen
*Euglena gracilis Klebs, 36
Eunuchs, 211–12
Euphemisms, sexual, English and Latin, 197–98
Eustachi, Bartolomeo, 167
*Exocrine glands, 241
Eyeball muscles, 172

Fabricius, Johann Christian, 89; on bees, 117; on dragonflies, 92; on earwigs, 98
Fairy shrimps, 75
*Fallopian tube, 211
Fallopio, Gabriello, 211
*Falx cerebri, 147
Farting. See Flatulence
*Feces, 185
*Fenestra vestibuli, inner ear, 253
Ferns. See Pteridophyta
*Fertilize, 203
Fibers of Purkinje, heart, 231
Fibrin, 59
*Fibrinogen, 59
*Filament (botany), 26
*Finally, 6
Fire, as element, 217
Fish lice, 77
Fish sauce, Roman, and etymological links with name for bone of big toe, 139
*Flagellata (class of Protozoans), 36
*Flatulence, 175
*Flavonol, 219
Fleas, 108–10
Flukes, 44–45. See also Trematoda
*Follicles, hair, 261. See also Skin
*Foramen magnum, 127

*Foramina, for spinal nerves, 153–54
*Foraminifera (phylum in Protozoa), 37
*Forceps (as pronged tail of earwig), 97
*Formica (trade name), 116
*Formicidae (ant family), 116
*Fornication, 201
Fracastoro, Girolamo, 204–205
*Frequency, 257
Fruitflies, 112
*Fundamentum, 192
*Fundus of stomach, 191
*Fungi, 27

Galangine (flavonol in bee glue), 118
Galen: adaptations of Hippocratic works, 276; on anatomy by analogy, 276; on gymnastics, 160; on leeches, 59. *Affected parts,* and injury to nerve of voice linked with back injury, 259–60. *Anatomical Procedures,* on calf of a leg, 165; on the carotid arteries, 233; on diastole of heart, 229; on Herophilus' duodenum, 193; on muscles of chewing, 171; on palmaris longus muscle, 160; on recurrent laryngeal nerve, 258–59. *Blood in the Arteries,* on double-ligature experiment demonstrating arterial blood, 178. *Crisis Days,* on chyme, 192. *Doctrines of Hippocrates and Plato,* on carotid arteries, 233; on mechanics of vision, 250; on muscles of breathing, 175. *Introduction to the Bones,* on the anklebone, 138; on a shallow joint socket, 36. *On the Natural Faculties,* on food altered into blood, 222; on powers of attraction and repulsion, 220. *On Prognosis,* on origins of speech, 258. *On Seed,* on the epididymus, 212. *Use of Breathing,* on purposes of breathing, 176. *Use of Parts,* on bones of palm of hand, 133; on carotid arteries, 233; on mouth of windpipe, 177; on muscle dividing thorax from abdomen, 179; on nerves to muscles of larynx, 259; on "point of the elbow," 132; on the term *hydatis,* 45; *Variations Among Pulses,* on systole, 229
*Gallbladder, 194
Gastric secretions, observed by Beaumont, 222
*Gastritis, 191
*Gastrolith, 191
*Gastrology, 191

*Gastropoda, 61–63
*Gastrotrichia (phylum), 53–54
Generation of Animals, by Aristotle, 25; on women, 26
*Genetics, 238–39
*Geniculate body, brain (visual impulse conveyor), 253
*Genus, 27
*Geography, 224
*Geology, 224
*Geophagy, 224
*Geoponics, 224
George III of England, and porphyria, 221
Ginkgo. *See* Gymnospermae
Gladius (Roman short sword), resembles sternum, 131
*Glaucoma, 220
*Glomerulus, kidney, 195
*Glottis, 177
*Glucose, 228
*Glycerin, 228
*Goiter, 243. *See also* Endocrines, thyroid
*Gonorrhea, 205–207
*Gradient, pressure, 229–30
Grape beetle, 107
Grasses, 15
Grasshoppers, 93–94
*Gravid, 202
*Gravitas, 202
*Grylloblattodea (insect order), 92
Gyllenhall, Leonhard, 89
*Gymnospermae, 28
*Gymnostomatida (order in Cilophora), 38

Hagen, Hermann August, on lacewings, 105
*Halogen, 227
*Halophyte, 227
*Hamstringing, 166
Harvey, William, 176; on closed circulation, 228; *De motu cordis* (*Movement of the Heart*), 213–16; on systole and diastole, 229
*Heart, 232
Heart valves, 229–30; *semilunar, 230
Heat (Greek *thermon*), 25
Heel bone. *See* Bones, tarsal
*Helix, 238
*Hemaglobin, 218
*Hematin, 218
*Hematite, 218
*Hematocrit, 218
*Hematology, 218

*Hemiptera (insect order), 103–104
*Hemophilia, 208, 218
*Hemorrhoids, 194
*Hepatic, 194
*Hepatitis, mimicked by whipworm infestation, 49
Hercules (Greek Herakles) and name *Hydrozoa, 39
*Hermaphrodites among gastrotrichs, 53
Hermit crabs, 81
Hernia, 225; inguinal, in Byzantine Greek, 110
Herodotus, *Histories*, on Cheops (Khufu), 109; on fish scales, 113
Herophilus: on the brain, 144–45; on the duodenum, 193; on medical terms, 145
*Herpes, genital, 207
Hesiod, *Theogony*, on Iris, 251–52
*Heterometric autoregulation, 230–31
*Heteroptera (insect suborder), 104
*Hexapoda (insects), 73, 85–119
*Hilum, 179–80
*Hippocampus, in limbic system, 148
Hippocratic writings: *Aphorisms*, on "scales" of butterflies, 112. *Fractures*, on setting fracture of humerus, 125. *Joints*, on sheath of the spinal cord, 106. *Nature of Man*, on the four humors, 217
*Hirudin, as anticoagulant, 59
*Hirudinea (class of Annelids: leeches), 58–59
*Histology, 164
Hittite, ultimate origin of "piss," 187
Hoeppli, R., on ancient knowledge of elephantiasis and guinea worms, 51
Holophyra nigricans Lauterborn, 38
*Homeostasis, 148
Homer: *Iliad*, on Iris as messenger among gods, 251. *Odyssey*, on "fishing nets," 95; on one-seeded wheat, 16
Homo sapiens, 32
*Homosexuality, 209
Honey, 118
Hookworms, 50
*Hormones, 238; *adrenaline, 244 (*see also* *Epinephrine); *adrenocorticotropic (ACTH), 242; *aldosterone, 244; calcitonin, 243; *epinephrine (*see also* *Adrenaline), 244; *estrogen, 245; *follicle-stimulating (FSH), 242–43; *glucagon, 245; *hydrocortisone, 244; *insulin, 245; *luteinizing (LH), 243; *melanocyte-stimulating (MSH), 242;

*melatonin, 246; *oxytocin, 243; *parathyroid (PTH), 243; *progesterone, 246; *prolactin, 243; *serotonin, 246–47; *somatotropic (STH), 242; thymosins, 246; *thyroid-stimulating (TSH), 242; *thyroxin, 243
Horseflies, 111–12
Horsetails. *See* Pteridophyta
Hot (quality), 217
"Housemaid's knee," 226
Humerus. *See* Bones
Humoral pathology, 221
Humors (blood, phlegm, yellow bile, black bile), 217; in Hippocratic *Nature of Man*, 217
Hunter, John, 247
Huxley, Thomas Henry, 42; on barnacles, 78; on crayfish and lobsters, 80
*Hydatid cysts, 45–46
*Hydremia, 225
*Hydrocele, 225
*Hydrogen, 225
*Hydrogogue, 225
*Hydrolysis, 190
*Hydrorrhea, 225
*Hydrosalpinx, 225
*Hydrotherapy, 225
*Hydrothionemia, 225
*Hydrozoa, 39–40
*Hygroblepharic, 226
*Hygroma, 226
*Hygrometer, 226
*Hygrophilia (genus of Asian herbs), 226
*Hygroscope, 226
*Hygrostomia, 226
*Hygrothermograph, 226
*Hymen, 210
*Hymenoptera (insect order), 114–19
*Hymenostomatida (order of Cilophora), 38
*Hypaxial, 9
*Hypertonic properties of honey, 118
*Hypothalamus, 148

*Identify, 6
*Ilium (intestine), 193
*Imago (in insect metamorphosis), 87
*Importance, 6
*Incisors. *See* Teeth
*Increasing(ly), 9
*Incus, auditory ossicle, 253
*Infibulation, 137
Inflections, 269–70

Ingrassia, Giovanni Filippo, 167
Inguinal hernia, 110
*Insects, 73; numbers of species, 34
*Insemination, 202–203
*Intercourse, 201
*Intestine, 192–94
*Intrinsic, 257
*Iodine, 221; and thyroxin, 243
Iris, useful rhizome, 252
*Iris of eye, 251–52. *See also* Uvea
Isidore of Seville: on plant names, 22; on solifuges, 122
*Isopoda (sowbugs, pillbugs), 78–79
*Isoptera (termites), 98–99
*Isthmus faucium, 191

Jamestown, first lasting English settlement in America, 20
Japanese, Latinized for ginkgo, 28
Japanese beetles, 106–107
Japanese giant spider crab, 81
*Jejunum, 193
Jellyfish, 40–41
*Jimson weed, 20–21
*Joint, 163; ball-and-socket, 134
Junebugs (beetles), 106
Juvenal, *Satires*: on feces as "scum," 185; on *micturition, 186

Kamel, Georg Josef, 94
Katydids, 93–94
*Ketone, 240
Kidney, 194–95
Kidney worms, 49
*Kinesiology, 164
Kinēsis (Greek) as "movement," 25
King crabs, 81
*Kinorhynchia (phylum), 54
Kirby, William, 88
Koinē Greek, 23
Kraseis (Greek) as "balances" in humoral theory, 236
Kubrick, Stanley, 206

*Labyrinth of inner ear, 253
Lacewings, 105
*Lachrymal glands, 241
*Lactation, 184
*Lamellibranchiata, 63–64. *See* Pelecypoda
Langerhans, Paul, 245
Lankford, Charles, 11
*Larva (in insect metamorphosis), 87

*Larynx, 177
Latin: as "common tongue" in Renaissance, 23–24; Renaissance, and medical terms in English, 214–16; and Romance languages, 10–11
Latreille, P. A.: on Hexapoda, 90; on silverfish, 91
Latrodectus mactans L. (black widow spider), 119–20
Lauterborn, E., 38
Lavoisier, Antoine: on "carbon" as element, 189; on water not an element, 176, 225
Leach, W. E., 104
Leafhoppers, 104
Leaf insects, 94–95
Leeches, 58–59; modern medical use, 59
Legal Latin: on eunuchs, 211; *Twelve Tables*, 198
Lemche, Henning, 60
*Lens of eye, 252
*Lepidoptera (insect order), 112–14
Lesbianism, 209
*Leukocytes, 247
Lice, human, 101–102
*Lichen, 27–28
*Ligament, 162
*Limbic system, 148
*Limpets, 61–62
*Lingual frenulum, 189
*Lingula (genus of Brachiopoda), 56
Linnaeus, Carl: on American grape beetles, 107; on the *Argonauta argo*, 68; on "bugs" (Hemiptera), 103; on butterflies and moths, 112; on chicken lice, 100–101; on the dandelion, 18; on *Datura* spp., 20–21; on the false stag beetle, 108; on *Hymenoptera, 114; on insects, 89–90; on the Monarch butterfly, 114; on the Phoenician murex, 65; seven-level classification system (1758), 35; on sexual parts of plants in classification, 26; on the "shipworm," 65; on the silkworm, 113; *Species Plantarum*, 1st ed. (1753), 15–16; *Systema Natura*, 10th ed. (1758), 16, 32; on termites, 98; on *Venus mercenaria*, used for wampum, 64; on the whipworm, 49
*Lipase (pancreatic enzyme), 194
*Liver, 194
Liverworts, *See* Bryophyta
Lobsters, 80
Locust, desert, 93

INDEX 297

Logos (Greek), as "purpose," 25
Loins, 128
*Long, 5
*Longitudinal, 8
"Long vowel sound," 269
Loxosceles spp. (brown recluse spiders), 121
*Lucanidae (stag beetles), 107–108
Lucretius, *De rerum natura*, on "spiritus," 180–81
Lumbricus spp. (earthworms), 57–58
"Lunar rainbow," iris is (Aristotle), 252
*Lung, 178–79
*Lutein, 219
Lyme Disease, 123
*Lymph, 247

*Macrocosm, 240
*Macroscopic, 240–41
Magellan, Ferdinand, 65
Maggots, fly larvae, 110–11
Maize, 15; from Hispaniolan Taino, 17
Majno, Guido, on bee glue, 118
*Malacology, 60
*Malacostrata (subclass of Crustacea), 78–81
*Malaria, 37, 111
*Malleus, auditory ossicle, 253
*Mallophaga (insect order), 100–102
*Maltose, 190–91. See also Ptyalin
Mandrake, 21
Mantids, praying, 96–97
Mantis shrimps, 78
*Manure, 186
Martial, *Epigrams*: on infibulation, 137; on shit, 187; use of *nasus*, 126
*Mastigophora (class of Protozoa), 36–37
*Masturbation, 204
Matthew, on fornication, 201
Mayflies, 91
*Meat, 184–85
*Meatus, external auditory, 253
*Mediastinum, 179
Medical English, illustrated by Harvey's Latin, 213–15
*Medulla oblongata, 147–48
*Medulla spinalis, 153
Medusas (among jellyfish), 40
Meissner's corpuscles, 261
Meissner, Georg, 261
*Melancholia, 219
*Melissa, 118

Mencken, H. L., 196–97
*Meninges, 146
Metabolē (Greek) as "change," 25
*Metabolism, 239, 241
Metamorphosis, among insects, 86–87
*Methionine (amino acid), 59
*Mica, 116
*Microbiology, 36, 240
*Microscopic, 240
Micturition, 186
Midbrain, 148
*Milk, 184
*Millipedes, 82–83; defense with hydrogen cyanide, 71
Mites, 122–23
*Mitral valve of heart, 229
*Molars. See Teeth
*Molecule, 238
*Mollusca (phylum), 59–69
Monocotyledons. See Angiospermae
*Monoplacophora (class of Molluscs), 60
Mores (sing. *mos*.), 183
Morphology, 3
Mosquitoes, 111
Mosses, 28. See also Bryophyta
Mothballs, 89
Mother-of-Pearl (limpet shells), 62
Moths, 112–14
Mountain sickness, 224
Mouse, analogy to muscle, 159–60
*Mouth, 189
Muscle, *fusiform belly of, 162
Muscles: *arrector pili, 261; *auricularis anterior, superior, and posterior, 171; *biceps femoris, 166; *buccinator, 171; *compressor naris, 171; *corrugator, 171; *deltoid, 169; eyeball, 172; *fascial layer, 163; *flexors, 163; *gastrocnemius, 165–66; *gemellus superior and inferior, 170; *gluteus maximus, medius, and minimus, 170; *intercostales, 170; *latissimus dorsi, 169; *levator palpebrae superioris, 171; *levator scapulae, 169; *masseter, 171; *obturator internus and externus, 170; *occipitofrontalis, 170; *orbicularis oculi, 171; *palmaris longus, 159–60; papillaries of the heart, 229; *pectoralis major and minor, 170; *piriformis, 170; *platysma, 171; *popliteus, 166; *quadratus femoris, 170; *rhomboideus minor and major, 169; *ri-

sorius, 171–72; *sartorius, 166–67; *semispinalis capitis, 168; *semitendinosus, 166; *serratus anterior, 169; *splenius capitis, 169; *stapedius, 167; *sternocleidomastoid, 168; *subclavius, 169; *teres minor and major, 169; *trapezius, 168
*Musculus (Latin), various meanings, 159
Mushrooms. See Thallophyta
*Mygalomorphs (proper name for tarantulas), 120
*Myology, 164
*Myrmecology, 116

*Naris (Latin), nose, 126–27
*Nasopharynx, 177
Nautilus spp., 67–68
Neanderthal at Shanidar, Iraq, 14
*Necrotic lesions, 121
Neilands, John, 11
*Nematoda (phylum), 47–52
*Nematophora (phylum), 52
*Nemertea (phylum), 46–47
Nerves: *axillary, 156; *cranial, optic chiasma, 252; *median and branches, 156; *parasympathetic, 154; *peripheral, 153; *plexus, 155; recurrent laryngeal, demonstrated by Galen, 259; spinal roots (*radices), 154; *sympathetic, 154; *synapse, 164
*Nervus (Latin), various meanings, 145
*Neuron (Greek), 142
*Neuropathology, 12–13
*Neuroptera (insect order), 104–105
Newman, E., on the Japanese beetle, 107
Nicander, Theriaca: on centipedes, 84; on snake scales, 113
Nicot, Jean, 22. See also Tobacco
Nightshades, 21–22
Nitzsch, C. L., 100
*Nose, 177
Nose (*naris), 126–27
*Nous (Greek), 143
Novocain. See Procaine hydrochloride
*Nucleus, 238
*Nudibranchiata (suborder of Molluscs), 62
Nymphal casts, cicadas, 104

*Obliquus inferior. See Muscles, eyeball
*Obliquus superior. See Muscles, eyeball
Obsidian (volcanic glass), 129

Octopus, 67
*Oculist, 220
*Odonata (insect order), 91–92
*Officinale drugs in nineteenth century, 18
*Oligochaeta (annelid class), 57–58
*Onomastic, 12
*Onychophagia, 74
*Onychophora (class of arthropods), 73–74
*Ophthalmologist, 220
*Optic chiasma, 149
Optic nerve. See Cranial nerves
*Optics, 252
Ordinal numbers, 263
Oribasius, on leeches (quoting Antyllus), 59
*Orthoptera (insect order), 93–94
*Osmosis, 230
Ossicles, auditory, 253
*Osteology, 124
*Ostracoda (subclass of Crustacea), 76
*Ovary, 211
Ovid: Metamorphoses, transformations, 86; Tristia, on spiritus, 180
*Oxygen, 225
*Oxymoron, 227–28
*Oxytocin, 202; as parturifacient, 227. See also Hormones
Oysters, 64

Pacini, Filippo, 261
Pacinian corpuscles, 261
*Palate, 257
*Paleontology, 74; and Aristotelian zoological syllogisms, 33
*Pancreas, 194
*Papillae, 189
*Papillary muscles of the heart, 229
*Paramecium, 38
*Parietal pleura, 179
*Parotid gland. See Salivary glands
*Parthenogenesis, among gastrotrichs, 54
*Parturient, 202
Pasteur, Louis, on plague bacillus, 109
Paulus, Julius, quoted in Justinian's Digest, on spiritus, 181
*Pauropoda (Myriapod class), 84
*Pelecypoda (class of Molluscs), 63–65
*Pelvis, renal, 195
*Penicillin, 205
*Penis, 211
*Pentekonter, 267

INDEX

*Pepsin (digestive enzyme), 192
*Perilymph of inner ear, 253
*Peristalsis, 192; mentioned, 57
*Permian period, 74
Persius, on "back of the head," 126
*pH, 118
*Pharmakon (Greek), 222
*Pharynx, 151
*Phasmida (insect order), 94–95
Philumenus, on solifuges, 122
Phlegm, as humor, 217
*Phlegmatic, 218
*Pholas (genus of Mollusca, rock borers), 66
*Phonation, 256
*Phycocyanin (botany), 27
*Phyla, 27
*Physics, 143
*Physis (Greek), 25
Picric acid, 227
Pillbugs, 79
Pines. See Gymnospermae
Pinworms, 50
*Piss, 186–88
*Pissabed, 187
*Pisspot, 187
*Pissprophet, 187
*Pistil, 26
Plagues, of locusts, 93
*Planaria worms, 44
*Plankton, 54
Plant species, numbers of, 34
*Plasmodium spp. and malaria, 37, 111
Plato: on intelligence in brain, 26; on seat of intellect, 143. Timaeus, on muscle dividing thorax from abdomen, 179; on taste and flavors, 223; on taste and smell, 227
*Platyhelminthes (phylum), 44–46
Plautus, on triticum (wheat), 15
Pliny the Elder, Natural History: on agricultural metaphors from Aristotle, especially progesterone, 246; on animals with hard shells, 75; on the coxendix (hipbone), 130; entomon translated into Latin's insectum, 73; on honey as a preservative, 118; on lobsters, 80; on *lumbus, 128; on plant names, 22; on shellfish yielding the Phoenician purple, 65; on "soft-shelled nuts," 59; on worms and maggots, 42–43
*Plumatella (genus in Bryozoa), 55–56

*Pneuma (Greek), 175
*Pollen, 26
*Pollination, 203
Pollux, Onomasticon: on the Atlas bone, 127; on bones of palm of hand, 133; on coccyx, 129; on epistropheus bone, 128; "hunting net" applied to Dictyoptera, 95; on knuckles, 135; on proglottids of tapeworms, 45
*Polychaeta (class of Annelids), 57
*Polypeptide, 59
*Polyplacophora (class of Molluscs), 60
Pomponius, Sextus, quoted in Justinian's Digest, on spiritus, 181
*Pons of brain, 148
Popilius, gens, and name for Japanese beetle, 107
*Porifera, 38–39
*Pornography, 209–10
*Porphyria, 221
Potato, Irish, 21
*Powder, 10
*Pregnancy, 202
*Prehistoric, 6
Prelog, Vladimir, 11
Priapism, 54
*Priapulida (phylum), 54
*Proboscis, 46
Procaine hydrochloride, 150
Procopius, History of the Wars, on bubonic plague, 109–10
*Prophylactic, 203–204
*Prophylaxis, 115
*Propolis, 118
*Prostate gland, 210, 212
*Prostitution, 210
Prothrombin, 59
*Protista, 34–35
*Protozoa, 34, 36
*Psocoptera (insect order), 100
*Psychē (Greek), 25
*Psychology, 226
*Psychoalgia, 226
*Psychroesthesia, 226
*Psychrotherapy, 226
*Pteridophyta, 28
Ptolemy I and II, and Alexandria, 144
*Ptyalin. See Salivary glands
*Pubes, 131
*Pulmonary, 179
*Pupa, in insect metamorphosis, 87
*Pupil of eye, 252

Purkinje, Johannes Evangelista, 231
*Pylorus, 192
*Pyrogen, 224
*Pyromania, 224
*Pyrophobia, 224
*Pyrosis, 224
*Pyrotechnics, 224
*Pyrotic, 224

Qualities (four), 217; the cold, 226; the dry, 226–27; the hot, 226; the wet, 225–26
Quintus Smyrnaeus, *Posthomerica* (Fall of Troy), on Achilles' fatal heel wound, 165–66

*Radiolaria (phylum of Protozoa), 37
Radius. *See* Bones
Rag worms, 57
*Ramus, dexter and sinister, of pulmonary artery, 234
Ray, John, 94
*Rectum, 194
*Rectus inferior. *See* Muscles, eyeball
*Rectus lateralis. *See* Muscles, eyeball
*Rectus medialis. *See* Muscles, eyeball
*Rectus superior. *See* Muscles, eyeball
"Renal" words, 195
*Resonator, 257–58
*Respiration, 180–81
*Retina of eye, 251
*Rhabdites, rhabdoms, rhabdomyoma, rhabdomyosarcoma, 43
*Rhizopoda (class of Protozoa), 37
*Rhododendron, 17, 19–20
*Rhythm, 230
Ribbonworms, 46–47. *See also* Nemertea
*Riboflavin, 219
Ribonucleic acid (RNA), 239. *See also* Riboflavin
Ricketts, Howard T., 102
Rocky Mountain spotted fever, 123
*Roseola, 220
*Rotifera (phylum), 52–53
Ruffini, Angelo, 262
Ruffini's corpuscles, 262
Rufinus, on plant names, 22

St. Martin, Alexis, 222
*Salivary glands, 189–91
Salvarsan. *See* Arsphenamine
Sandhoppers, 79

Sappho, 209, 221
*Sarcodina (class of Protozoa), 37
Sawflies, 118
Scallops, 65
*Scaphopoda (class of Molluscs), 63
*Scatology, 187
*Scatoma, 187
*Scatoscopy, 187
*Schistosomiasis, 44–45
*Schyphozoa, 40–41
*Sclera of eye, 252
*Scolex of tapeworms, 45
Scorpions, 121
Scribonius Largus, *Compositiones*: on bee glue, 118; on respiration, 180
"Sea gooseberries," 42
Sea hares, 62
Sea slugs, 62
*Season, 6
Seaweeds. *See* Thallophyta
*Sebaceous glands, 241, 261
*Secrets, 6
Seed shrimps, 76
*Semen, 202–203
Semicircular canals, inner ear, 253–54. *See also* Labyrinth
*Semilunar valves, heart, 230
*Semipermeable membrane, 230
*Sepia, 67
*Septal wall, heart, 231
*Sesamoid bones, 126
Shanidar, Neanderthal site (30,000 B.C.), 14
Shieldbugs, 104
Shinbone. *See* Bones, tibia
Shipworms, 65–66
*Shit, 186–87
Shoulder blade, 131
*Siderophores, 11
*Sigmoid colon, 194
Silk, 113
Silverfish (insects), 91
Simpson, George Gaylord, on classification, 35
*Sinoatrial node, heart, 231
*Siphonaptera (insect order), 108–10
*Skeleton, 125
Skin, 260–62
*Slaved, 6
Slugs, 61
Snails, 61
Snakeflies, 105

INDEX   301

"Social insects," 114–18
Socrates, 143
*Solanaceae, 21–22. *See also* Nightshades
*Solenogasters, Aplacophora among molluscs, 61
*Solifuges, 122
*Solution, 230
*Somatogenic, 217
*Soma words, 217
Soranus, *On Bandages,* on "thōrax" as chest bandage, 128
Soul (*psychē*), 25
Sowbugs, 79
*Species, 27
*Sperm, 203
*Sphecidae (wasp family), 115
*Sphincter (pyloric), 192
Spiders, 119–21
Spinal cord. *See* Medulla spinalis
*Spiritus, 180–81; in legal Latin, 181
Spirochete, causing Lyme Disease, 123; *spirochete of syphilis, 205
*Spleen, 194; as organ of lymph system, 247
Sponges, 38–39
*Sporozoa (class of Protozoa), 37
Springtails (insects), 91
Squids, 67
Stag beetles, 107–108
*Stamen, 26
*Stapes, auditory ossicle, 253
Starling equilibrium in heart, 230
*Stercoraceous, 187
*Sterol, 240
*Stirrup, 167
*Stomach, 191
*Strange, 5
*Style (botany), 26
Sublingual gland. *See* Salivary glands
Submandibular gland. *See* Salivary glands
*Suctorida (order of Cilophora), 38
*Sudorific drug, 261. *See also* Sweat glands
Suetonius, *Augustus,* on the *coxendix* (hipbone), 130
*Sugar, 190
*Sulcus medianus linguae, 189
*Summer, 10
Superlative forms, adjectives, 273
Sylvius, Franciscus, 147
*Symbiosis, 28
*Symphyla (class of Myriapods), 84
*Synapses of nerves, 164

*Synovial membrane, 163
*Syphilis, 204–205
*Systemic circulation, 235
Systole of heart, 229, 230
Sweat glands, 261

*Table, 6
Tacitus, *Annals,* on the *sacrum,* 128
*Tactile sensations, 249
Tapeworms, 45–46
Tarantulas, 120–21
Taxonomy, defined by Simpson, 30
Teeth, 188
Teleology, 25
*Tendo calcaneus, 165
*Tenthredinide (sawflies), 118
*Teredo navalis L., wood-boring "shipworm," 65–66
*Terminal conducting fibers, heart, 231
*Termites, 98–99
*Testis or testicle, 211–12
*Testosterone, 240
*Tetragnatha (solifuges), 122
*Thalamus, 148
Thales of Miletus, 142; on water as primordial element, 216
*Thallophyta, 27–28
Theocritus, *Idylls,* on the praying mantis, 96
Theophrastus of Eresus: on plant names, 22. *Enquiry into Plants* (HP), 26; on snowflakes, 113; on thrips, or woodboring insects, 102; on wood-boring "shipworm," 65. *On Odors,* on tastes and flavors, 223. *On Stones,* on coal/charcoal, 111
*Theridiidae (cobweb weaver spiders), 119
*Thermanesthia, 226
*Thermochemistry, 226
*Thermoneurosis, 226
Thermos bottles, 226
*Thermotherapy, 226
*Thorax, 9
Thornapple, 20–21. *See also* Jimsonweed; *Datura stramonium* L.
Threadworms, 49–50
Thrips (insect order), 102–103
*Thrombin, 59
Thymus, as organ of lymph system, 247. *See also* Endocrines; Hormones
*Thyroid cartilage, 177
*Thysanoptera (insect order), 102–103

*Thysanura (insect order), 90–91
Ticks, 122–23
Tobacco, 21–22
Tomato, as aphrodisiac, 21
*Tongue, 189
Tooth (*dens), 188
Tooth shells, 63
*Trachea, 178
*Trematoda (class of Platyhelminthes), 44–45
*Trichella, 48–49
*Tricuspid valve, heart, 229
*Tridacna (genus of giant clams), 64
*Trilobites, 74–75
*Triticum spp. (wheats), 15–16
*Trypanosoma (protozoans), 111–12
*Trypsin (pancreatic enzyme), 194
*Tryptophan (amino acid), 59
Tsetse flies, 112
*Tube, 8
*Tularemia, 111
"Tumblebugs" (dung beetles), 108
*Tumulus, 6
*Turbellaria (class of Platyhelminthes), 44
*Tympanic: cavity, 167; membrane, 253. See also Eardrum
*Typhus, 101

Ulna. See Bones
Ulpian: on eunuchs, 211; on money belt (ventralis), 154; quoted in Justinian's Digest, on dardanarius as "speculator," adapted as name for large hermit crab, 81
*Ureter, 195
*Urethra, 195
*Urine, 186
*Uropygia (whipscorpions), 122
*Uterus, 210–11
*Utricle of inner ear, 253–54
*Uvea of eye, and parts, 251–52

*Vacuum, 257
*Vagina, 211
van Leeuwenhoek, Antony, on rotifers, 53
Varro, Marcus Terentius: Agriculture, on lobsters, 80; De lingua Latina, on fundulum, 191
*Vascular mucous membrane, 177–78
*Vein, 8, 234
*Veinule, 234
*Vena cava, 234

Venereal diseases, 204–206
*Venery (two derivations), 204
*Ventricle of heart, 229
*Venus mercenaria L. (clams), 64
Vergil: Aeneid, on Palinurus (Aeneas' helmsman) as name for genus of spiny lobsters, 80; on sacred objects, 128. Eclogues, on cicadas, 104. Georgics, on mice, 158–59; on sacred objects, 128
Vermes, according to Linnaeus, 42
*Vermiform appendix, 193–94
"Vermin," 43
*Vespidae (wasp family), 115
*Vessel(s), 9
*Vibration, 257
Villars, D., 16
Vinegaroons, 122. See also Uropygia
*Virus, 205
*Visceral pleura of lungs, 179
*Vitreous humor of eyeball, 252
Vitruvius, On Architecture: on nares, 127; on "resonation," 258
"Vocal" words, 256
Volar interosseous. See Nerves, *median, and Nerves, branches
*Vulva, 210

Walker, E. M., on Grylloblattodea (insect order), 92
Walkingsticks (insects), 94–95
Wampum, from marine clams, 64
Wasps, 115
Water, as element, 216–17
Waterbug, giant, 103–104
Water closet (WC), 185
Waterstriders (among Hemiptera), 103
Watson, James D., 236
Weber, G. H., 18
Webspinners (insect order), 99
Westwood, J. O., on Chinese cranefly, 110
Wet (quality), 217
Wheat (American), 14–16. See also Corn
Whipworms, 49
White blood cells. See Leukocytes
Windscorpions, 122. See also Solifuges
Women as "deformed men," according to Aristotle, 26
Wrist bones. See Bones, ossa carpi
Wucherer, Otto, 50
Wyclif, John, 1388 English translation of Bible, 187–88

*Xanthophyll, 219
*Xeransis, 227
*Xeroderma, 227
*Xerophagia, 227
*Xerophthalmia, 227
*Xerostomia, 227
Xerox (trade name), 226

Yellow bile, as humor, 217
"Yellow" words, 219
Yersin, A. E. J., on plague bacillus, 109

Zinsser, Hans, on typhus, 102
*Zoraptera (insect order), 99